Case Studies in Gastrointestinal Tract Disorders

Case Studies in Gastrointestinal Tract Disorders

Editor: Olivia Harris

AMERICAN
MEDICAL PUBLISHERS
www.americanmedicalpublishers.com

AMERICAN
MEDICAL PUBLISHERS
www.americanmedicalpublishers.com

Cataloging-in-Publication Data

Case studies in gastrointestinal tract disorders / edited by Olivia Harris.
p. cm.
Includes bibliographical references and index.
ISBN 979-8-88740-600-8
1. Gastrointestinal system--Diseases. 2. Gastrointestinal system--Diseases--Diagnosis.
3. Gastrointestinal system--Examination. 4. Gastrointestinal system--Diseases--Treatment.
I. Harris, Olivia.
RC816 .G37 2023
616.33--dc23

American Medical Publishers,
41 Flatbush Avenue,
1st Floor, New York,
NY 11217, USA

ISBN 979-8-88740-600-8 (Hardback)

Contents

Preface

Gastrointestinal tract disorders refer to a wide spectrum of medical conditions that affect the organs and structures involved in the digestion and absorption of food. The gastrointestinal tract, often referred to as the digestive system, comprises the esophagus, stomach, small intestine, large intestine, rectum and anus. Disorders of the gastrointestinal tract can lead to abdominal pain, bloating, diarrhea, constipation, nausea, vomiting and gastrointestinal bleeding. Some common gastrointestinal tract disorders are gastroesophageal reflux disease (GERD), peptic ulcers, gastritis, inflammatory bowel disease, irritable bowel syndrome (IBS) and colorectal cancer. The diagnostic process for such disorder may involve a combination of patient history assessment, physical examination, laboratory tests, endoscopy, colonoscopy and tissue biopsies. These diagnostic tools help identify the underlying cause and determine the most appropriate treatment approach. This book contains some path-breaking studies on gastrointestinal tract disorders. It will provide comprehensive knowledge to the readers.

Various studies have approached the subject by analyzing it with a single perspective, but the present book provides diverse methodologies and techniques to address this field. This book contains theories and applications needed for understanding the subject from different perspectives. The aim is to keep the readers informed about the progresses in the field; therefore, the contributions were carefully examined to compile novel researches by specialists from across the globe.

Indeed, the job of the editor is the most crucial and challenging in compiling all chapters into a single book. In the end, I would extend my sincere thanks to the chapter authors for their profound work. I am also thankful for the support provided by my family and colleagues during the compilation of this book.

Editor

1

Atypical Presentation of Acquired Hypoganglionosis in a Patient Taking Clozapine

Catherine Gisi,[1] Anamaria Munteanu,[2] Lawrence Ku,[1] Samuel French,[2] Michael Fleischman,[3] and Viktor Eysselein[3]

[1]*Department of Internal Medicine, Harbor-UCLA Medical Center, Torrance, CA, USA*
[2]*Department of Pathology, Harbor-UCLA Medical Center, Torrance, CA, USA*
[3]*Department of Internal Medicine, Division of Gastroenterology, Harbor-UCLA Medical Center, Torrance, CA, USA*

Correspondence should be addressed to Catherine Gisi; ckulaga@dhs.lacounty.gov

Academic Editor: Shiro Kikuchi

Acquired hypoganglionosis (HG) is a rare enteric gastrointestinal neuromuscular disorder previously associated with chronic inflammation that can lead to constipation, ileus, and even death. There is little known about the pathophysiology of acquired hypoganglionosis, and it is unclear if medications are related to the development of the disease. Clozapine is an atypical antipsychotic used to treat refractory schizophrenia that is well known for its side effects including agranulocytosis and gastrointestinal dysmotility. This is an unusual case of acquired hypoganglionosis in a patient with anticholinergic toxicity on clozapine therapy.

1. Introduction

Normal gastrointestinal motility depends on appropriate enteric nervous system signaling and coordinated smooth muscle contraction [1]. The enteric nervous system is the largest and most intricate component of the peripheral nervous system. The myenteric (Auerbach's) and submucosal (Meissner's) plexuses contain the majority of neurons and ganglia in the gastrointestinal tract [2]. Acquired hypoganglionosis (HG) is a rare gastrointestinal neuromuscular disease characterized by a decreased number of ganglia in the myenteric and submucosal plexuses [3, 4]. In contrast to congenital hypoganglionosis, such as in Hirschsprung's disease, the acquired form presents in adolescence or in adulthood. Histopathology characteristically demonstrates thickened muscularis mucosa and muscularis propria with decreased numbers of myenteric ganglia [3]. There are multiple theories regarding the pathophysiology of HG. It is primarily thought to be caused by chronic inflammation in the colon [3]. No medications have yet been associated with development of the disease. Differential diagnosis of acquired hypoganglionosis includes chronic intestinal pseudo-obstruction, rare enteric myopathies (mutations of the ACTG2 gene), Hirschprung's disease, Chagas disease, enteric neuropathies, and Waardenburg–Shah syndrome [5, 6].

Clozapine is an atypical antipsychotic that is regarded as the most effective treatment for refractory schizophrenia. Despite its efficacy, clozapine remains a third-line medication due to its side effects, including agranulocytosis and severe constipation leading to ileus, gastrointestinal necrosis, and perforation [7]. In January 2020, the FDA strengthened its warning that clozapine-related ileus can lead to serious complications. A review by Cohen et al. reported the case-fatality rate for clozapine-related lower gastrointestinal hypomotility to be 15–27.5%, which is about 7 times that of clozapine-related agranulocytosis [8]. Another review reports a mortality rate of 43.7% due to clozapine-induced ileus from cumulative case reports [9]. Though the mechanism is unknown, it is postulated that clozapine causes constipation due to its anticholinergic, serotonergic, and antihistaminergic properties, similar to other antipsychotics [10].

Presented is a case of acquired hypoganglionosis found in a patient with severe ileus in the setting of the anticholinergic toxicity attributed to clozapine.

2. Case Report/Case Presentation

A 45-year-old Caucasian male with a history of schizoaffective disorder and chronic constipation was brought to the emergency department for acute encephalopathy. He was somnolent and unresponsive to questions. His home medications included a total of 1,200 mg of clozapine daily. It is unclear how long he was taking this dose. He was also taking risperidone, propranolol, linaclotide, benztropine, alprazolam, and diphenhydramine. The patient's medical team could not determine exactly how many years the patient had been taking clozapine, but family and the patient's medical team indicated that he was started on the clozapine therapy years ago in his adulthood. He had never been diagnosed with ileus or other complications of constipation. He had no surgical history. On arrival, the patient was febrile to 38.5°Celsius and tachycardic but otherwise hemodynamically stable. Initial abdominal examination was soft, nontender, mildly distended with reduced bowel sounds.

Laboratory studies showed a clozapine level of 735 mcg/L and norclozapine level of 449 mcg/L (reference value normal 25–440 mcg/L). Other labs were unremarkable except for a hemoglobin level of 11.8 g/dL. Cerebrospinal fluid, blood cultures, and urine cultures were negative. Computed tomography (CT) of the head without contrast was unremarkable. He was found to have significant urinary retention on bladder ultrasound. Given the negative infectious workup and his clinical presentation, along with his multitude of medications with anticholinergic side effects, a working diagnosis of anticholinergic toxicity was made, and the patient's home clozapine was held.

On hospital day 2, he developed bilious emesis and physical exam revealed a soft, distended, and tympanic abdomen that was mildly tender. Abdominal CT showed a large stool burden diffusely in the small and large intestines without obvious transition points that was concerning for ileus. The patient underwent aggressive medical therapy including frequent tap water enemas and polyethylene glycol administered via nasogastric tube and per rectum. He remained NPO (nulla per os) and underwent intermittent nasogastric tube suctioning. Large amounts of stool were evacuated, but the patient continued to have bilious vomiting. Repeat abdominal CT showed fecalization of stool in the small intestine and dilatation of the proximal and rectosigmoid colon to 8.4 cm and 7 cm, respectively, without a clear transition point. The patient was transferred to the intensive care unit and treated with two doses of intravenous neostigmine with significant evacuation of stool. Repeat abdominal CT demonstrated bowel without stool but with significantly worsened dilatation. The patient underwent total colectomy with end ileostomy. Given the remarkable dilatation of the rectum, there was concern that primary ileorectal anastomosis would have led to an inadequate functional outcome, and the decision was made to perform an end ileostomy. The patient recovered rapidly to his mental and functional baseline postoperatively with resumption of normal bowel movements.

Given the patient's severe psychiatric symptoms refractory to other medications, a multidisciplinary meeting with psychiatry was held and it was decided to slowly restart the patient on clozapine with monitoring of symptoms and drug levels. Clozapine was titrated slowly with close monitoring for side effects. The repeat serum clozapine and norclozapine levels were 433 mcg/L and 121 mcg/L, respectively. There was no recurrence of systemic clozapine toxicity or symptoms of gastrointestinal dysmotility at these lower levels.

Full-thickness sections from the ileum (Figure 1), cecum (Figure 2), appendix, colon, sigmoid, and rectum (Figures 3 and 4) were obtained and stained with hematoxylin and eosin (H&E), calretinin, and for S-100, a neuronal marker. Final pathologic diagnosis showed hypertrophy of the colonic muscularis propria in the rectum, sigmoid, and cecum. There was focal loss of muscularis propria in the proximal colon. Though there were some ganglia present in the myenteric and submucosal plexuses, they were only focally present in the proximal colon and appendix. Sections from the ileum showed similar muscle hypertrophy and focally absent ganglia in both plexuses consistent with acquired HG.

3. Pathology

Full-thickness sections from the ileum, cecum, appendix, colon, and rectum were obtained and stained with hematoxylin and eosin (H&E) and for S-100, a neuronal marker.

Final pathologic diagnosis showed hypertrophy of the colonic muscularis propria in the rectum, sigmoid, and cecum. There was focal loss of muscularis propria in the proximal colon. Though there were some ganglia present in the myenteric and submucosal plexuses, they were only focally present in the proximal colon and appendix. Sections from the ileum showed similar muscle hypertrophy and focally absent ganglia in both plexuses. Findings were consistent with acquired hypoganglionosis.

4. Discussion

There are approximately 100 reported cases of isolated HG distinct from Hirschsprung's disease in the literature in the last 40 years, and only a few of those cases were in Caucasian adults [3, 11]. It is also associated with considerable morbidity and mortality [5, 11]. The prevalence of the disease is difficult to quantify because diagnosis is made on histology, which requires examination of full-thickness bowel sections [5]. Immunohistochemistry stains for acetylcholinesterase, S-100, interstitial cells of Cajal, silver, and lactate dehydrogenase are essential in making the diagnosis [11]. It is distinctly different from congenital HG (Hirschsprung's disease), which is diagnosed in children with characteristic contiguous aganglionic segments that start at the anal sphincter and extend proximally [2].

Chronic inflammation in the colon and lower gastrointestinal tract is a common theme unifying theories behind the pathophysiology of acquired HG [3]. Infections, autoimmune diseases, and inflammatory bowel diseases have all been postulated as etiologies of chronic inflammation leading to gut mucosal breakdown and formation of autoantibodies to ganglion cells [3]. Though antipsychotics have

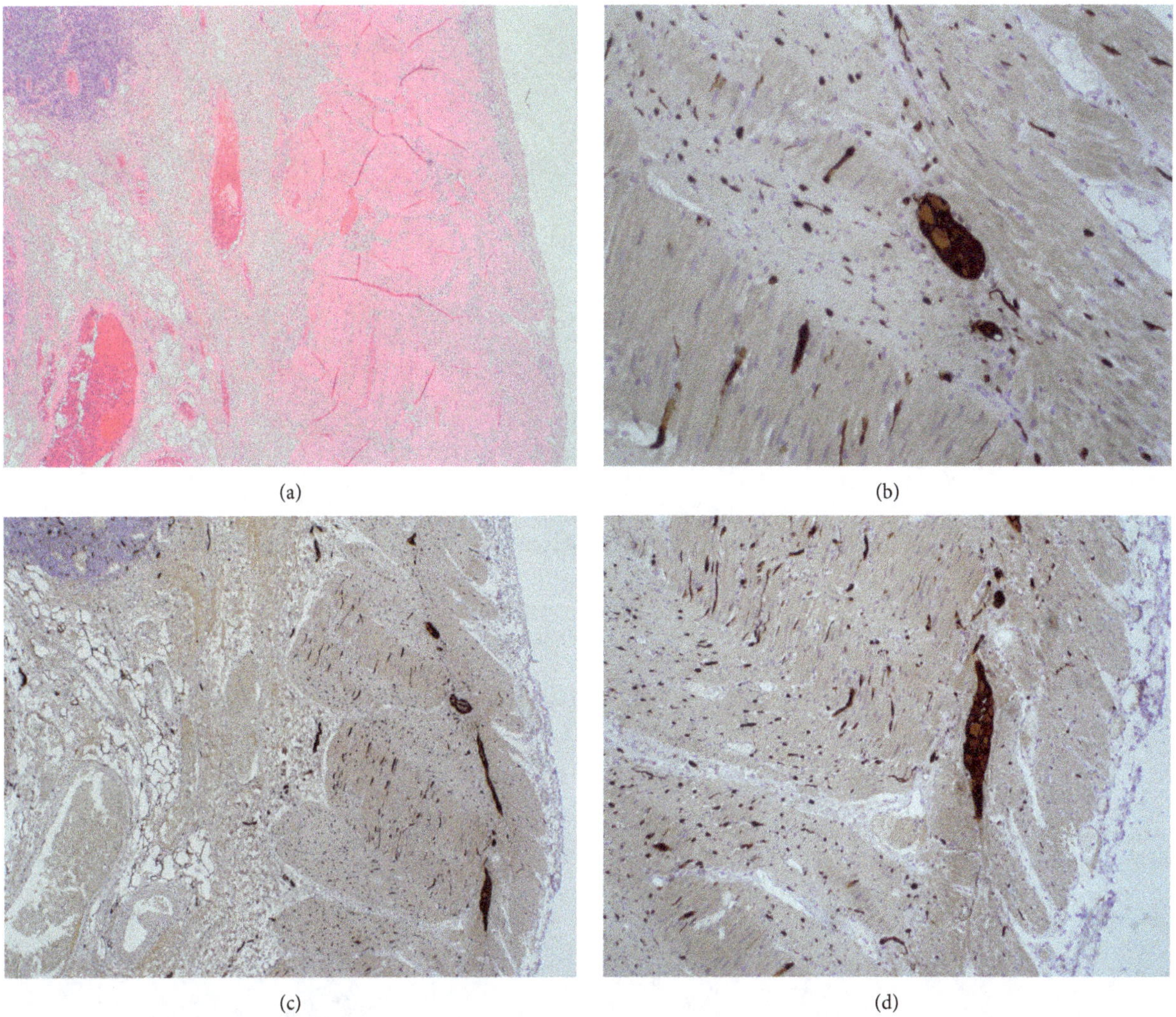

FIGURE 1: Ileum. (a) Hypertrophy of muscularis propria (magnification 10x, H&E). (b) Focally absent ganglion cells (magnification 20x, S100). (c) Auerbach's plexus highlighted in dark brown (magnification 10x, S-100). (d) Numerous ganglion cells in some areas (magnification 20x, S100).

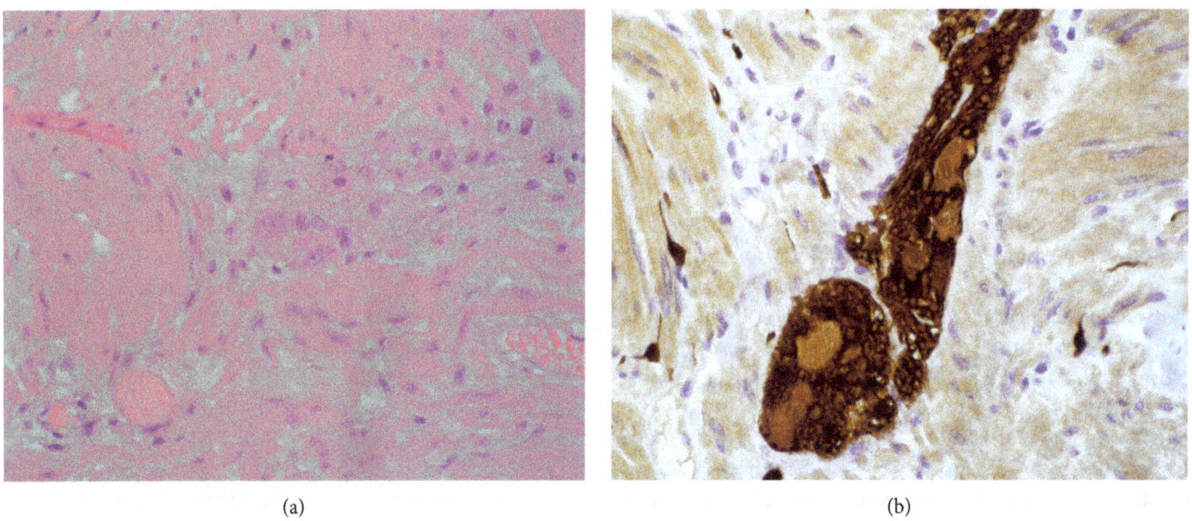

FIGURE 2: Cecum. (a) Reduced ganglion cells (magnification 40x, H&E). (b) Reduced ganglion cells (magnification 40x, S100).

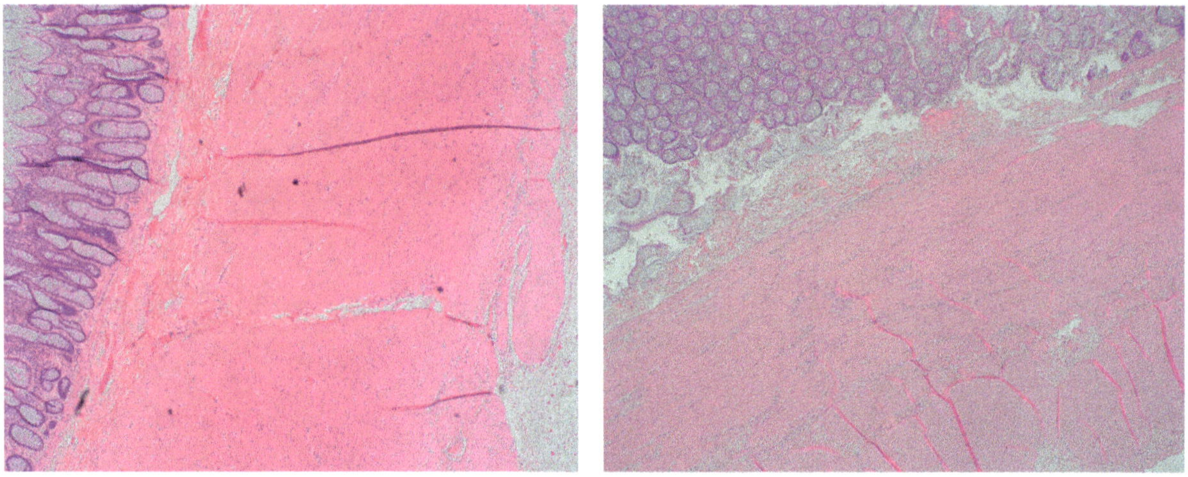

(a) (b)

Figure 3: Hypertrophy of the muscularis propria in rectum and sigmoid sections. (a) Rectum (magnification 10x, H&E). (b) Sigmoid colon (magnification 10x, H&E).

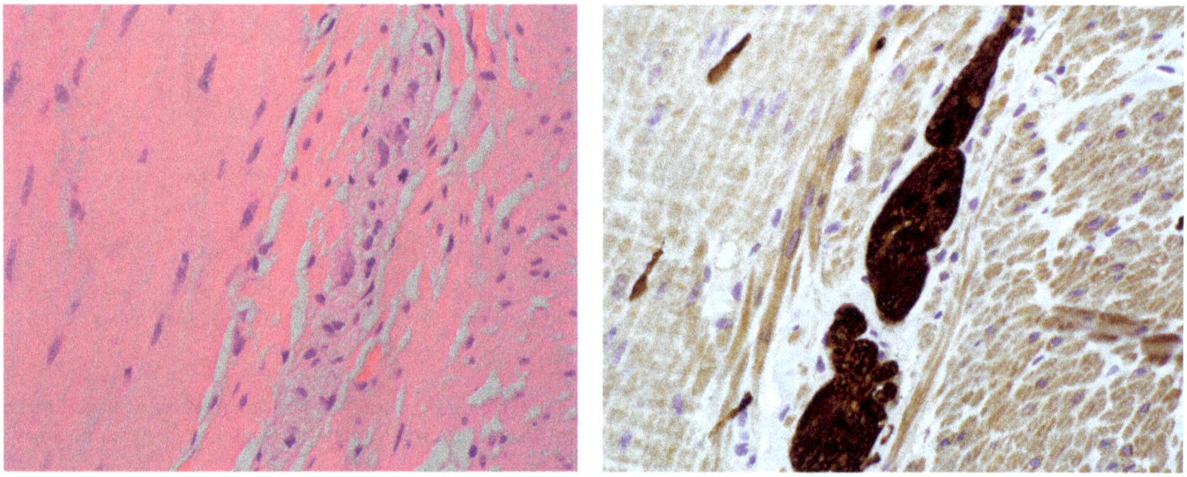

(a) (b)

Figure 4: Sigmoid colon. (a) Focally absent ganglion cells (magnification 40x, H&E). (b) Focally absent ganglion cells (magnification 40x, S100).

prominent anticholinergic effects and have been known to cause constipation and diarrhea, they have not been previously linked to inflammation [9].

It has been reported that acute infection may dramatically increase the serum concentration of clozapine through downregulation of cytochrome *P*450 enzymes during inflammation and infection [12]. In this case, no obvious signs of infection were found, but similar cases of severe ileus in the setting of clozapine may warrant close investigation into possible concurrent infections. There are various data on the optimal therapeutic serum levels of clozapine and its more active metabolite, norclozapine [13, 14]. Serum levels between 350 and 1000 mcg/L have been associated with greater efficacy and less toxicity, though patients may experience toxicity at various levels, and titration should be individualized with careful monitoring of side effects and symptoms [14]. In this patient, initial higher levels of clozapine and its metabolite, norclozapine, were associated with severe side effects, which were no longer present when clozapine was stopped. With careful titration and monitoring, the patient achieved lower serum concentrations of clozapine without suffering severe side effects, though this is difficult to interpret because he was postcolectomy.

The Naranjo scale is a validated scoring system for estimating the probability of an adverse drug reaction. In this case, the Naranjo score is 7, indicating a probable adverse drug reaction [15].

Very few cases of acquired HG have been reported, but the typical presentation of the disease is severe adult-onset ileus with significant colonic distension resulting in colonic necrosis, perforation, and curative colectomy. Pathology in this case did not show classic signs of chronic inflammation but was consistent with the typical clinical and histopathologic presentation of acquired hypoganglionosis. It also overlaps with the well-documented presentation of clozapine-related ileus. Despite a large body of literature on clozapine-related ileus, there is a scarcity of data describing the histopathology of this disease [16].

There are numerous reports of fatal clozapine-related ileus in the literature [17]. It is thought that clozapine significantly reduces gastrointestinal motility primarily by affecting the peripheral muscarinic anticholinergic activity via the M3 receptors in the gut wall [7]. Clozapine is three times more likely to cause constipation than other antipsychotics [5]. One recent study demonstrated that 82% of patients taking clozapine had dysmotility in at least one region of the GI tract, with more than half of those patients experiencing multiregional dysmotility [18].

In this case, the patient had suffered from constipation for most of his adult life. He had no known history of severe constipation as an adolescent, making congenital aganglionosis unlikely. Given the prevalence of clozapine-induced dysmotility and his severe manifestations of constipation later in adulthood, it is likely that his constipation was caused by years of clozapine and antipsychotic use. The mechanism of clozapine-induced constipation is unknown and difficult to study. One challenge is obtaining tissue for analysis from patients who suffer from clozapine-related dysmotility and ileus. Colon biopsies are relatively invasive and difficult to obtain. It is possible that many patients taking clozapine have acquired hypoganglionosis but remain undiagnosed because tissue analysis and special stains for ganglionic cells are rarely performed. In this case, this patient would have remained undiagnosed if he had not had catastrophic complications and a subsequent colectomy. More research is needed to determine the pathophysiologic mechanism behind clozapine-induced ileus and the possibility that it is related to acquired hypoganglionosis.

Authors' Contributions

Catherine Gisi, MD, was involved in conception, data acquisition, interpretation, and drafting of the manuscript.

Acknowledgments

The authors thank Harbor-UCLA Department of Internal Medicine, Division of Gastroenterology, and Harbor-UCLA Department of Pathology for the support.

References

[1] K. M. Sanders, S. D. Koh, S. Ro, and S. M. Ward, "Regulation of gastrointestinal motility-insights from smooth muscle biology," *Nature Reviews Gastroenterology & Hepatology*, vol. 9, no. 11, pp. 633–645, 2012.

[2] S. Krishnamurthy and M. D. Schuffler, "Pathology of neuromuscular disorders of the small intestine and colon," *Gastroenterology*, vol. 93, no. 3, pp. 610–639, 1987.

[3] A. M. Kwok, A. B. Still, and K. Hart, "Acquired segmental colonic hypoganglionosis in an adult Caucasian male: a case report," *World Journal of Gastrointestinal Surgery*, vol. 11, no. 2, pp. 101–111, 2019.

[4] T. Taguchi, K. Masumoto, S. Ieiri, T. Nakatsuji, and J. Akiyoshi, "New classification of hypoganglionosis: congenital and acquired hypoganglionosis," *Journal of Pediatric Surgery*, vol. 41, no. 12, pp. 2046–2051, 2006.

[5] M. Y. Aldossary, A. Privitera, O. Elzamzami, N. Alturki, and K. Sabr, "A rare case of adult-onset rectosigmoid hypoganglionosis," *American Journal of Case Reports*, vol. 19, pp. 557–561, 2018.

[6] M. Rao and M. D. Gershon, "Enteric nervous system development: what could possibly go wrong?," *Nature Reviews Neuroscience*, vol. 19, no. 9, pp. 552–565, 2018.

[7] A. Shirazi, B. Stubbs, L. Gomez et al., "Prevalence and predictors of clozapine-associated constipation: a systematic review and meta-analysis," *International Journal of Molecular Sciences*, vol. 17, no. 6, p. 863, 2016.

[8] D. Cohen, J. P. A. M. Bogers, D. Van Dijk, B. Bakker, and P. F. J. Schulte, "Beyond white blood cell monitoring," *The Journal of Clinical Psychiatry*, vol. 73, no. 10, pp. 1307–1312, 2012.

[9] D. Cohen, "Clozapine and gastrointestinal hypomotility," *CNS Drugs*, vol. 31, no. 12, pp. 1083–1091, 2017.

[10] H. L. Philpott, S. Nandurkar, J. Lubel, and P. R. Gibson, "Drug-induced gastrointestinal disorders," *Frontline Gastroenterology*, vol. 5, no. 1, pp. 49–57, 2013.

[11] T. C. Deroche, S.-Y. Xiao, and X. Liu, "Histological evaluation in ulcerative colitis," *Gastroenterology Report*, vol. 2, no. 3, pp. 178–192, 2014.

[12] K. Raaska, V. Raitasuo, M. Arstila, and P. Neuvonen, "Bacterial pneumonia can increase serum concentration of clozapine," *European Journal of Clinical Pharmacology*, vol. 58, no. 5, pp. 321-322, 2002.

[13] J. C. Ellison and R. L. Dufresne, "A review of the clinical utility of serum clozapine and norclozapine levels," *Mental Health Clinician*, vol. 5, no. 2, pp. 68–73, 2015.

[14] A. Stark and J. Scott, "A review of the use of clozapine levels to guide treatment and determine cause of death," *Australian & New Zealand Journal of Psychiatry*, vol. 46, no. 9, pp. 816–825, 2012.

[15] C. A. Naranjo, U. Busto, E. M. Sellers et al., "A method for estimating the probability of adverse drug reactions," *Clinical Pharmacology and Therapeutics*, vol. 30, no. 2, pp. 239–245, 1981.

[16] C. A. Janecek, B. C. Morson, S. G. Meuwissen, N. W. Schipper, J. Lindeman, and C. J. Meijer, "Histopathological evaluation of colonic mucosal biopsy specimens in chronic inflammatory bowel disease: diagnostic implications," *Gut*, vol. 32, no. 12, pp. 1514–1520, 1991.

[17] M. T. Osterman, C. Foley, and I. Matthias, "Clozapine-induced acute gastrointestinal necrosis: a case report," *Journal of Medical Case Reports*, vol. 11, no. 1, 2017.

[18] S. Every-Palmer, S. J. Inns, E. Grant, and P. M. Ellis, "Effects of clozapine on the gut: cross-sectional study of delayed gastric emptying and small and large intestinal dysmotility," *CNS Drugs*, vol. 33, no. 1, pp. 81-91, 2019.

2

Bleeding Meckel's Diverticulum in a 33-Year-Old Female Diagnosed with Video Capsule Endoscopy and a Technetium-99 m Pertechnetate Scan with a Favorable Response to H_2 Blocker and PPI

Gregor Krstevski, Urim Isahi, and Vladimir Andreevski

University Clinic of Gastroenterohepatology, Medical Faculty, Ss. Cyril and Methodius University, Boulevard Mother Teresa 17, Skopje 1000, North Macedonia

Correspondence should be addressed to Gregor Krstevski; gregor.krstevski@medf.ukim.edu.mk

Academic Editor: Haruhiko Sugimura

Meckel's diverticulum is a true diverticulum consisting of all three layers of the small intestine resulting from incomplete regression of the vitelline duct. While it is often benign, it can present with serious complications such as intussusception, ulceration, torsion, hemorrhage, obstruction, inflammation, and fistula formation. Although it typically presents in infancy and early childhood, it can also manifest much later into adulthood. We report a case of Meckel's diverticulum complicated by significant bleeding in a 33-year-old female patient. Diagnosis was accomplished with video capsule endoscopy and a technetium-99 m pertechnetate scan. The patient responded well to acid suppression, initially with an H_2 blocker and later with a PPI (proton pump inhibitor), and remained asymptomatic for nearly four months in the interim to definitive surgical treatment. Microscopic examination of the resected diverticulum confirmed the presence of ectopic gastric mucosa. A PubMed literature search revealed several similar cases of Meckel's diverticulum complicated by hemorrhage with a favorable response to H_2 blockers and PPIs. While surgical resection remains the mainstay of definitive treatment, medications aimed at acid suppression can delay the need for urgent surgery, allow for diagnostic assessment, and optimize conditions for elective surgical treatment.

1. Introduction

Meckel's diverticulum is the most common congenital anomaly of the gastrointestinal tract. It is a true diverticulum that results from incomplete regression of the omphalomesenteric, also known as the vitelline duct. Although it is often benign, it can cause complications, and these include intussusception, ulceration, torsion, hemorrhage, obstruction, inflammation, and fistula formation. The rule of 2s has traditionally been used to characterize this condition, referring to a population prevalence of 2%, typically located within 2 feet proximal to the ileocecal valve; symptomatic lesions largely present prior to the age of 2, and their length is often approximately 2 inches (5 cm). Nonetheless, Meckel's diverticulum can remain silent and become symptomatic in adulthood [1]. We report a case of Meckel's diverticulum complicated by significant bleeding in an adult female diagnosed with video capsule endoscopy and confirmed with a technetium-99 m pertechnetate scan that responded well to acid suppression in the interim prior to surgical resection.

2. Case Report

Our patient is a 33-year-old female that presented with a three-day history of abdominal pain, malaise, and maroon-colored loose stools. She noted bloating and nonspecific abdominal pain localized in the periumbilical region and epigastrium. During the previous day, she had experienced a syncopal episode at her place of employment with spontaneous return of consciousness. Subsequent laboratory testing revealed anemia with erythrocyte count 2.6×10^{12}/L, hemoglobin 82 g/L, and hematocrit 23.3%, and urgent upper gastrointestinal endoscopy did not display a bleeding lesion. The patient reported no pertinent past medical history and did not take NSAIDs or blood thinners. She reported no allergies to food or drugs and did not smoke cigarettes, drink alcohol, or use illicit drugs. Family history was positive in her father for hemorrhoids and in her aunt for a duodenal ulcer. On physical examination, blood pressure was 120/70 mmHg, pulse was 70/min, and palpation elicited light pain in the left hemiabdomen. Digital rectal examination showed maroon-colored stool. Additional laboratory testing showed leukocytosis 20.1×10^{9}/L, prothrombin time 14.3 seconds, INR 1.33, serum amylase 148 U/L, and a normal level of urea, thrombocytes, proteins, and electrolytes. The patient was admitted and transfused with two units of packed red blood cells. She was also treated with an NPO regimen, intravenous fluids, continuous octreotide infusion, and H_2 blocker. Following treatment, the patient's condition stabilized and no new bloody stools were noted. Laboratory values also trended towards normal. Abdominal ultrasound and repeat upper gastrointestinal endoscopy showed no abnormalities. Lower gastrointestinal endoscopy permitted evaluation up to 10 cm proximal to the ileocecal valve and displayed no significant abnormalities. Video capsule endoscopy (using PillCam SB capsule, Given Imaging, Yoqneam, Israel) demonstrated the presence of a solitary diverticulum in the distal half of the ileum, a finding suggestive of Meckel's diverticulum. Images can be found in Figure 1.

MR enterography did not show any abnormalities; however, abdominal scintigraphy with Technetium-99 m pertechnetate revealed abnormal accumulation of the radioisotope in the distal ileum in correlation with the presence of ectopic gastric mucosa (Figure 2).

The patient was maintained on PPI for nearly four months and remained asymptomatic, with stable hemoglobin and no new episodes of gastrointestinal bleeding. She then underwent laparoscopic surgery, and the diverticulum was resected. The surgical specimen, which showed a diverticulum contralateral to the mesentery, was then sent for histopathologic analysis. The relevant macroscopic and microscopic findings detailed in the pathology report are summarized in Table 1. At high magnification (x200) of the area of gastric mucosa, parietal cells with a deeply eosinophilic cytoplasm in comparison to the mucinous and chief cells are seen (Figure 3).

3. Discussion

In summary, this is a case of Meckel's diverticulum in a 33-year-old female patient with significant bleeding and a resultant profound, life-threatening anemia. As noted above, Meckel's diverticulum is a vestigial remnant of the omphalomesenteric duct. It develops in the fourth week of gestation and serves as a connection between the loops of the primitive gut and the yolk sac. It normally obliterates by the tenth week of gestation; however, it can persist even into adulthood. There are several distinct entities that arise from persistence of the vitelline duct. An umbilicoileal fistula occurs when the duct remains entirely patent. In the case of persistence of the distal portion at the umbilicus, it is termed an umbilical sinus. Persistence of the middle portion results in the formation of fluid-filled cysts termed enterocystomas. The most common anomaly is nonobliteration of the proximal segment in continuity with the small intestine, forming what is known as Meckel's diverticulum. It is a true diverticulum consisting of all three layers of the small intestine [2].

The first description of this condition by Johann Friedrich Meckel dates more than 200 years back. In-depth understanding and definition of the embryological origins, histological constitution, and span of complications have been defined since. As pluripotent cells line the vitelline duct, ectopic tissue is a typical feature of Meckel's diverticulum. Gastric mucosa is most common; however, duodenal, colonic, pancreatic, Brunner's glands, and hepatobiliary and endometrial mucosa can also be found. Of importance is that silent or asymptomatic Meckel's diverticula are less likely to contain ectopic tissue [3–5].

Most studies place the true incidence of this abnormality between 0.6% and 4% and the male to female ratio of symptomatic disease at 1.5–4:1. More than half of symptomatic cases requiring surgery occur in children, and the most common complications are obstruction, hemorrhage, and inflammation. This holds true in both the pediatric and adult populations, with obstruction accounting for a higher proportion in children when compared to adults. Bleeding can result from erosion of the adjacent intestinal mucosa by gastric mucosal secretions in the manner of peptic ulceration. Bleeding can also occur in the setting of strangulation, torsion, or intussusception, and these are commonly accompanied by pain. Obstruction can be caused by intussusception, volvulus, herniation, diverticulitis, bowel loop entrapment, and phytobezoar formation. Meckel's diverticulum has a greater neoplastic potential than the remainder of the ileum, and the mean age for Meckelean cancers is 60. Inflammation is another important complication, and it can lead to perforation. The mechanism generally includes blockage of the opening of the diverticulum by food, foreign bodies, large microorganisms such as parasites, and enteroliths. Consequent perforation leads to peritonitis, and the presentation is very similar, if not indiscernible, to acute appendicitis [3–5].

Diagnosis is particularly challenging in adults as Meckel's diverticulum is very rare and mimics an array of differing pathologies [4]. Conventional techniques such as x-ray, ultrasound, CT, and barium studies have limited diagnostic value as the findings are nonspecific. For example, a plain abdominal x-ray may show pneumoperitoneum in the case of perforation or bowel distention proximal to the site of obstruction. Ultrasound may show bowel wall thickening, focal findings that suggest an abscess, or the presence of anomalous vessels via use of Doppler. These findings may raise suspicion, but do not pinpoint to the exact diagnosis. Imaging with labelled red blood cells and angiography of the abdominal blood vessels (the superior

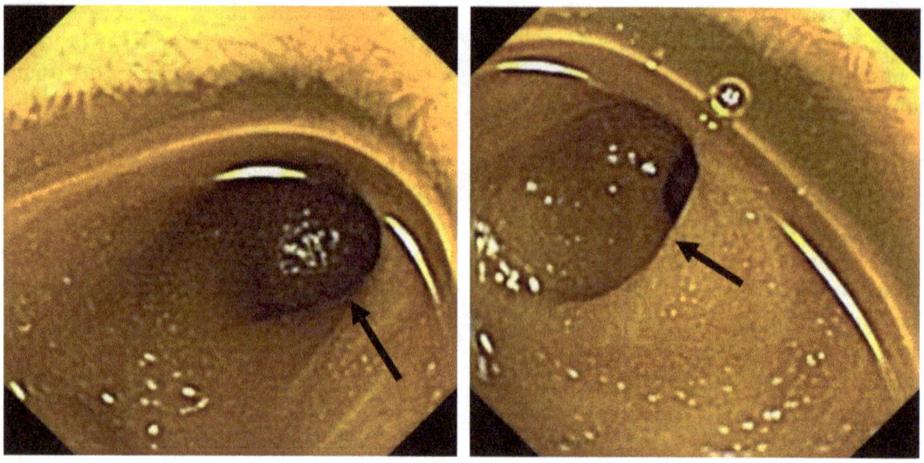

Figure 1: Video capsule endoscopy demonstrated a solitary diverticulum (indicated by black arrows) in the distal half of the ileum.

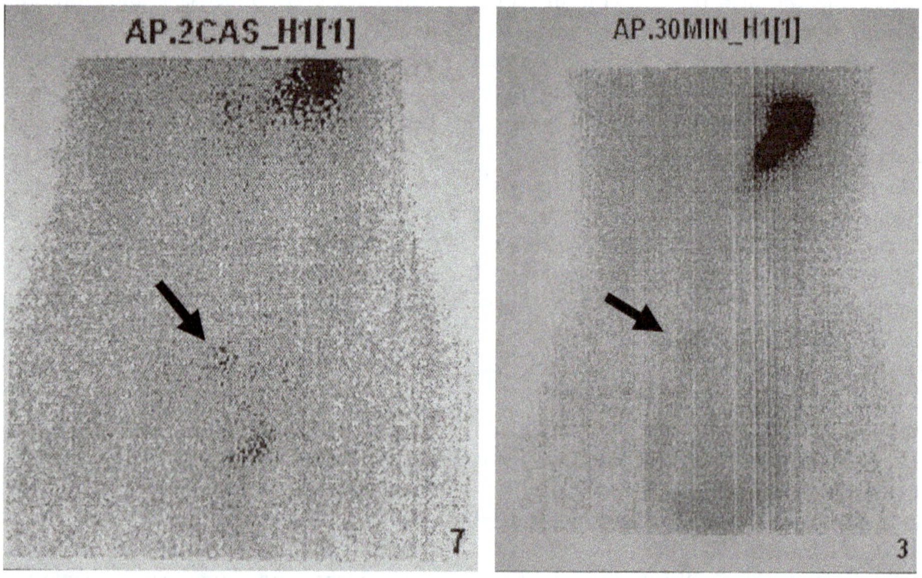

Figure 2: Abdominal scintigraphy with 99 m Tc pertechnetate (Meckel scan) showed abnormal accumulation of the radioisotope indicating the presence of ectopic gastric mucosa. The black arrows point to the areas of abnormal accumulation.

Table 1: Pathology report of the resected tissue.

Macroscopic findings	We received a partially longitudinally resected segment of the small intestine with a total length of 5 cm, perimeter of 3.5 cm, and mural width of 0.4–0.8 cm. The contour of the small intestinal mucosa is regular, while in a zone of approximately 2.2 × 2 cm contralateral to the mesentery, there is a semicircular widening of the lumen, a diverticulum, with thinning of the wall to 0.4–0.5 cm, and flattened and hyperaemic mucosa. The width of the wall in the remaining part is 0.6–0.8 cm
Microscopic findings	In part, the structure of the small intestinal wall has a regular histologic architecture, with scant chronic inflammatory infiltrate in lamina propria, while in part, the lumen is covered by gastric mucosa with a moderate and, in some places, accentuated chronic inflammatory infiltrate in lamina propria with the presence of many eosinophils and multifocal mucinous metaplasia. There are small foci of cystic glandular dilation and an atrophic appearance of the mucosa. Parietal cells with a deeply eosinophilic cytoplasm are detected. In places, the inflammatory infiltrate spreads to the submucosa, where it has a much lesser intensity. In the part of the diverticular widening, there is thinning of the muscle layer of the wall of the diverticulum
Conclusion	The findings correlate with Meckel's diverticulum with gastric mucosa and signs of chronically active inflammation. The resection margin shows regular small intestinal structure except for the presence of a discrete inflammatory infiltrate in lamina propria

mesenteric artery in particular) has greater use as it can pinpoint the exact location of hemorrhage [5, 6]. However, studies demonstrate that angiography is only effective when bleeding exceeds 0.5 ml/min [4]. CT and MR enterography can also provide a good means for the examination of irregularities within the intestinal lumen, wall, and

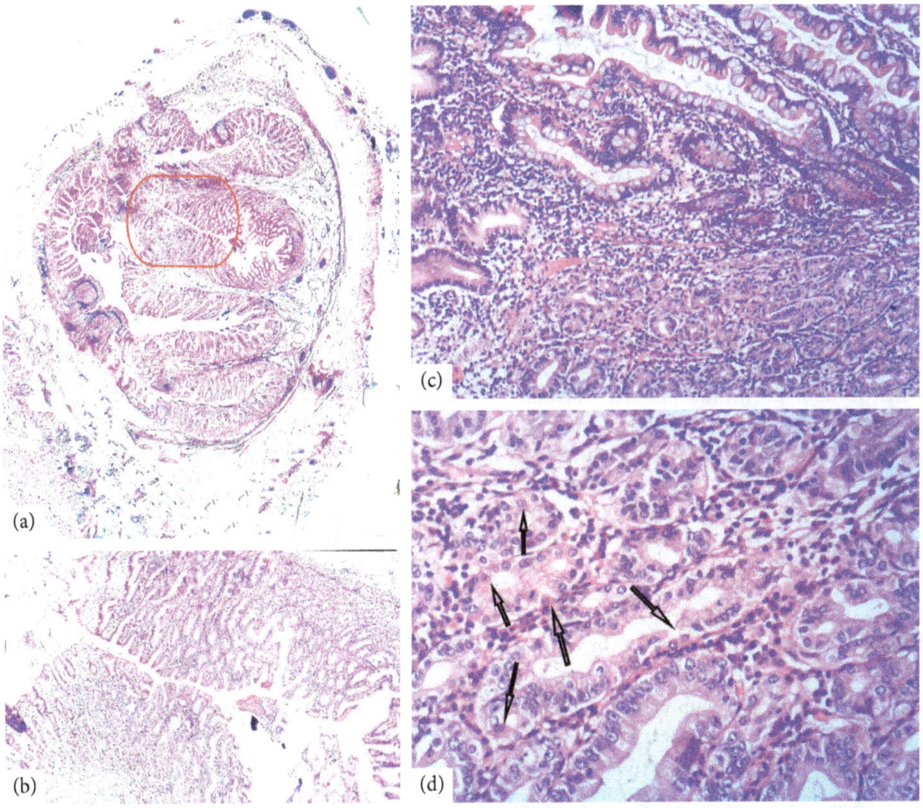

FIGURE 3: (a) HeEo (x5): cross section of the diverticulum. Gastric mucosa is delineated with a red line. (b) HeEo (x40): the section with gastric mucosa at higher magnification. (c) HeEo (x100): margin between intestinal (upper half) and gastric mucosa (lower half). (d) HeEo (x200): some of the parietal cells in the gastric mucosa (arrows), with a deeply eosinophilic cytoplasm as opposed to the mucinous and chief cells.

surroundings. The special diagnostic value of the technetium-99 m pertechnetate scan is in the radioisotope's proclivity to gastric mucosa, which is why it has been termed the Meckel scan. The rate of false negatives can be reduced by administering pentagastrin or an H_2 blocker prior to the scan. These agents increase uptake and decrease the release of the radioisotope by gastric mucosa, respectively. A more novel approach to diagnosing Meckel's diverticulum is direct visualization via capsule endoscopy and anterograde and retrograde double balloon enteroscopy. These allow for more precise localization and characterization of the lesion. Nevertheless, Meckel's diverticulum is most commonly discovered incidentally during surgical interventions for unrelated conditions [5, 6].

Management of incidentally discovered Meckel's is controversial. The lifetime incidence of complications of Meckel's diverticula is approximated at 4–6%. While surgical resection may prevent future adverse events, surgery in itself carries a risk for immediate and delayed complications. When incidentally discovered intraoperatively, weighted risk scores can be applied to reach a decision. Factors that increase the risk for future complications provide support for resection: age (<45 or <50 depending on the author), male gender, lesions 2 cm or longer, broad based, the presence of abnormal tissue, and attached fibrous bands [5]. The surgeon should take into account the patient's comorbidities, other intraoperative strains and complications, and an initial poor prognosis. Therefore, resection of an intraoperatively and incidentally discovered Meckel's diverticulum is largely at the operator's discretion [4–6].

The most common ectopic tissue found in Meckel's diverticula is gastric mucosa. Secretions from these cells can damage and erode adjacent intestinal mucosa, closely resembling peptic gastric and duodenal ulceration. Proton pump inhibitors block the H+/K+ ATP proton pump, thereby inhibiting the final process of acid production and secretion that is mediated by gastrin, H_2, and cholinergic pathways. H_2 blockers specifically act on H_2-dependent acid generation and secretion [7]. It is theorized that acid secretion from Meckel's diverticula that contain ectopic gastric mucosa can be suppressed by the use of PPIs and H_2 blockers, thereby preventing mucosal damage. Using PubMed, we performed a literature search and looked for articles containing the term Meckel's diverticulum in combination with PPIs, pantoprazole, omeprazole, lansoprazole, H_2 blockers, ranitidine, famotidine, and cimetidine. The resulting lists of articles were then carefully assessed, with the majority focusing on the use of H_2 blockers in increasing the sensitivity of the technetium-99 m pertechnetate scan. Several case reports discussing the use of PPIs and H_2 blockers as treatment modalities for Meckel's diverticulum were identified, and an additional article published in the American Journal of Gastroenterology was identified by using Google search. The relevant details of each case are listed in Table 2. A study by Schonsberg et al.

Table 2: Identified cases of Meckel's diverticulum treated with acid suppression.

Author and year	Presentation and diagnostic work-up	Medication	Outcome
1. Kirkpatrick A. R., 1978 [8]	A 27-year-old male with abdominal pain, gross bloody stool, and pallor, diagnosed using the Tc-99 m scan. The patient initially refused surgery due to financial reasons	Cimetidine 300 mg 4x/day per os.	Hemoglobin stabilized, and symptoms resolved for three months. Bleeding recurred upon stopping medication, and surgery was performed
2. Colins, J. C. Jr., 1980 [9]	A 26-year-old female with rectal bleeding and abdominal pain. Initial diagnosis was made with barium studies; it was confirmed with the Tc-99 m scan	Cimetidine initially i.v. and then per os.	There was no further bleeding. Elective surgery was performed 10 days later. Microscopic examination reiterated the diagnosis
3. Selker H. P., 1983 [10]	A 23-year-old male with postprandial infraumbilical pain, stool occult blood, and microcytic hypochromic anemia. Barium studies demonstrated a large ileal diverticulum; the Meckel scan was normal	Cimetidine 400 mg 4x/day per os.	Medication was stopped, and bleeding recurred. Cimetidine was restarted with good response, and surgery was performed five days later. Microscopic examination confirmed the diagnosis and demonstrated gastric-like mucosa
4. Xinias I. et al., 2012 [11]	An 8-year-old boy with bright red stools, eventually diagnosed with wireless capsule endoscopy	Ranitidine 6 mg/kg of body weight 2x/day per os.	Maintained symptom free for six months, after which surgery was performed. Microscopic examination confirmed the diagnosis
5. Dashan A., 2006 [12]	A 9-year-old boy with overt gastrointestinal bleeding. Diagnosis was made with isotope scanning	Pantoprazole 40 mg/day i.v.	Symptoms resolved, and surgery was performed 4 days after initial presentation
6. Ottaviano L. F. et al., 2016 [13]	A 72-year-old female with beta-thalassemia trait presented with weakness and anemia. Double-balloon enteroscopy found midileal diverticulum with adjacent ulcer	PPI	The patient refused surgery, and at 7 months' follow-up, hemoglobin remained stable with no new episodes of melena or overt GI bleeding
7. Ottaviano L. F. et al., 2016 [13]	An 80-year-old male with abdominal pain and anemia. CT showed distal small-intestinal wall thickening, and video capsule endoscopy demonstrated an ulcer. Double-balloon enteroscopy showed a nonbleeding jejunal angioectasia (treated with argon plasma coagulation) and ulcerated midileal mucosa surrounding a small diverticulum	PPI	Symptom resolution up to study date
8. Manning R. J., 1987 [14]	A 25-year-old male with copious gastrointestinal bleeding	Cimetidine 300 mg 4x/day and ranitidine 150 mg 3x/day per os.	Despite two H2 blockers and aggressive i.v. fluid and blood replacement, bleeding persisted, and emergent surgery was performed. Meckel's diverticulum was found intraoperatively and confirmed microscopically

discussing two cases of Meckel's diverticulum that presented with enterorrhagia and were managed with H_2 blockers was not included as the full text of the study was inaccessible and an attempt at contacting the authors to obtain it was unsuccessful.

Temporary symptom resolution was accomplished with acid suppression in seven of the eight identified cases of bleeding Meckel's diverticulum. Albeit in two of the cases (6 and 7), the diagnosis was highly likely, it was not confirmed with an isotope scan or microscopically. Moreover, case 7 showed the presence of a jejunal angioectasia that was not bleeding at the moment of double-balloon enteroscopy and was treated with argon plasma coagulation. In case number 8, the patient had persistent copious bleeding despite intense acid suppression and ectopic gastric mucosa later being demonstrated microscopically. This suggests that acid suppression with PPIs or H_2 blockers may be useful in many cases of bleeding Meckel's diverticulum with ectopic gastric mucosa in the interim to definitive surgical treatment.

4. Conclusions

To conclude, this case demonstrates that Meckel's diverticulum can manifest with life-threatening blood loss even in the adult population. The practicing gastroenterologist should include this condition in the differential diagnosis of any case of obscure gastrointestinal bleeding and take the necessary diagnostic measures to confirm or exclude its presence. Acid suppression may favorably alter the disease course of Meckel's diverticulum when ectopic gastric mucosa is present, allowing for diagnostic work-up and optimizing conditions for definitive elective surgical treatment. Considering the fact that gastric mucosa is the most common type of ectopic tissue found in Meckel's diverticulum, PPI or an H_2 blocker should be administered when faced with obscure gastrointestinal bleeding.

References

[1] A. Stallion and J. M. Shuck, "Meckel's diverticulum," in *Surgical Treatment: Evidence-Based and Problem-Oriented*, R. G. Holzheimer and J. A. Mannick, Eds., Zuckschwerdt, Munich, Germany, 2001, https://www.ncbi.nlm.nih.gov/books/NBK6918/.

[2] N. K. Kuwajerwala, Y. J. Silva, V. S. Kanthimathinathan, M. R. Villalba, A. Mohammed, and J. Geibel, *Meckel Diverticulum*, 2021, https://emedicine.medscape.com/article/194776.

[3] C. C. Hansen and K. Søreide, "Systematic review of epidemiology, presentation, and management of meckel's diverticulum in the 21st century," *Medicine*, vol. 97, no. 35, Article ID e12154, 2018.

[4] J. Sagar, V. Kumar, and D. K. Shah, "Meckel's diverticulum: a systematic review," *Journal of the Royal Society of Medicine*, vol. 99, no. 10, pp. 501–505, 2006.

[5] S. Kuru and K. Kismet, "Meckel's diverticulum: clinical features, diagnosis and management," *Revista Espanola de Enfermedades Digestivas: Organo Oficial de La Sociedad Espanola de Patologia Digestiva*, vol. 110, no. 11, pp. 726–732, 2018, PMID: 30032625.

[6] V. K. Kotha, A. Khandelwal, S. S. Saboo et al., "Radiologist's perspective for the meckel's diverticulum and its complications," *The British Journal of Radiology*, vol. 87, no. 1037, Epub 2014 Feb 17. PMID: 24611767; PMCID: PMC4075535, Article ID 20130743, 2014.

[7] J. R. Pisegna, "Pharmacology of acid suppression in the hospital setting: focus on proton pump inhibition," *Critical Care Medicine*, vol. 30, no. 6 Suppl, pp. S356–S361, 2002.

[8] R. A. Kirkpatrick, "Cimetidine and meckel's diverticulum," *Annals of Internal Medicine*, vol. 88, no. 6, pp. 846-847, 1978, PMID: 307357.

[9] J. C. Collins Jr., "Hemorrhage from a meckel's diverticulum: one case with heterotopic gastric mucosa treated with cimetidine," *Archives of Surgery*, vol. 115, no. 1, pp. 83-84, 1980, PMID: 6965344.

[10] H. P. Selker, "Cimetidine and cryptic "dyspepsia meckeli"," *JAMA: The Journal of the American Medical Association*, vol. 249, no. 10, p. 1266, 1983 PMID: 6827698.

[11] I. Xinias, A. Mavroudi, M. Fotoulaki, G. Tsikopoulos, A. Kalampakas, and G. Imvrios, "Wireless capsule endoscopy detects meckel's diverticulum in a child with unexplained intestinal blood loss," *Case Reports in Gastroenterology*, vol. 6, no. 3, pp. 650–659, 2012 Sep, Epub 2012 Oct 18. PMID: 23139657; PMCID: PMC3493004.

[12] A. Dahshan, "Bleeding meckel diverticulum responds to intravenous pantoprazole," *Southern Medical Journal*, vol. 100, no. 3, p. 334, 2007 PMID: 17396746.

[13] L. F. Ottaviano, Y. Cui, E. Quintero, J. M. Buscaglia, and J. Carlos, "Suspected meckel's diverticulum as cause of gastrointestinal bleeding in elderly adults," *American Journal of Gastroenterology*, no. p S1369, p. 111, 2016.

[14] R. J. Manning, "Failure of H2 blocker therapy in a case of hemorrhage from a meckel's diverticulum," *Journal of Clinical Gastroenterology*, vol. 9, no. 2, p. 242, 1987 PMID: 3494758.

3

Ovarian Crohn's Disease: A Case Report and Review of the Literature

Hamza Mohammed,[1] Rana Bokhary,[2] Mohammed Nassif,[3] and Mahmoud Mosli[1]

[1]*Departments of Medicine, King Abdulaziz University, Jeddah, Saudi Arabia*
[2]*Departments of Pathology, King Abdulaziz University, Jeddah, Saudi Arabia*
[3]*Departments of Surgery, King Abdulaziz University, Jeddah, Saudi Arabia*

Correspondence should be addressed to Mahmoud Mosli; mmosli@kau.edu.sa

Academic Editor: Haruhiko Sugimura

We present to you a rare case of Crohn's disease involving the ovary in a 28-year-old nulligravida Eritrean patient. This is considered a rare manifestation of Crohn's disease that is believed to be due to fistulization between the ovary and intestines.

1. Introduction

Crohn's disease (CD) is an inflammatory bowel disorder (IBD) that is progressive in nature, resulting in certain complications such as fistulization or stricture formation that once developed may require surgical intervention [1]. The clinical picture of CD includes gastrointestinal symptoms such as abdominal pain, weight loss, and diarrhea [2], in addition to systemic manifestations such as joint pain and skin involvement [3, 4]. The age group for CD varies from childhood to older age groups, but it is most commonly diagnosed between 15 and 30 years of age [4]. The prevalence of CD worldwide and in Saudi Arabia has been increasing over the past 30 years. The most commonly affected site in CD is the ileo-cecal region [5].

There are no firm diagnostic features for CD but typical signs include perianal fistulas, large skin tags or abscesses on physical examination [6], small bowel involvement, mucosal ulceration, cobble stoning, narrowing, obstruction, and fistulas seen on cross-sectional imaging [6], as well as ileo-cecal valve stenosis, cobble stoning, ulcerations, strictures, and fistulas seen endoscopically [6]. Histopathological features suggestive of CD include noncaseating granulomas and transmural lymphoid aggregates, which are often only noticeable after examining a resected part of the bowel [6]. Differentiating CD from intestinal tuberculosis remains a diagnostic challenge and often results in a delay in the diagnosis and treatment [7, 8]. Both CD and intestinal TB can result in fistulization into adjacent organs, commonly into other small or large bowel segments, the urinary bladder, the vagina, or even to the skin. There are also reports of fistulization into the stomach and duodenum [9–11]. Here, we present a case of a young female presenting with a rare complication of CD, which involved the ovary.

2. Case Presentation

A 28-year-old single nulligravida Eritrean patient presented in 2013 to the emergency department with right lower quadrant pain for 3 weeks. Her pain started gradually; it was colicky and throbbing in nature and radiated to her right leg. The pain was aggravated by fatty and spicy food, occurred on and off, and was partially alleviated by painkillers. The pain was associated with nausea, vomiting, bloating, alternating diarrhea and constipation, and episodes of bleeding per rectum. The patient had her first menstrual period when she was 11; she had regular cycles for 7 days until recently, as her period lasted only for 3 days in the two cycles preceding her presentation, with increased premenstruation pain. She reported that she had no weight loss, no loss of appetite, no night sweats, but had palpitations while her other systems were unremarkable. She only complained of eczema and her past surgical history was of an anal fistula in 2010; she had no blood transfusion and no known food or drug allergies, and she is a nonsmoker. Her younger sister was known to have ileal Crohn's disease.

She was diagnosed in the ER with appendicitis and underwent emergency appendectomy. After appendectomy, she continued to complain of continuous abdominal discomfort. In March of 2017, the patient returned to the hospital due to recurrence of pain associated with loss of appetite. A CT scan of the abdomen revealed a right adnexal mass inseparable from a thickened and stenosed distal ileum. An exploratory lower midline laparotomy was done that revealed an abscess in the right side of the abdomen in the vicinity of the distal part of the small intestines along with ovarian swelling. She underwent abscess drainage and right ovarian cystectomy only, as the ileum itself was inflamed but with no fat creeping and was not fibrotic, indicating that it itself was not diseased but showed signs of inflammation due to proximity to the diseased ovary. The patient tolerated the procedure well, had an uneventful hospital stay, and was discharged from the hospital three days later.

The histopathological examination of the right ovarian mass revealed infiltration of the ovarian stroma by a mixture of inflammatory cells composed of lymphocytes, plasma cells, neutrophils, and histiocytes, with formation of multiple microabscesses. Collections of epithelioid histiocytes with formation of granulomas were also noted. Some of these granulomas showed central suppuration. There was no evidence of malignancy. Ziehl-Neelsen and Grocott's methenamine silver stains were performed and found to be negative for acid-fast *Bacilli* and fungal organisms. The final pathological impression was of a diffuse multifocal necrotizing granulomatous inflammation that was consistent with CD (see Figure 1).

3. Discussion and Review of the Literature

There are 18 reported cases of ovarian CD in the literature. Gawron et al. reported a case in 2017 that described a 27-year-old nulligravida patient that was known to have CD who presented with fever, pelvic pain, and a palpable mass. Transabdominal ultrasound confirmed this mass to be located in the right iliac fossa, and hence, a tubo-ovarian abscess was suspected. As a result, the patient underwent diagnostic laparoscopy; a right-sided oophorectomy was performed and upon examining the surgical sample, a granuloma was identified and was suggestive of CD [12].

In August 2016, a total of three cases of ovarian CD were also reported, there were pelvic abscesses documented in the first two cases because of fistulization with the terminal ileum, and an ovarian abscess was noticed in the third case as a consequence of disease adjacency [13]. Rindos et al. reported in 2015 on a 35-year-old nulligravida patient known to have CD who was also diagnosed with ovarian involvement; this was believed by the authors to have started from an ovario-intestinal fistula [14].

Yabushita et al. also presented a case of ileal/ovarian cystoma fistula due to CD. A 22-year-old woman was diagnosed at the age of 20 in the hospital with CD of the large and small intestine; she had right lower abdominal pain and thus was admitted for investigations; GI contrast studies showed no fistulas but CT examination suspected an intestinal ovarian cyst fistula. Surgery was performed and revealed that the ovarian cyst became a lump with the ileum and was diagnosed as ileo-ovarian fistula; partial resection of the ileum and resection of the appendix were performed [15].

Ouakaa-Kchaou et al. reported a case of a 32-year-old Caucasian female that presented with a 1-day history of lower right quadrant abdominal pain that was associated with vomiting and fever; the patient was medically and surgically free with no family history of IBD; a diagnosis of acute appendicitis was in consideration; therefore, the patient was referred to surgery; during laparotomy, a thickened segment of the terminal ileum was adherent to the right edematous enlarged ovary with direct fistulization seen between them accompanied by an ovarian abscess with an ileo-ileal fistula, which led to the suspicion of CD. This led the surgeon to perform an en bloc right salpingo-oophorectomy with a standard ileo-cecal and ileo-ileal fistula resection. On histopathology, a section of the small intestine showed patchy mucosal ulceration, submucosal fibrosis, lymphoid aggregation, fissure ulcers, and transmural inflammation, while the right ovary showed extensive necrotizing inflammation with multinucleated giant cells and epithelioid consistent and confirming CD. Tuberculosis, actinomycosis, and malignancies were excluded. The patient is reportedly doing well after 4 years of follow-up and treatment with azathioprine [16].

Andreani et al. described a case of an ovary with an intact capsule that was macroscopically abnormal in a 28-year-old female patient complaining of a 1-year history of lower abdominal pain, weight loss of 9 kg, and unformed stools. The patient was medically and surgically free and had a negative family of IBD, and her general examination and abdominal examinations were negative [17].

Monneuse et al. reported a case of a 37-year-old female patient diagnosed with CD who came complaining of lower abdominal pain on admission. A right ovarian cyst was associated with inflammatory changes of the pelvis and involved the terminal ileum and sigmoid and was detected by an abdominal gynecologic ultrasound [18].

McCluggage et al. reported four cases of ovarian granulomas that were related to CD. Three of the four cases had similar features, two of them with granulomas that had central suppuration with microabscess formation. The author described them as having fissure ulcerations, lined by inflammatory granulation tissue that extended from the ovarian surface into the parenchyma, and vegetable materials were also identified. In the fourth case that involved the left ovary, the ovarian cortex had several small, well circumscribed, and nonnecrotizing granulomas [19].

Allen and Calvert reported a case of a 58-year-old female patient presented with lower abdominal pain and diarrhea leading to a right hemicolectomy for CD; the patient was symptom-free for 23 years; during her presentation, the disease had recurred and led to the resection of 17 cm of the ileum. 5 years later, the patient had multiple short Crohn's related strictures with fistulas and abscesses into the pelvis; two areas of the ileum measuring 10 cm and 20 cm were excised; one year

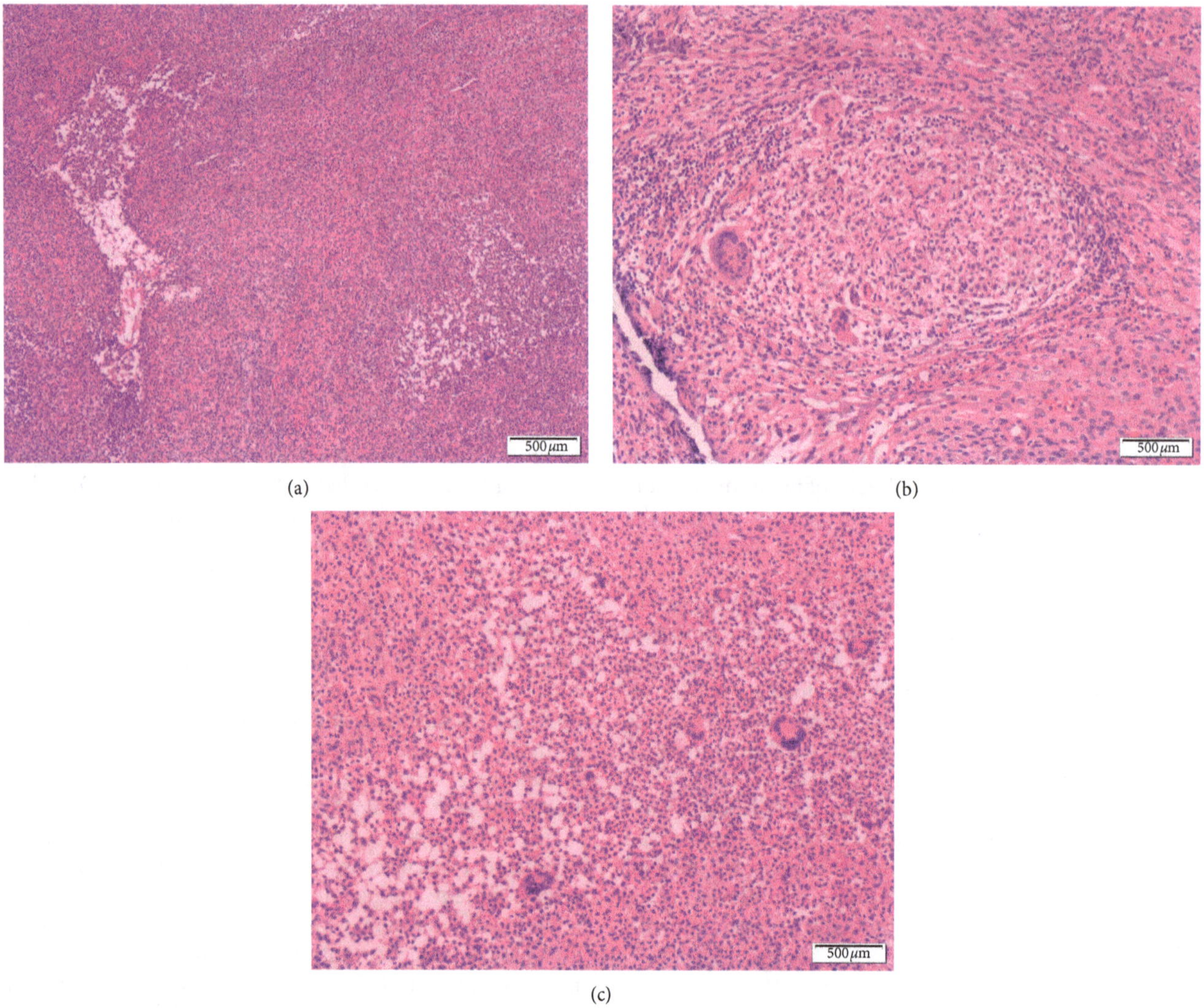

FIGURE 1: Histopathological findings in the resected ovarian mass. (a) Low-power view showing diffuse mixed inflammatory infiltrate of the ovarian stroma with the formation of a microabscess "on the left side of the figure" and a suppurative granuloma "on the right side of the figure" (H&E, ×40). (b) A nonnecrotizing granuloma composed of epithelioid histiocytes, few multinucleated giant cells, and a thin rim of lymphocytes (H&E, ×100). (c) Another epithelioid granuloma with central suppurative inflammation composed of numerous neutrophils (H&E, ×100).

later, the patient presented with lower abdominal pain and subacute obstruction. The patient was unsuccessfully treated with several courses of steroids and azathioprine, leading to further investigations that showed a short area of Crohn's ileitis and two strictures. The patient underwent a stricturoplasty and a further segment of the ileum next to an inflammatory mass surrounding the ovary was excised; postoperatively, the patient did well. The resected tubo-ovarian mass weighed 48 grams measuring 5 x 5 x 3 cm; it was pale with irregular areas of necrosis. Histology showed florid necrotizing and suppurative and nonsuppurative granulomatous salpingo-oophritis, due to fistulization from the adherent bowel. Multiple acute abscesses and fragments of vegetable material were found, adjacent to the fallopian tube and between these areas were many granulomas same as the ones found in Crohn's ileitis [20].

Goldberg et al. described that vesicular fistulas and salpingitis are rare complications of CD after presenting a case of oophoro-vesicular-colonic fistula secondary to CD. Interestingly, the patient reported that during menstruation, she experienced bleeding from the bladder. A single stage oophorectomy, sigmoid resection, and repair of the fistula were done; the patient had complete resolution of her symptoms and preservation of fertility [21].

Honore presented a case of a 30-year-old nulliparous woman who complained of nonspecific symptoms, diagnosed radiologically to have distal ileitis suggesting of CD; the patient had a partial ileo-colectomy along with excision of the adherent right adnexa. Suppurative oophoritis was found in relation to an ileo-ovarian fistula and a noncaseating granulomatous inflammatory response similar to what was observed in the ileum [22].

Frost et al. reported a case of a 26-year-old black female who complained of abdominal pain for 1 year; the patient was diagnosed clinically with cystic ovaries and underwent an exploratory laparotomy that revealed ileo-cecal CD with multiple adhesions to the bowel, peritoneum, and right adnexa; a biopsy of the right ovary and an appendectomy were performed. The ovary showed multiple cysts lined by granulosa cells with scattered epithelioid granulomas beneath the serosal surface [23].

Brooks and Wheeler reported a case of a 30-year-old female patient that was known to have CD who underwent resection of the bowel and adherent adnexa. Granulomatous salpingitis, oophoritis, and enterocolitis were identified histologically. A few features that were not usual for CD included the presence of an adnexal mass and florid atypical proliferation of the tubal epithelium that are similar to the changes that can be seen in tuberculous salpingitis [24].

In this case report, we present a case of ovarian CD, a rare complication that is likely a result of direct fistulization between the bowel and the ovary. As presented, similar cases were previously reported by authors from the United States, Canada, the United Kingdom, Europe, Tunisia, and Japan. Similar to many of these reported cases, our patient presented as a case of acute abdomen that was misdiagnosed as appendicitis and led to surgery. After persistence of symptoms postoperatively, the diagnosis was questioned and an exploratory laparotomy was performed and revealed an enlarged ovary. Following resection of the ovary, the histopathological examination revealed features consistent with CD.

4. Conclusions

Crohn's disease is a progressive disease that can result in fistulization between the bowel and other organs. Involvement of the ovary in females with Crohn's disease is a rare complication that can be missed on initial presentation. A high index of suspicion and careful examination of histological specimens are needed to accurately reach the diagnosis. Management should be individualized but surgical intervention is usually required.

References

[1] B. Lo, M. K. Vester-Andersen, I. Vind et al., "Changes in disease behaviour and location in patients with Crohn's disease after seven years of follow-up: a Danish population-based inception cohort," *Journal of Crohn's and Colitis*, vol. 12, no. 3, pp. 265–272, 2017.

[2] G. Tomasello, M. Scaglione, M. Mazzola et al., "CROHN'S disease and extraintestinal granulomatous lesions," *Journal of Biological Regulators & Homeostatic Agents*, vol. 32, no. 32, pp. 7–11, 2018.

[3] A. Fatemi, H. H. Jazi, M. H. Emami, A. Kazemizadeh, H. Tavakkoli, and A. Smiley, "Relationship between articular and nonarticular manifestations in inflammatory bowel diseases," *Journal of Research in Medical Sciences*, vol. 21, 2016.

[4] N. Bernett and K. Krishnamurthy, *Cutaneous Crohn Disease Courtney*, Stat Pearls, Treasure Island, FL, USA, 2020.

[5] I. A. Al-Mofleh and N. A. Azzam, "Crohn's disease. Increasing trend in Saudi Arabia," *Saudi Medical Journal*, vol. 34, no. 11, pp. 1105–1113, 2013.

[6] A. Bousvaros, D. A. Antonioli, A. Bousvaros et al., "Differentiating ulcerative colitis from Crohn disease in children and young adults: report of a working group of the north American society for pediatric gastroenterology, hepatology, and nutrition and the crohn's and colitis foundation of America," *Journal of Pediatric Gastroenterology and Nutrition*, vol. 44, no. 5, pp. 653–674, 2007.

[7] M. Almadi, "Distinguishing between Crohn's disease, tuberculosis, and lymphoma: still in murky waters," *Saudi Journal of Gastroenterology*, vol. 20, no. 4, p. 205, 2014.

[8] M. A. Almadi, S. Ghosh, and A. M. Aljebreen, "Differentiating intestinal tuberculosis from Crohn's disease: a diagnostic challenge," *The American Journal of Gastroenterology*, vol. 104, no. 4, p. 1003, 2009.

[9] H. L. Reynolds Jr and T. A. Stellato, "Crohn's disease of the foregut," *Surgical Clinics of North America*, vol. 81, no. 1, pp. 117–135, 2001.

[10] H. So, B. D. Ye, Y. S. Park et al., "Gastric lesions in patients with Crohn's disease in Korea: a multicenter study," *Intestinal Research*, vol. 14, no. 1, pp. 60–68, 2016.

[11] T. Zuiki, Y. Meguro, H. Kumano et al., "Successful management of a colo-duodenal fistula in a patient with crohn's disease using a double lumen gastro-jejunostomy tube," *Case Reports in Gastroenterology*, vol. 8, no. 2, pp. 162–168, 2014.

[12] I. Gawron, L. Chmura, D. Adamek, K. Skotniczny, K. Pityński, and A. Ludwin, "Laparoscopic intervention in acute crohn's disease involving an ovary," *Journal of Minimally Invasive Gynecology*, vol. 24, no. 6, pp. 1040–1045, 2017.

[13] D. Giuseppe Ribaldone, L. Conti, A. Resegotti, and M. Astegiano, "Adnexal localization of Crohn's disease and recurrent massive ovary cysts," *Revista Española de Enfermedades Digestivas*, vol. 108, no. 8, pp. 525-526, 2016.

[14] N. Rindos, A. Ecker, G. Carter, and S. Mansuria, "Crohn's disease with ovarian granuloma: a case report and review of the literature," *Journal of Minimally Invasive Gynecology*, vol. 22, no. 5, pp. 914–916, 2015.

[15] Y. Yabushita, H. Kimura, H. Yamamoto et al., "A case of ileo-ovarian fistula in Crohn's disease," *The Japanese Journal of Gastroenterological Surgery*, vol. 45, no. 3, pp. 340–344, 2012.

[16] A. Ouakaa-Kchaou, H. Elloumi, A. Kochlef et al., "Ovarian Crohn's disease," *Journal of Crohn's and Colitis*, vol. 4, no. 6, pp. 705-706, 2010.

[17] S. M. Andreani, H. H. Dang, D. P. Edwards, M. K. Baig, M. Khan, and J. G. Payne, "Ovarian Crohn's disease: contiguousor metastatic?," *Inflammatory Bowel Diseases*, vol. 12, no. 11, pp. 1091-1092, 2006.

[18] O. Monneuse, F. Pilleul, L. Gruner, X. Barth, and E. Tissot, "MRI evaluation in a rare case of crohn's disease complicated by abscess of the ovary," *Gastroentérologie Clinique et Biologique*, vol. 30, 2006.

[19] W. G. McCluggage and D. C. Allen, "Ovarian granulomas: a report of 32 cases," *Journal of Clinical Pathology*, vol. 50, no. 4, pp. 324–327, 1997.

[20] D. C. Allen and C. H. Calvert, "Crohn's ileitis and salpingo-oophoritis," *The Ulster Medical Journal*, vol. 64, no. 1, p. 95, 1995.

[21] S. D. Goldberg, R. R. Gray, K. I. Cadesky, and R. L. Mackenzie, "Oophorovesicular-colonic fistula: a rare complication of Crohn's disease. Canadian journal of surgery," *Journal canadien de chirurgie*, vol. 31, no. 6, pp. 427-428, 1988.

[22] L. H. Honoré, "Combined suppurative and noncaseating granulomatous oophoritis associated with distal ileitis (Crohn's disease)," *European Journal of Obstetrics & Gynecology and Reproductive Biology*, vol. 12, no. 2, pp. 91–94, 1981.

[23] S. S. Frost, M. P. Elstein, F. Latour, and J. L. A. Roth, "Crohn's disease of the mouth and ovary," *Digestive Diseases and Sciences*, vol. 26, no. 6, pp. 568–571, 1981.
[24] J. J. Brooks and J. E. Wheeler, "Granulomatous salpingitis secondary to Crohn's disease," *Obstetrics and Gynecology* vol. 49, no. 1 suppl, pp. 31–33, 1977.

4

Bouveret Syndrome: A Rare Case of Instance and Treatment in a Younger Patient

Kevin J. Yang[1] **and C. K. Chang**[2]

[1]*University of California, Berkeley, CA, USA*
[2]*Kaiser Permanente, Oakland, CA, USA*

Correspondence should be addressed to C. K. Chang; ck.chang@kp.org

Academic Editor: Olga I. Giouleme

Bouveret syndrome, a specific form of gallstone ileus, is the obstruction of the gastric outlet by a gallstone, which can enter the duodenum through a fistula. While the average age of individuals with Bouveret syndrome is 74 years, our patient was 42 years of age at the time of operation, significantly younger than the average patient afflicted with this condition. In the treatment of our patient's condition, the operation conducted entailed a partial duodenectomy, gastrojejunostomy, cholecystectomy, common bile duct exploration, extraction of bile duct stones, and insertion of a t-tube in the bile duct. The patient was found to be in healthy condition upon check-up six months after the operation. The outcome of our case suggests that younger Bouveret patients can safely undergo multiple surgical procedures in the treatment of Bouveret syndrome. Our case also suggests that a cholecystectomy and the removal of the obstructing gallstone can both be carried out within one operation, although coupling these two procedures in one operation might be riskier for patients within the normal age range of Bouveret syndrome. We also suggest that fistula repair be carried out for younger Bouveret patients in particular and that the patient be subjected to a CT scan in the diagnosis of Bouveret syndrome when this condition is suspected.

1. Case Presentation

Bouveret syndrome, a specific form of gallstone ileus, is the obstruction of the gastric outlet by a gallstone, which can enter the duodenum through a fistula. Bouveret syndrome most often occurs in individuals of advanced age; 74 years old is the average age of Bouveret syndrome patients [1]. This report summarizes and discusses the treatment of Bouveret syndrome in a patient who is 42 years of age at the time of operation, well below the age of the average Bouveret syndrome patient.

The patient is a 42-year-old female who presented with a gastric outlet obstruction. A CT scan showed a 2.5×5 cm stone in the duodenal bulb with a cholecystoduodenal fistula (Figures 1 and 2). An upper endoscopy was performed which showed a large gallstone in the duodenal bulb, causing complete obstruction of the duodenum. The gallstone could not be removed endoscopically. Surgical exploration identified a large stone in the duodenum which could not be mobilized proximally or distally. A cholecystectomy was performed, confirming the presence of the large cholecystoduodenal fistula identified in the CT scan. The fistula was 3 cm in diameter. A partial duodenectomy, a gastrojejunostomy, a cholecystectomy, and a common bile duct exploration with extraction of multiple common bile ducts stones were performed. A t-tube was placed into the bile duct after bile duct exploration. A follow-up t-tube cholangiogram was performed four weeks after the operation, revealing no strictures or additional stones. The t-tube was removed at six weeks after the operation. The patient was found to be in healthy condition upon check-up six months after the operation.

2. Discussion

At 42 years of age, our patient is well below the age of 74, the average age of individuals who are treated for Bouveret syndrome [1]. Our patient affords the unique opportunity to

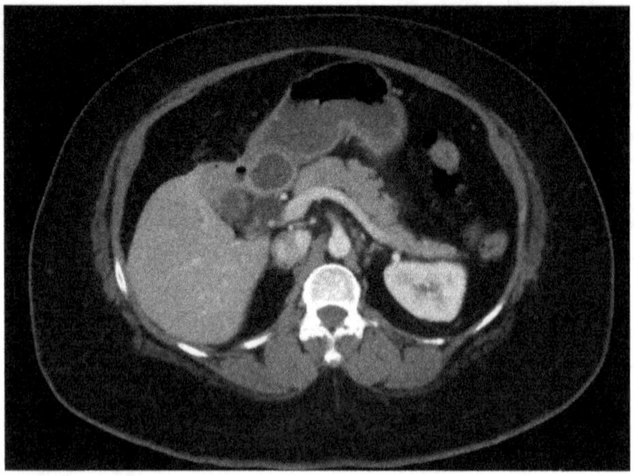

FIGURE 1: CT scan showing a large stone in the duodenum and a cholecystoduodenal fistula.

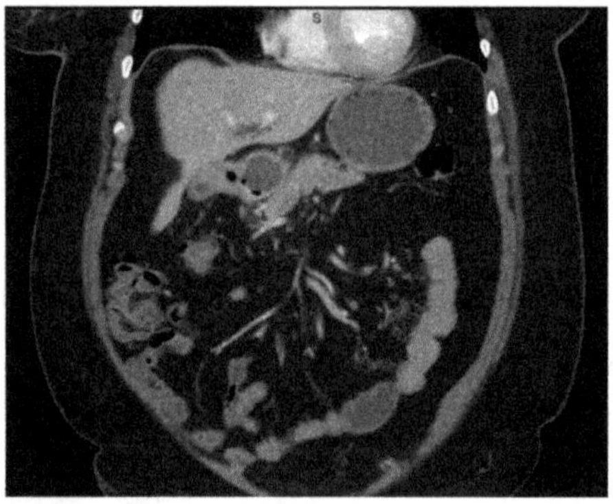

FIGURE 2: Addition CT scan showing a large stone in the duodenum and a cholecystoduodenal fistula.

examine the treatment of a younger individual afflicted by this condition.

Existing literature warns against carrying out anything beyond an enterolithotomy in the treatment of Bouveret syndrome if endoscopic methods fail, as the advanced age of most Bouveret patients and the conditions associated with advanced age most often render these patients poor surgical candidates [2]. Such a conclusion suggests that younger Bouveret patients should be able to safely undergo multiple procedures in one surgery, but this is not self-evident and requires more support. Our patient underwent five major procedures (partial duodenectomy, gastrojejunostomy, cholecystectomy, bile duct exploration, and the extraction of stones in the common bile duct) within one surgery and is in good health as of six months after the operation, with no complications between the operation and the time of writing. As such, the outcome of our case supports the statement that younger Bouveret patients can safely undergo multiple surgical procedures in the treatment of Bouveret syndrome, a course of action which can reduce the risk of gallstone recurrence [2].

Our case corroborates several existing trends in the literature concerning the surgical treatment of Bouveret syndrome in the context of a younger patient. The current literature suggests that one of the most effective, if not the most effective, imaging technique to diagnose Bouveret syndrome is the CT scan [1, 3–5]. In the diagnosis of our patient, the CT scan successfully revealed both a large stone within the duodenal bulb and its associated cholecystoduodenal fistula. As such, our case, alongside the aforementioned existing literature, demonstrates that the CT scan is an efficacious means by which to diagnose Bouveret syndrome. Furthermore, reviews of the literature have stated that endoscopy, while being the least invasive (and therefore most desirable) method to remove a Bouveret syndrome gallstone, is rarely successful [6, 7]. We, too, were unable to remove the gallstone endoscopically, necessitating full surgical intervention. Thus, while it remains that endoscopic methods may be useful as a diagnostic tool, surgeons presented with the task of treating Bouveret syndrome should be prepared to remove the gallstone surgically.

Our case may have implications with regards to the ongoing debate over whether or not to carry out fistula repair when addressing Bouveret syndrome via surgical intervention [3, 5–7]. Evidence against fistula repair includes the fact that Bouveret syndrome patients who did not undergo fistula repair have lower mortality rates and the theory that such fistulas will close spontaneously [5, 7]. Evidence in favor of fistula repair includes reduction in the chance of a number of postoperative complications, such as the recurrence of gallstone ileus and cancer risk [3]. In our particular case, fistula repair was carried out, with positive results evidenced by the healthy condition of the patient six months after the operation. This course of action was taken considering the age of the patient; being much younger than most patients afflicted with Bouveret syndrome, our patient would most likely have a much lower chance of mortality associated with fistula repair than that expressed in the literature, as this mortality rate is based on a patient population with a much higher mean age. Moreover, our patient's young age means that she would be at a greater risk of developing those problems associated with a persisting fistula, as this fistula would persist in our patient for the entire duration of the patient's life before death if spontaneous closure of the fistula does not occur. These factors lead us to recommend that fistula repair be carried out in the surgical treatment of Bouveret syndrome in younger patients.

Furthermore, our case may have implications with regards to an ongoing debate over the treatment of the broader condition of gallstone ileus. The present controversy in the literature is over whether to remove the obstructing gallstone and perform a cholecystectomy in one surgery or in two separate surgeries [8]. In our case, these two procedures were carried out within one surgery with positive results, lending support to a "one surgery" approach. However, additional studies of cases are necessary to lend such a statement reasonable credibility, especially considering the fact that our patient is well below the age of the average gallstone ileus patient [9].

Our recommendations fall in line with the successful treatment of Bouveret syndrome in patients below the age of 50. Those cases documenting a cholecystectomy performed this procedure within the same operation as the removal of the gallstone, with successful results [10–13]. Furthermore, all cases of patients below the age of 50 carried out a fistula repair, again with successful results [10–14]. As such, our case, alongside the existing literature regarding treatment in younger patients, shows that younger patients indeed can accept the greater surgical pressures associated with these approaches.

Our case offers the rare opportunity to study the successful treatment and outcome of a Bouveret syndrome patient whose age is far below that of the average patient afflicted by this condition. Existing literature finds that the old age of most Bouveret patients makes them unfit to undergo numerous surgical procedures in the treatment of Bouveret syndrome; however, the inverse of this conclusion, that a younger Bouveret patient is fit for a greater number of procedures within one surgery, lacks support in the existing body of literature. Our case lends support to the statement that a young patient can undergo a more elaborate set of procedures in the treatment of this condition. With regard to two present controversies in the literature, we recommend performing cholecystectomy in the same surgery as the gallstone removal when cholecystectomy is deemed necessary and to carry out fistula repair when treating young Bouveret patients. Lastly, we recommend employing a CT scan to diagnose Bouveret syndrome when this condition is suspected.

References

[1] M. S. Cappell and M. Davis, "Characterization of Bouveret's syndrome: a comprehensive review of 128 cases," *The American Journal of Gastroenterology*, vol. 101, no. 9, pp. 2139–2146, 2006.

[2] F. Alemi, N. Seiser, and S. Ayloo, "Gallstone disease: cholecystitis, mirizzi syndrome, bouveret syndrome, gallstone ileus," *Surgical Clinics of North America*, vol. 99, no. 2, pp. 231–244, 2019.

[3] A. S. Lowe, S. Stephenson, C. L. Kay, and J. May, "Duodenal obstruction by gallstones (bouveret's syndrome): a review of the literature," *Endoscopy*, vol. 37, no. 1, pp. 82–87, 2005.

[4] Y. A. Masannat, "A rare complication of a common disease: Bouveret syndrome, a case report," *World Journal of Gastroenterology*, vol. 12, no. 16, pp. 2620-2621, 2006.

[5] V. K. Mavroeidis, D. I. Matthioudakis, N. K. Economou, and I. D. Karanikas, "Bouveret syndrome-the rarest variant of gallstone ileus: a case report and literature review," *Case Reports in Surgery*, vol. 2013, Article ID 839370, 6 pages, 2013.

[6] J. K. Bhama, J. W. Ogren, T. Lee, and W. E. Fisher, "Bouveret's syndrome," *Surgery*, vol. 132, no. 1, pp. 104-105, 2002.

[7] I. Doycheva, A. Limaye, A. Suman, C. E. Forsmark, and S. Sultan, "Bouveret's syndrome: case report and review of the literature," *Gastroenterology Research and Practice*, vol. 2009, Article ID 914951, 4 pages, 2009.

[8] Y. B. Yu, Y. Song, J. B. Xu, and F. Z. Qi, "Bouveret's syndrome: a rare presentation of gastric outlet obstruction," *Experimental and Therapeutic Medicine*, vol. 17, no. 3, pp. 1813–1816, 2019.

[9] V. Scuderi, V. Adamo, M. Naddeo, W. Di Natale, L. Boglione, and S. Cavalli, "Gallstone ileus: monocentric experience looking for the adequate approach," *Updates in Surgery*, vol. 70, no. 4, pp. 503–511, 2018.

[10] M. Mengual-Ballester, M. P. Guillén-Paredes, M. J. Cases-Baldó, M. L. García-García, and J. L. Aguayo-Albasini, *Hemorragia Digestiva y Obstrucción Intestinal Alta Como Presentación del Síndrome de Bouveret. (Spanish)*, vol. 79, no. 6, Mexico City, Mexico, 2011, https://search.ebscohost.com/login.aspx?direct=true&db=edb&AN=73471614&site=eds-live.

[11] D. S. Kalwaniya, S. V. Arya, S. Guha et al., "A rare presentation of gastric outlet obstruction (GOO)—the Bouveret's syndrome," *Annals of Medicine and Surgery*, vol. 4, no. 1, pp. 67–71, 2015.

[12] A. Iñíguez, J. M. Butte, J. M. Zúñiga, F. Crovari, and O. Llanos, "Síndrome de bouveret: resolución endóscopica y quirúrgica de cuatro casos clínicos/bouveret syndrome: report of four cases," *Revista Médica de Chile*, vol. 136, no. 2, pp. 163–168, 2008.

[13] S. K. Venkatesh, M. S. Thyagarajan, R. B. Gujral, and A. Gupta, "Sonographic diagnosis of Bouveret's syndrome," *Journal of Clinical Ultrasound*, vol. 31, no. 3, pp. 163–166, 2003.

[14] L. Mejia, "Bouveret's syndrome presenting as upper GI bleed in a young female," *The American Journal of Gastroenterology*, vol. 98, no. 9, p. S131, 2003.

5

Case Report: An Obscure Presence of Gastroduodenal Involvement in a Newly Diagnosed Ileocolic Crohn's Disease Patient

Clive Jude Miranda, Murad Hayatt Ali, Muddasir Ayaz, Yousef Soofi, and Thomas Christopher Mahl

Department of Gastroenterology, University at Buffalo, 955 Main Street, Buffalo 14203, New York, USA

Correspondence should be addressed to Clive Jude Miranda; clive.miranda91@gmail.com

Academic Editor: Hirotada Akiho

Whereas typical Crohn's disease is confined to the terminal ileum and presents with abdominal pain and diarrhea, gastroduodenal manifestations of Crohn's disease are rare, with often asymptomatic patient presentations and inconclusive diagnostic testing. It is, however, a more severe form of Crohn's disease and thus warrants treatment with steroids and biologics much earlier than its ileocolonic counterpart. We present the case of a young, otherwise healthy, male with newly diagnosed ileocolonic Crohn's disease with concurrent gastroduodenal involvement that initially failed management with biologic agents. We discuss the clinical manifestations and often obscure pathology of gastroduodenal Crohn's disease and highlight the necessity of performing a concurrent esophagogastroduodenoscopic evaluation on newly diagnosed ileocolonic Crohn's disease to assess the presence of upper gastrointestinal involvement.

1. Introduction

Crohn's disease (CD) is an idiopathic, multisystem, inflammatory disease with an etiology intertwined by environmental, microbial, and genetic factors characterized by transmural and segmental involvement of the gastrointestinal (GI) tract, anywhere from the mouth to the anus [1]. Afflicted patients experience episodes of remission and relapse throughout the course of their lives, with the most common complaints including epigastric pain, nausea, vomiting, and weight loss. The disease is most definitively diagnosed with endoscopic evaluation, with aphthous, longitudinal ulcers, and cobblestoning being typical endoscopic findings, and noncaseating granulomas being a hallmark of pathology [2, 3].

Gastroduodenal CD affects 0.5–4% of all CD patients [4], with the majority of such patients having concurrent involvement of the colon with isolated gastroduodenal involvement accounting for less than 0.07% of all CD patients [5, 6]. Pathology is more obscure in the upper GI tract, and noncaseating granulomas are not necessarily needed for confirmatory diagnosis. Though many patients are asymptomatic, gastroduodenal involvement indicates a more severe form of CD and thus warrants steroidal treatment and biological agents earlier in the disease course. Most patients respond well to medical therapy, with surgery indicated for perforation, bleeding, or significant structural disease causing obstructive complications. Here, we present a case of a healthy, young male presenting with new onset gastroduodenal Crohn's disease with concurrent colonic involvement that responded well to biological therapy. We aim to describe the often obscure endoscopic and pathological features associated with gastroduodenal CD and highlight the importance of including upper endoscopy in newly diagnosed ileocolonic CD patients.

2. Case Presentation

A 30-year-old male with no prior medical history presented to the Emergency Departmentfor ongoing hematochezia with watery diarrhea, cramping abdominal pain, vomiting, and poor intake for the past 3 months resulting in an unintentional 30 lb

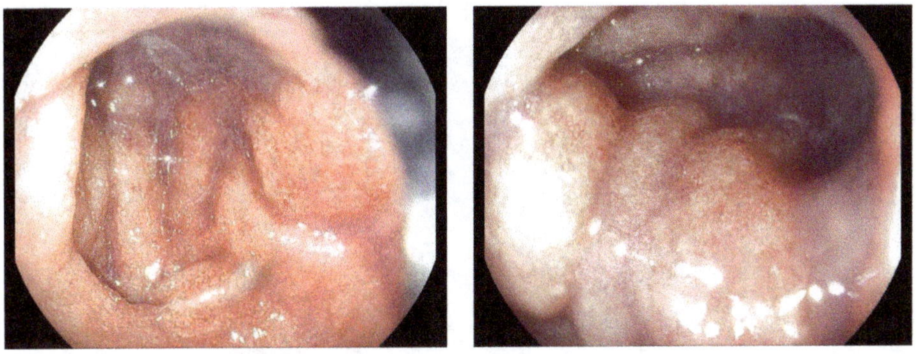

(a) (b)

FIGURE 1: Diffuse ulceration and friability in the rectum and sigmoid colon.

weight loss. He worked as a plumber and denied any family history of inflammatory bowel disease. Upon presentation, temperature was elevated at 100.4F with a leukocytosis of 12,000/mm^3 with neutrophilic predominance. CRP was elevated at 50, stool lactoferrin was positive and calprotectin was 2562. CT angiography showed thickening of the left hemicolon from mid-transverse to rectosigmoid colon with diffuse reactive adjacent mesenteric lymph nodes, suggestive of acute colitis.

Colonoscopy was notable for multiple, nonbleeding, round, and shallow ulcers measuring between 3-7 mm with extensive inflammation and loss of vascularity throughout rectum. Extensive erythema, friability, and shallow ulcerations were noted extending from the anus up to 22 cm, at which point the procedure was aborted due to significant inflammation and the inability to traverse the rectum (Figures 1(a) and 1(b)). Subsequent pathology showed chronic and active colitis with plasma cells and crypts full of neutrophils, consistent with a definitive diagnosis of Crohn's disease (Figure 2). The Crohn's disease activity index (CDAI) score was between 220–450, consistent with moderate-to-severe Crohn's disease. Esophagogastroduodenoscopy showed multiple nonbleeding, round, clean-based, and shallow ulcers ranging between 3–7 mm in the duodenal bulb and the 1st and 2nd parts of the duodenum (Figures 3(a)–3(c)). Pathology showed fragments of duodenal mucosa with focal ulceration and acute inflammation with surface epithelium replaced by neutrophils and plasma cells, as well as moderately chronic, focally active gastritis with negative *H pylori*, establishing a diagnosis of gastroduodenal Crohn's disease (Figure 4). The patient was started on solumedrol and discharged on prednisone, mesalamine enemas, and pantoprazole with follow-up withplans to start infliximab. The patient missed his follow-up and presented 10 days later with diffuse abdominal pain, bilious emesis, and 10–12 episodes of bloody diarrhea daily. White count was 17,900/mm^3 with ESR 71, CRP 51.59, and calprotectin 3327. CT A/P showed wall thickening and a mild inflammatory fat stranding adjacent to the left colon, now involving the splenic flexure and rectum with increasing inflammatory changes since last admission. The patient was switched to IV methylprednisolone in-house and discharged on prednisone with outpatient adalimumab infusions. This medication switch was made due to an easier home administration regimen, given concerns about noncompliance. He was seen a month later and was doing well with no symptoms. He was then started on azathioprine. His CRP and ESR remained normal, and we suspect his disease is currently under control. The patient was unfortunately lost to follow-up, and subsequent upper and lower endoscopies could not be carried out to evaluate clinical remission.

3. Discussion

Symptomatic gastroduodenal CD accounts for approximately less than 4% of all patients affected by CD, with most patients presenting with concurrent large bowel involvement [4]. Our patient presented with CD involving the gastric antrum, the proximal duodenum, and most of the colon with poor response to steroids and mesalamine, returning with an exacerbation. However, subsequent adalimumab and azathioprine therapy resulted in a significantly improved response.

Current literature is bereft of controlled studies assessing the efficacy of medication for the treatment of CD in the upper gastrointestinal tract and, as a result, treatment is based on a combination of distal disease activity and clinical experience [7]. Aside from acid suppression and corticosteroids for flares, emerging cases of biological therapy with antitumor necrosis factor-alpha (TNFα) medications have recently yielded promising results, with both infliximab and adalimumab showing clinical effectiveness in complicated CD patients [8–11]. One key prospective trial showed that, among 19 patients with gastroduodenal CD, 72.7% of those treated with infliximab or adalimumab biological therapy resulted in mucosal healing at 12 weeks post-treatment compared to 12.5% of patients given conventional therapy [12]. Our patient never followed up for infliximab therapy, resulting in his returning with an exacerbation. Our decision to then begin adalimumab therapy was based on our impression that adalimumab would prove a better medication due to easier home administration and its comparable efficacy to infliximab in studies on small bowel CD treatments [13, 14]. This proved successful as he maintained remission for the months to follow. This approach advocates for either infliximab or adalimumab as the initial

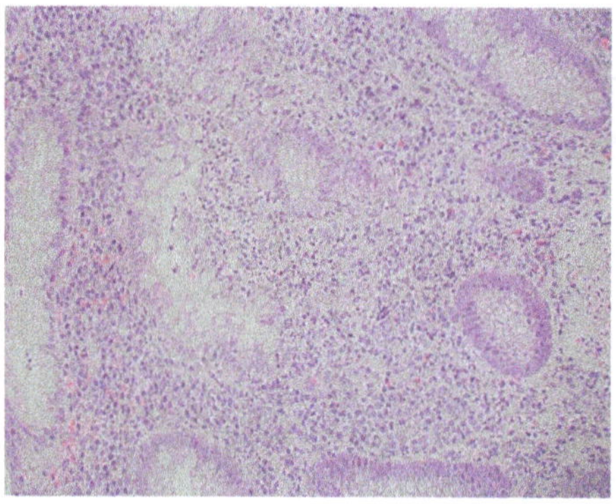

FIGURE 2: Rectal mucosa with chronic active inflammation with plasma cells and neutrophilic crypts consistent with Crohn's disease, 200x.

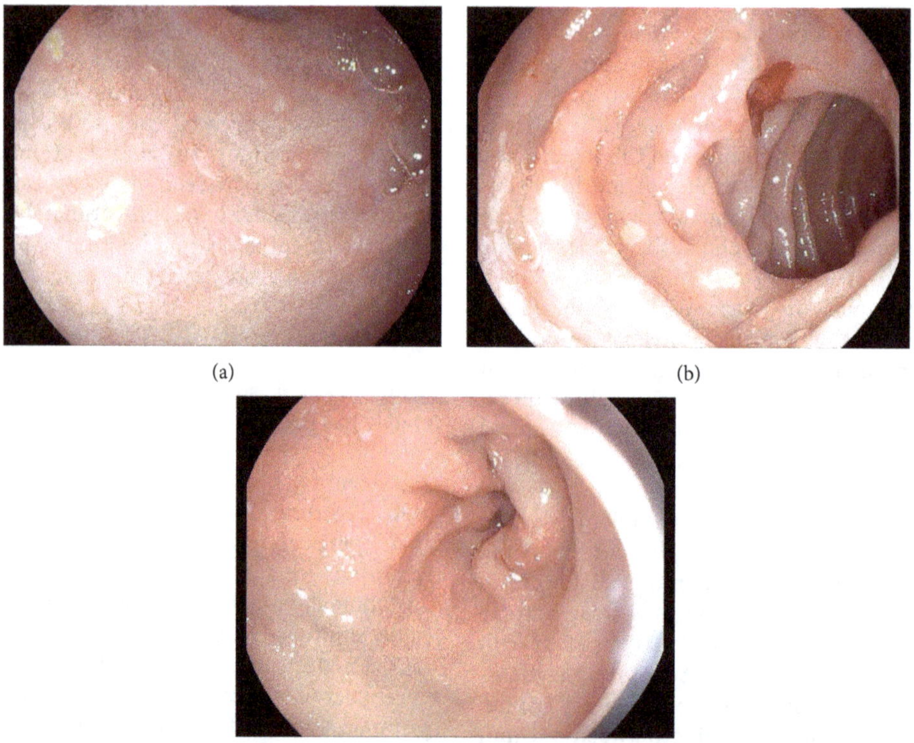

(a) (b)

(c)

FIGURE 3: Duodenal bulb, 2nd portion of the duodenum, and gastric antrum with multiple erosions and ulcerations.

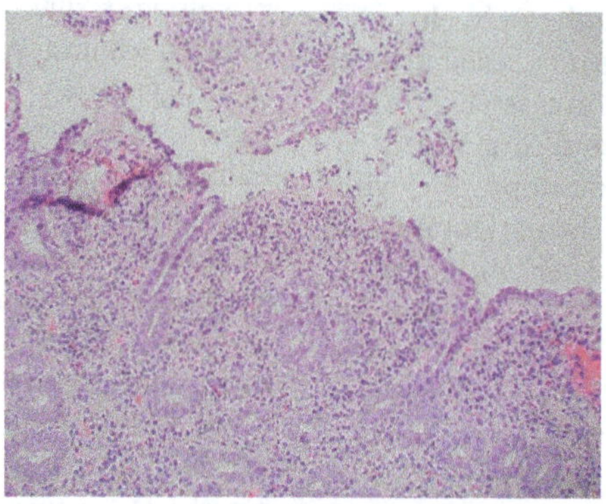

FIGURE 4: Duodenal mucosa with active erosive chronic duodenitis, villous blunting and surface epithelium replaced by neutrophils consistent with duodenal Crohn's disease, 200x.

anti-TNF medication, with clinical judgement and patient factors determining the drug of choice.

It was the concurrent presence of abdominal pain and emesis that prompted an EGD in our patient which then identified findings consistent with gastroduodenal CD. However, as the disease is often asymptomatic in adults, an EGD is not routinely performed in this population to investigate possible IBD pathology. This results in many CD lesions of the upper GI tract being missed and discovered only later in the disease course if symptoms clinically warrant an upper endoscopy by the overseeing gastroenterologist. The European Crohn's and Colitis Organisation (ECCO) consensus recommends investigation of the small bowel in a newly diagnosed distal-CD patient to determine the extent of upper GI involvement [15]. In a prospective study of 119 adults with new or previously known CD, 16% of patients were found to have upper GI CD, with 63% of them being asymptomatic at the time [13]. Sakuraba et al. performed a retrospective study of 138 distal-CD patients who underwent EGD for any upper GI symptoms, with a significant finding of 51.3% of patients having CD-specific lesions of the upper GI tract [16]. This emphasizes the importance of including routine upper endoscopy in the diagnostic evaluation of ileocolonic CD patients in order to investigate the presence, distribution, and severity of gastroduodenal involvement.

It bears mentioning that CD is a difficult condition to treat, with vast financial resources being used to research and develop more efficacious therapies. The current consensus for moderate-to-severe CD is the use of biologics early in the disease course to decrease the risk of steroid usage, hospitalizations, and surgeries and to increase quality of life [17]. The categories of current available biologics for CD include anti-TNFα agents, anti-integrins, and anti-interleukin (IL) 12–23. However, emerging and recently approved therapies for CD have yielded significant headway in disease management. Risankizumab is a monoclonal antibody directed against the p19 subunit of IL-23 that has recently been approved by the Food and Drug Administration for moderate-to-severe Crohn's disease. Ustekinumab inhibits both IL-12 and IL-23 and has also been effective in the induction and remission of moderate-to-severe Crohn's disease [18] since 2016. Going further back, vedolizumab is an anti-integrin biologic approved in 2014 for treating moderate-to-severe Crohn's disease. Several other janus kinase (JAK) inhibitor, antitrafficking agents, and sphingosine-1-phosphate receptor modulator therapies are currently in development for the more efficacious treatment of CD [19].

Despite EGD and biopsy being the gold standard for diagnosing gastroduodenal CD, both endoscopy and histopathology may often yield nonspecific results which then may cast doubt to establishing a definitive diagnosis. One therefore needs to be vigilant when suspecting gastroduodenal CD by combining these findings with clinical acumen, as the diagnosis warrants early intervention with biological treatment to promote and/or maintain remission. Endoscopic findings range from edema, enanthem, and longitudinal/irregular/serpiginous erosions to "cobblestoning," mucosal nodularity, duodenal stenosis/"notching," and a "bamboo-joint-like" appearance [7, 20, 21]. Affected areas are frequently confined to the antrum, pylorus, and proximal duodenum with the proximal stomach usually spared [22]. Histological findings also vary and range from nonspecific focal inflammatory changes, acute and chronic inflammation, and focal gastritis to lymphoid aggregates, epithelioid granulomas, and duodenitis with or without granulomas. Due to such variability and the focal distribution of disease presentation, biopsies should be performed in both endoscopically normal and abnormal areas. While noncaseating granulomas are nearly pathognomonic for CD, their absence does not rule out gastroduodenal pathology. They are most frequently located in the stomach rather than in the duodenum, with their presence reported between 7%–87.7% and 0–49% in those areas, respectively [21]. Focal gastritis in the absence of *H. pylori* has also been described in several studies as suggestive of gastric CD, located more frequently in the antrum [23, 24]. Other studies further note that even chronic *H. pylori* negative gastritis has been reported at high frequences in CD patients to establish a gastroduodenal disease component [13, 25]. Our patient did not have granulomas identified on EGD. However, his nonspecific biopsy findings of focal gastritis and ulceration, along with macroscopic findings of multiple shallow ulcers on endoscopy, were sufficient to establish the diagnosis of gastroduodenal involvement of CD. We again emphasize the importance of concurrent, early endoscopic evaluation in CD patients to assess for upper GI involvement, as the presence of positive findings warrants the initiation of more aggressive medical and/or surgical interventions. Furthermore, the frequent obscurity in identifying gastroduodenal CD encourages the integration and amalgamation of clinical, endoscopic, histological, and radiological findings along with practitioners' clinical experience and gestalt in order to establish a confirmatory diagnosis of this disease.

Data Availability

The case report data, including pathology, hospital course, and cited studies used to support the findings of this study are included within the article and are also available from the corresponding author upon request. The personal protected patient information used to support the findings of this study is restricted by the University at Buffalo Institutional Review Board in order to protect patient privacy. Data are available from the primary author clive.miranda91@gmail.com for researchers who meet the criteria for access to confidential data.

References

[1] E. V. Loftus, "Update on the incidence and prevalence of inflammatory bowel disease in the United States," *Gastroenterology and Hepatology*, vol. 12, no. 11, pp. 704–707, 2016.

[2] S. Nikolaus and S. Schreiber, "Diagnostics of inflammatory bowel disease," *Gastroenterology*, vol. 133, no. 5, pp. 1670–1689, 2007.

[3] G. Van Assche, A. Dignass, J. Panes et al., "The second European evidence-based consensus on the diagnosis and management of Crohn's disease: definitions and diagnosis," *Journal of Crohn's and Colitis*, vol. 4, no. 1, pp. 7–27, 2010.

[4] H. L. Reynolds and T. A. Stellato, "Crohn's disease of the foregut," *Surgical Clinics of North America*, vol. 81, no. 1, pp. 117–135, 2001.

[5] S. B. Ingle, G. P. Pujari, Y. G. Patle, and B. S. Nagoba, "An unusual case of Crohn's disease with isolated gastric involvement," *Journal of Crohn's and Colitis*, vol. 5, no. 1, pp. 69-70, 2011.

[6] C. Gottlieb and S. Alpert, "Regional jejunitis," *American Journal of Roentgenology*, vol. 38, pp. 881–883, 1937.

[7] A. M. Pimentel, R. Rocha, and G. O. Santana, "Crohn's disease of esophagus, stomach and duodenum," *World Journal of Gastrointestinal Pharmacology and Therapeutics*, vol. 10, no. 2, pp. 35–49, 2019.

[8] Y. L. Kim, Y. S. Park, E. K. Park et al., "Refractory duodenal Crohn's disease successfully treated with infliximab," *International Researchers*, vol. 12, no. 1, p. 66, 2014.

[9] M. Odashima, M. Otaka, M. Jin et al., "Successful treatment of refractory duodenal Crohn's disease with infliximab," *Digestive Diseases and Sciences*, vol. 52, no. 1, pp. 31-32, 2007.

[10] S. Gaggar, J. Scott, and N. Thompson, "Pyloric stenosis associated Crohn's disease responding to adalimumab therapy," *World Journal of Gastrointestinal Pharmacology and Therapeutics*, vol. 3, no. 6, p. 97, 2012.

[11] A. Tursi, "Duodenal Crohn's disease successfully treated with adalimumab," *Endoscopy*, vol. 43, no. S 02, p. E22, 2011.

[12] M. L. Annunziata, R. Caviglia, L. G. Papparella, and M. Cicala, "Upper gastrointestinal involvement of Crohn's disease: a prospective study on the role of upper endoscopy in the diagnostic work-up," *Digestive Diseases and Sciences*, vol. 57, no. 6, pp. 1618–1623, 2012.

[13] Y. Bouhnik, F. Carbonnel, D. Laharie et al., "Efficacy of adalimumab in patients with Crohn's disease and symptomatic small bowel stricture: a multicentre, prospective, observational cohort (CREOLE) study," *Gut*, vol. 67, no. 1, pp. 53–60, 2018.

[14] J. D. Doecke, F. Hartnell, P. Bampton et al., "Infliximab vs. adalimumab in Crohn's disease: results from 327 patients in an Australian and New Zealand observational cohort study," *Alimentary Pharmacology & Therapeutics*, vol. 45, no. 4, pp. 542–552, 2017.

[15] F. Gomollón, A. Dignass, V. Annese et al., "3rd European evidence-based consensus on the diagnosis and management of Crohn's disease 2016: Part 1: diagnosis and medical management," *Journal of Crohn's and Colitis*, vol. 11, no. 1, pp. 3–25, 2017.

[16] A. Sakuraba, Y. Iwao, K. Matsuoka et al., "Endoscopic and pathologic changes of the upper gastrointestinal tract in Crohn's disease," *BioMed Research International*, vol. 2014, pp. 1–6, Article ID 610767, 2014.

[17] E. Klenske, C. Bojarski, M. Waldner, T. Rath, M. F. Neurath, and R. Atreya, "Targeting mucosal healing in Crohn's disease: what the clinician needs to know," *Therap Adv Gastroenterol*, vol. 12, Article ID 175628481985686, 2019.

[18] B. G. Feagan, W. J. Sandborn, C. Gasink et al., "Ustekinumab as induction and maintenance therapy for Crohn's disease," *New England Journal of Medicine*, vol. 375, no. 20, pp. 1946–1960, 2016.

[19] B. Al-Bawardy, R. Shivashankar, and D. D. Proctor, "Novel and emerging therapies for inflammatory bowel disease," *Frontiers in Pharmacology*, vol. 12, Article ID 651415, 2021.

[20] S. B. Ingle, B. D. Adgaonkar, N. P. Jamadar, S. Siddiqui, and C. R. Hinge, "Crohn's disease with gastroduodenal involvement: diagnostic approach," *World Journal of Clinical Cases*, vol. 3, no. 6, pp. 479–483, 2015.

[21] Y. Nomura, K. Moriichi, M. Fujiya, and T. Okumura, "The endoscopic findings of the upper gastrointestinal tract in patients with Crohn's disease," *Clin J Gastroenterol*, vol. 10, no. 4, pp. 289–296, 2017.

[22] C. H. Kefalas, "Gastroduodenal Crohn's disease," *Baylor University Medical Center SAVE Proceedings*, vol. 16, 2003.

[23] M. H. D. Magalhães-Costa, B. R. D. Reis, V. L. A. Chagas, T. Nunes, H. S. P. Souza, and C. Zaltman, "Focal enhanced gastritis and macrophage microaggregates in the gastric mucosa: potential role in the differential diagnosis between Crohn's disease and ulcerative colitis," *Arquivos de Gastroenterologia*, vol. 51, no. 4, pp. 276–282, 2014.

[24] G. Oberhuber, A. Püspök, C. Oesterreicher et al., "Focally enhanced gastritis: a frequent type of gastritis in patients with Crohn's disease," *Gastroenterology*, vol. 112, no. 3, pp. 698–706, 1997.

[25] A. Sonnenberg and R. M. Genta, "Low prevalence of Helicobacter pylori infection among patients with inflammatory bowel disease," *Alimentary Pharmacology & Therapeutics*, vol. 35, no. 4, pp. 469–476, 2012.

6

Management of Refractory Gastrointestinal Bleeding in Hereditary Hemorrhagic Telangiectasia with Bevacizumab

Muaaz Masood,[1] **Michael Coles**,[1] **and Humberto Sifuentes**[2]

[1]*Department of Internal Medicine, Medical College of Georgia at Augusta University, Augusta, Georgia, USA*
[2]*Department of Gastroenterology and Hepatology, Medical College of Georgia at Augusta University, Augusta, Georgia, USA*

Correspondence should be addressed to Muaaz Masood; mmasood@augusta.edu

Academic Editor: Olga I. Giouleme

Hereditary hemorrhagic telangiectasia (HHT) is an autosomal dominant disorder resulting in vascular malformations of several organs including the pulmonary, cerebral, and gastrointestinal systems. One sequela is recurrent gastrointestinal (GI) bleeding. Bevacizumab (Bev) is emerging as an effective treatment of recurrent gastrointestinal bleeding in HHT. Bev is a recombinant monoclonal antibody that inhibits vascular endothelial growth factor (VEGF), an integral part of angiogenesis.

1. Introduction

Hereditary hemorrhagic telangiectasia (HHT), also known as Osler–Weber–Rendu syndrome, is an autosomal dominant disorder which is characterized by the abnormal formation of blood vessels [1]. HHT affects approximately 1 in 5000 individuals in North America [2]. Its prevalence has been underreported due to variable penetrance [3].

Several genetic mutations have been identified in HHT [4]. The most common mutations are in *ENG*, *ACVRL1*, and *SMAD4* which encode proteins that are part of the transforming growth factor beta (TGF-β) pathway in vascular endothelial cells [2]. Studies have demonstrated that patients with HHT have abnormal levels of TGF-β and vascular endothelial growth factor (VEGF) which are key players in angiogenesis [3, 5]. Mutations in these pathways result in abnormal vessel development and arteriovenous malformations (AVMs) [6].

AVMs can be present in mucocutaneous membranes (i.e., lips, tongue, buccal mucosa, or fingers) as well as in the lungs, brain, and GI tract [5]. Bleeding of AVMs is common and typically presents as epistaxis or symptoms related to iron deficiency anemia [3]. Recurrent GI bleeding is present in up to one-third of patients [7]. These patients often fail to respond to conventional treatments [8].

Bevacizumab (Bev) is a recombinant monoclonal antibody that inhibits VEGF [9]. Bev is emerging as an efficacious treatment for recurrent GI bleeding in patients with HHT [5, 9–14]. We present a case of a 67-year-old Caucasian female with a history of HHT, GI AVMs, and multiple admissions for recurrent GI bleeding who failed conventional therapy and had an excellent clinical response to Bev infusions.

2. Case Presentation

A 67-year-old Caucasian female with a history of HHT with GI AVMs and no pulmonary or hepatic AVMs required multiple hospital admissions for recurrent gastrointestinal bleeding. In one calendar year, the patient had 8 admissions for gastrointestinal bleeding and required a total of 14 units of packed red blood cells (pRBC) transfused. Endoscopic evaluation showed recurrent gastric, duodenal, jejunal, and colonic AVMs (Figures 1–3) which were treated with argon plasma coagulation. The patient was tried on tranexamic acid and aminocaproic acid without improvement. She was started on Bev 5 mg/kg every 2 weeks for a total of 6 infusions over 3 months. She had marked improvement in symptoms and a decrease in the frequency of bloody stools since induction. With regard to anemia, her hemoglobin

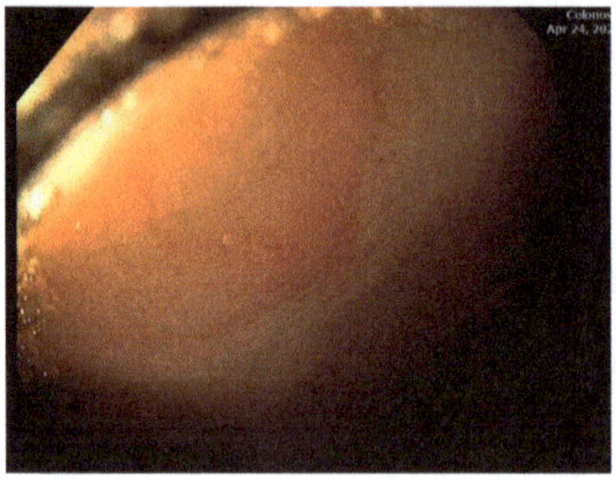

Figure 1: Arteriovenous malformation in the cecum.

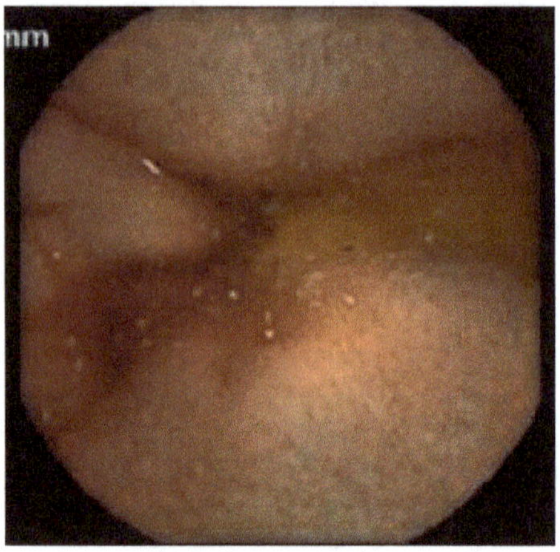

Figure 2: Intraluminal bleeding in the duodenum on video capsule endoscopy.

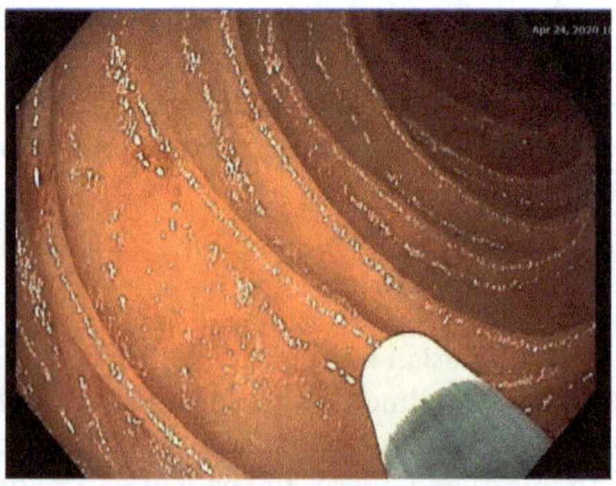

Figure 3: Two arteriovenous malformations in the jejunum.

level recovered to 13 g/dL from 9 g/dL after receiving the 6 Bev infusions. Her hemoglobin level remained at its peak of 13 g/dL for approximately 2 months. She had just one hospitalization for GI bleeding and required only one pRBC transfusion since induction with Bev. The plan is for Bev to be administered if the patient's hemoglobin decreased 1.5 g/dL from its peak. It was determined that the patient would likely require a dose of Bev once every 2 months with serial monitoring of her hemoglobin levels given the severity of her disease.

3. Discussion

HHT is a multisystemic disease which results from mutations in genes that regulate angiogenesis [5]. AVMs are a hallmark of the disease and can occur in the gastrointestinal, cerebral, pulmonary, and integumentary systems [1]. The most common symptoms include epistaxis, symptomatic anemia, GI bleeding, and mucocutaneous telangiectasias [3]. The diagnosis is clinical with three or more of the following features which must be present to establish the diagnosis: epistaxis, mucocutaneous telangiectasias, visceral AVMs, and a family history in a first-degree relative [2]. Genetic testing (i.e., SMAD4, ACVRL1, ENG, and GDF2) is not only performed for confirmation in individuals in whom there is a high suspicion for the disease but also may define the risk of various types of AVMs [4, 15]. A study by Canzonieri et al. explored the prevalence and distribution of telangiectasias in relation to their genotype. Patients with mutations in ENG (HHT-1), ACVRL1 (HHT-2), and SMAD4 (in association with juvenile polyposis syndrome) underwent endoscopic evaluation, and it was discovered that patients with ENG mutation (HHT-1) had a higher rate of multiple telangiectasias with a higher prevalence of telangiectasias in the duodenum [15]. Genetic testing in our patient was negative for ALK1, ENG, SMAD4, RASA1, and GDF2. However, our patient reported a childhood history of epistaxis. She also had a family history of GI bleeding and epistaxis in her father. Examination of the patient was notable for mucocutaneous telangiectasias on her lips and thumb. Endoscopic evaluation revealed recurrent GI AVMs.

AVMs in the GI tract typically occur in the stomach and duodenum and most commonly present as GI bleeding after 40 years of age [7]. AVMs in the liver are typically between hepatic arteries and portal veins and may manifest as symptoms of pulmonary or portal hypertension, heart failure, abdominal pain, or encephalopathy [16]. There may also be abnormalities in cardiac biomarkers or liver function tests [17]. HAVMs are more prevalent in patients with mutations in ACVRL1 (HHT-2) [18]. The current guidelines recommend screening for HAVMs with diagnostic imaging in patients who are symptomatic and in patients whom HHT is suspected or definite [17].

Recurrent GI bleeding in HHT is debilitating and is associated with a decreased quality of life [1]. Chronic bleeding episodes also result in increased healthcare costs, repeated hospital admissions, endoscopic interventions, and pRBC transfusions [8]. Repeated endoscopic ablation of GI AVMs is not recommended due to poor long-term results and complications [19].

Bev has established efficacy in the treatment of inflammatory disorders and in various cancers in which the mechanism of action is inhibition of tumor angiogenesis [20]. The use of Bev in HHT is off-label but is supported by evidence from several retrospective studies [10, 12, 21–23]. However, many of these studies have focused on epistaxis outcomes [7, 21, 22]. Data regarding the efficacy of Bev in GI bleeding have been limited yet promising. Recent studies have reported that the use of Bev in GI bleeding has led to significantly reduced RBC transfusion requirements, increased mean hemoglobin levels, and reduced GI procedures [9, 12–14]. A multicenter study, the inHIBIT-Bleed study, of 238 patients noted that one year of treatment with Bev resulted in an increase in mean hemoglobin by 3.2 g/dl, decrease in RBC units transfused by 82%, and decrease in iron infusions by 70% [24]. The findings of the present case are consistent with prior studies concerning the use of Bev to manage GI bleeding. Our case adds to the emerging body of literature on the efficacy of Bev for the management of recurrent GI bleeding in patients with HHT.

Although effective, Bev has common and often serious adverse effects (AEs) related to on-target mechanism of action, which may be present in up to 10% of patients [20]. AEs may include arterial thrombosis, hypertension, heart failure, massive GI tract hemorrhage, thromboembolic events, and nephrotic syndrome [20, 23]. Buscarini et al. noted that AEs of Bev affected females more than males with the most common AEs being arthralgias, headache, and proteinuria [25]. Our patient developed hypertension, arthralgias, and lower extremity edema. These AEs were mitigated by dose reduction of Bev to 2.5 mg/kg which is to be administered if the patient's hemoglobin decreased by 1.5 g/dL from its peak. It was determined that the patient would likely require a dose of Bev once every 2 months with serial monitoring of her hemoglobin levels given the severity of her disease.

4. Conclusion

In summary, clinicians must consider HHT in the differential for patients with recurrent GI bleeding and AVMs. We recommend the use of Bev in patients with HHT who do not respond to conventional treatment based on its potent efficacy as seen in our case. The AE profile is serious such that dose titration with careful monitoring for vascular complications is critical. Further studies are needed to explore optimal dosing, duration, and long-term safety of Bev.

References

[1] C. Grigg, D. Anderson, and J. Earnshaw, "Diagnosis and treatment of hereditary hemorrhagic telangiectasia," *The Ochsner Journal*, vol. 17, no. 2, pp. 157–161, 2017.

[2] K. Athena, A.-S. Hanny, and J. K. David, "Hereditary hemorrhagic telangiectasia: diagnosis and management from the hematologist's perspective," *Haematologica*, vol. 103, no. 9, pp. 1433–1443, 2018.

[3] S. B. Jackson, N. P. Villano, J. N. Benhammou, M. Lewis, J. R. Pisegna, and D. Padua, "Gastrointestinal manifestations of hereditary hemorrhagic telangiectasia (HHT): a systematic review of the literature," *Digestive Diseases and Sciences*, vol. 62, no. 10, pp. 2623–2630, 2017.

[4] J. McDonald and R. E. Pyeritz, "Hereditary hemorrhagic telangiectasia," in *GeneReviews (®)*, M. P. Adam, H. H. Ardinger, R. A. Pagon et al., Eds., University of Washington, Seattle, WA, USA, 1993.

[5] N. Epperla and W. Hocking, "Blessing for the bleeder: bevacizumab in hereditary hemorrhagic telangiectasia," *Clinical Medicine & Research*, vol. 13, no. 1, pp. 32–35, 2015.

[6] N. Garg, M. Khunger, A. Gupta, and N. Kumar, "Optimal management of hereditary hemorrhagic telangiectasia," *Journal of Blood Medicine*, vol. 5, pp. 191–206, 2014.

[7] R. Acharya, K. Portwood, and K. Upadhyay, "Hereditary hemorrhagic telangiectasia presenting as a recurrent epistaxis in an adolescent: a case report," *World Journal of Clinical Pediatrics*, vol. 10, no. 1, pp. 1–6, 2021.

[8] W. Brinjikji, C. P. Wood, G. Lanzino et al., "High rates of bleeding complications among hospitalized patients with hereditary hemorrhagic telangiectasia in the United States," *Annals of the American Thoracic Society*, vol. 13, no. 9, pp. 1505–1511, 2016.

[9] A. Lupu, C. Stefanescu, X. Treton, A. Attar, O. Corcos, and Y. Bouhnik, "Bevacizumab as rescue treatment for severe recurrent gastrointestinal bleeding in hereditary hemorrhagic telangiectasia," *Journal of Clinical Gastroenterology*, vol. 47, no. 3, pp. 256-257, 2013.

[10] T. Rosenberg, A. D. Fialla, J. Kjeldsen et al., "Does severe bleeding in HHT patients respond to intravenous bevacizumab? Review of the literature and case series," *Rhinology*, vol. 57, no. 4, pp. 242–251, 2019.

[11] J. Kochanowski, M. Sobieszczańska, S. Tubek, M. Żurek, and J. Pawełczak, "Successful therapy with bevacizumab in a case of hereditary hemorrhagic telangiectasia," *Human Vaccines & Immunotherapeutics*, vol. 11, no. 3, pp. 680-681, 2015.

[12] V. N. Iyer, D. R. Apala, B. S. Pannu et al., "Intravenous bevacizumab for refractory hereditary hemorrhagic telangiectasia-related epistaxis and gastrointestinal bleeding," *Mayo Clinic Proceedings*, vol. 93, no. 2, pp. 155–166, 2018.

[13] J. M. Fleagle, R. K. Bobba, C. G. Kardinal, and C. E. Freter, "Iron deficiency anemia related to hereditary hemorrhagic telangiectasia: response to treatment with bevacizumab," *The American Journal of the Medical Sciences*, vol. 343, no. 3, pp. 249–251, 2012.

[14] H. Bennesser Alaoui, M. Lehraiki, S. Hamaz, N. El Attar, N. Fakhreddine, and K. Serraj, "Bevacizumab: un nouveau succès dans la maladie de Rendu-Osler," *La Revue de Médecine Interne*, vol. 36, no. 9, pp. 623–625, 2015.

[15] C. Canzonieri, L. Centenara, F. Ornati et al., "Endoscopic evaluation of gastrointestinal tract in patients with hereditary hemorrhagic telangiectasia and correlation with their genotypes," *Genetics in Medicine*, vol. 16, no. 1, pp. 3–10, 2014.

[16] G. Garcia-Tsao, "Liver involvement in hereditary hemorrhagic telangiectasia (HHT)," *Journal of Hepatology*, vol. 46, no. 3, pp. 499–507, 2007.

[17] M. E. Faughnan, J. J. Mager, S. W. Hetts et al., "Second international guidelines for the diagnosis and management of hereditary hemorrhagic telangiectasia," *Annals of Internal Medicine*, vol. 173, no. 12, pp. 989–1001, 2020.

[18] C. Sabbà, G. Pasculli, G. M. Lenato et al., "Hereditary hemorrhagic telangiectasia: clinical features in ENG and ALK1 mutation carriers," *Journal of Thrombosis and Haemostasis*, vol. 5, no. 6, pp. 1149–1157, 2007.

[19] M. E. Faughnan, V. A. Palda, G Garcia-Tsao et al., "International guidelines for the diagnosis and management of hereditary haemorrhagic telangiectasia," *Journal of Medical Genetics*, vol. 48, no. 2, pp. 73–87, 2011.

[20] V. Gerriets and A. Kasi, *Bevacizumab*, StatPearls Publishing LLC., Treasure Island, FL, USA, 2020.

[21] H. Al-Samkari, A. Kritharis, J. M. Rodriguez-Lopez, and D. J. Kuter, "Systemic bevacizumab for the treatment of chronic bleeding in hereditary haemorrhagic telangiectasia," *Journal of Internal Medicine*, vol. 285, no. 2, pp. 223–231, 2019.

[22] N. P. Arizmendez, L. Rudmik, and D. M. Poetker, "Intravenous bevacizumab for complications of hereditary hemorrhagic telangiectasia: a review of the literature," *International Forum of Allergy & Rhinology*, vol. 5, no. 11, pp. 1042–1047, 2015.

[23] A. Guilhem, A.-E. Fargeton, A.-C. Simon et al., "Intra-venous bevacizumab in hereditary hemorrhagic telangiectasia (HHT): a retrospective study of 46 patients," *PLoS One*, vol. 12, no. 11, Article ID e0188943, 2017.

[24] A.-S. Hanny, S. K. Raj, G. P. Joseph et al., "An international, multicenter study of intravenous bevacizumab for bleeding in hereditary hemorrhagic telangiectasia: the InHIBIT-bleed study," *Haematologica*, 2020.

[25] E. Buscarini, L. M. Botella, L. M. Botella et al., "Safety of thalidomide and bevacizumab in patients with hereditary hemorrhagic telangiectasia," *Orphanet Journal of Rare Diseases*, vol. 14, no. 1, p. 28, 2019.

7

Parastomal Varices with Recurrent Bleeding in the Absence of Liver Cirrhosis

Jonathan Kopel ,[1] Rebeccah Baucom,[2] Samuel Campbell,[3] and Gregory L. Brower[4]

[1]*Texas Tech University Health Sciences Center School of Medicine, Lubbock, TX, USA*
[2]*Department of Surgery, Texas Tech University Health Sciences Center, Lubbock, TX, USA*
[3]*Department of Surgery Division of Vascular Surgery, Texas Tech University Health Sciences Center, Lubbock, TX, USA*
[4]*Department of Medical Education, Texas Tech University Health Sciences Center, Lubbock, TX, USA*

Correspondence should be addressed to Jonathan Kopel; jonathan.kopel@ttuhsc.edu

Academic Editor: Yoshifumi Nakayama

Gastrointestinal (GI) bleeding is a common problem in patients with portal hypertension. One of the most common causes of GI bleeding are varices (e.g., esophageal varices). In some instances, varices can develop between an intestinal stoma and the abdominal wall vasculature, known as parastomal varices. Specifically, parastomal varices are common in patients with a preexisting stoma and concurrent chronic portal hypertension. These patients often present with recurrent bleeding and may require regular transfusions. Herein, we report on a patient with parastomal varices and portal hypertension without hepatic cirrhosis. Given the high morbidity and mortality associated with surgical interventions, most clinical guidelines encourage observation and medical management of bleeding from parastomal varices. Among the nonsurgical interventions, manual compression and local maneuvers often successfully stop the bleeding. However, subsequent rebleeding from parastomal varices can remain a problem requiring additional treatment. Further research is needed to investigate appropriate medical or surgical alternatives for managing parastomal varices bleeding.

1. Introduction

Varices are a common cause of gastrointestinal (GI) bleeding in patients with portal hypertension [1]. In most cases, varices will develop in three primary locations: (1) the left gastric and esophageal veins, (2) the superior, middle, and inferior rectal veins, and (3) the paraumbical veins [2]. However, varices can also develop between an intestinal stoma and the abdominal wall vasculature, with the resulting parastomal varices being particularly common among portal hypertension patients [2]. Peristomal varices occur in 27%–50% of patients with portal hypertension and a preexisting stoma [3]. In most cases, parastomal varices appear as circumferential blue or purple subcutaneous rings extending from the mucocutaneous junction of the subcutaneous stomal skin and present with external bleeding, which may be life-threatening [3]. In this case report, we discuss a patient with parastomal varices and portal hypertension without known liver cirrhosis.

2. Case Report

A 56-year-old man presented to the emergency department with bleeding (>700 cc) around his colostomy site persisting for two days. The patient denied any pain with the bleeding, fever, chills, sweats, weakness, abdominal pain, nausea, vomiting, or diarrhea. The patient denied any history of smoking, alcohol, or any other substance abuse. The patient's surgical history included a remote colectomy with permanent colostomy for stage IV colon cancer and a subsequent colostomy revision and hernia repair (8 and 6 years, respectively, before this episode), after experiencing a massive bleed from a parastomal varices. The patient has a medical history of hypertension, hyperlipidemia, diabetes, hypothyroidism, colon cancer, obstructive sleep apnea, and obesity.

The patient's current medications upon presentation in the emergency department included pioglitazone, ipratropium bromide, insulin glargine, montelukast, levocetirizine, atorvastatin, azelastine, bisoprolol, levothyroxine, lisinopril, metformin, triamcinolone, and aspirin. The patient's blood pressure was 128/84 mmHg. The patient's white blood cell count was 3,970 cells/μL, platelet count was 119,000/μL, and red blood cell count was low at 4.080 million cells/uL. His hemoglobin and hematocrit levels were 13.7 g/dL and 39.2%, respectively. His sodium was below normal, and he was hypochloremic (135 mmol/L and 95 mmol/L, respectively), glucose was elevated at 313 mg/dL, and creatine was normal at 0.8 mg/dL. His liver function was normal, aside from slightly elevated alanine transaminase of 64 international units/L.

Given the recurrent bleeding over several days, surgery was consulted to evaluate the bleeding. No further bleeding was elicited, and the patient was discharged. However, the patient returned to the emergency department the next day reporting 50 cc of dark red blood while emptying his colostomy bag. Vascular surgery and gastroenterology were consulted. A right upper quadrant ultrasound demonstrated a gallstone, no pericholecystic fluid or wall thickening, and common bile duct diameter of 6 mm without intrahepatic biliary ductal dilatation. The liver measured 20 cm in length with the portal vein slightly dilated at 1.1 cm. Furthermore, the portal vein showed hepatopedal blood flow with a velocity of 14.6 cm/s. The liver echotexture was also hyperechogenic suggesting mild hepatic steatosis. Visualization of the pancreas was normal.

The colonoscopy performed through the stoma was without abnormality. EGD showed a normal esophagus without any esophageal varices and a normal duodenum; however, mild portal hypertensive gastropathy was found diffusely in the entire stomach. A CT scan of the abdomen showed the main portal vein to be slightly dilated measuring 14 mm. The superior mesenteric vein was also dilated measuring 15 mm. Mesenteric veins extending into the parastomal hernia were also dilated. As shown in Figure 1, the CT scan demonstrated a parastomal hernia with accompanying dilated parastomal varices. Given the lack of further bleeding, the patient was released and given instructions on how to reduce the risk of further bleeding from the parastomal varices. The patient subsequently had another episode of massive bleeding (>700 cc) occurring two years after the incident described herein, which resolved sponstaneously after the patient aggressively debrided the vascular erosion and applied manual compression. No rebleeding has occurred in the year since the last incident.

3. Discussion

Obstruction of the portal venous blood flow is a well-known mechanism leading to portal hypertension in between high- and low-pressure systemic venous systems [2,3]. Patients with portal hypertension who have a colostomy or ileostomy may develop collateral venous channels to the anterior abdominal wall forming parastomal varices [2]. In most instances, parastomal varices branch from mesenteric branches off the superior mesenteric vein [7]. In this case report, the patient had a history of stage IV colon cancer requiring the formation of a permanent colostomy. The patient subsequently developed parastomal varices with a parastomal hernia. As shown in Table 1, most patients with parastomal varices have a history of ulcerative colitis, carcinoma of rectum, carcinoma of urinary tract, liver cirrhosis, primary sclerosing cholangitis, or hepatitis. However, the patient in this case presented with a history of colon cancer with portal hypertension without known liver cirrhosis.

The bleeding from parastomal varices can be a slow venous ooze without a focal source or a pressurized spurting bleed [7]. The bleeding resulting from portal hypertension can be massive and cannot always be manually compressed [7]. When bleeding is focal, manual compression with a single-digit at the bleeding site or outside the stoma may provide temporary control [7]. The parastomal varices in this patient showed focal bleeding that was controlled by applying pressure using a cotton swab. Recent case reports have shown the use of percutaneous *N*-butyl-2-cyanoacrylate glue injection effectively stopped bleeding from parastomal varices [8]. However, injection of *N*-butyl-2-cyanoacrylate glue is not approved in the United States [1]. Other case reports have used a combination of sodium tetradecyl sulfate, ethanol, and saline to reduce the number of blood transfusions [1]. Polidocanol, 5% phenol, and nonselective beta-blockers have also shown some beneficial reduction in parastomal varices bleeding [1].

Despite being common in patients with a colostomy, many patients and physicians are unaware of parastomal varices and the frequency of bleeding [2,8]. Physicians are encouraged to remove any bandages or stoma appliance to examine the surrounding skin for a purplish hue around the stomal area, which suggests presence of parastomal varices [8]. However, only 25% of patients exhibit the purplish hue; physicians are encouraged to use Doppler ultrasound, contrast-enhanced CT, and portal vein venography to confirm the diagnosis for many patients with recurrent bleeding around the stoma site [2]. Furthermore, direct suture repair or stoma relocation is not recommended due to the high rate of recurrence (60%) [4].

Although no standard treatment for bleeding from parastomal varices has been established, the current report suggests that conservative management of parastomal varices using manual compression, with or without focal debridement, should be given consideration. However, because this approach frequently fails to effectively control the bleeding, several other treatment options have been used to treat parastomal varices, including nonoperative treatment, local operative treatment, surgical portosystemic shunts, embolization (transhepatic or transjugular), transjugular intrahepatic portosystemic shunt, and liver transplant [2]. In recent years, alternative surgical techniques, such as extraperitoneal tunneling, stapled ostomy creation, stoma-fascia fixation, and prophylactic mesh reinforcement, were used to prevent the development of parastomal varices [5]. A meta-analysis including 1,071 patients who had a

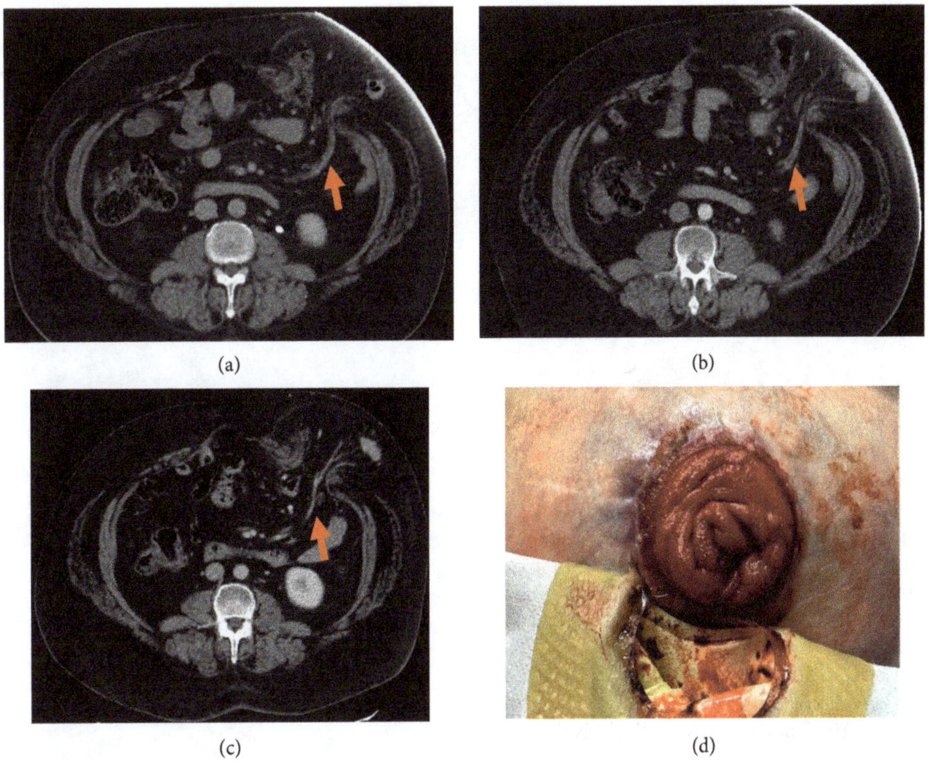

FIGURE 1: (a–c) Abdominal CT scans demonstrating dilated parastomal varices (red arrows). (d) Image depicting parastomal varices and hernia.

TABLE 1: Summary of parastomal varices risk factors, presentation, and treatment [4–6].

Patient risk factors	Surgical risk factors	Appearance	Clinical presentation	Treatment
(i) Obesity (ii) Malnutrition (iii) Advanced age (iv) Smoking (v) Collagen abnormalities (vi) Corticosteroid use (vii) Postoperative wound sepsis (viii) Ascites (ix) Abdominal distention (x) Chronic constipation (xi) Obstructive uropathy (xii) Chronic obstructive lung disease	(i) Inappropriate stoma site selection (ii) Oversized fascial trephine (iii) Excessive splitting and stretching of abdominal rectus muscle (iv) Epigastric nerve denervation (v) Emergency stoma creation	Circumferential blue or purple subcutaneous rings extending from the mucocutaneous junction of the subcutaneous stomal skin	(i) Peristomal esthetic complaints (ii) Discomfort (iii) Pain (iv) Bowel obstruction (v) Incarceration	(i) Prophylactic synthetic mesh placement (ii) *N*-Butyl-2-cyanoacrylate glue injection (iii) Single-digit compression (iv) Sodium tetradecyl sulfate (v) Polidocanol (vi) 5% phenol (vii) Nonselective beta-blockers (viii) Liver transplant (ix) Embolization (x) Transjugular intrahepatic portosystemic shunt

colostomy created using either the extraperitoneal versus intraperitoneal techniques found a lower rate of parastomal hernias in the extraperitoneal group [9].

If bleeding remains persistent or increases in severity, reducing portal hypertension using a transjugular intrahepatic portosystemic shunt (TIPS) effectively prevents most rebleeding events from parastomal varices [8]. Specifically, only 20% of patients with parastomal varices with a history of rebleeding continued to have bleeding after the TIPS procedure [2]. However, a TIPS procedure is contraindicated for patients with primary or metastatic liver cancer or for those with advanced liver cirrhosis. Currently, over 75% of patients with parastomal varices and bleeding are treated medically using nonselective beta-blockers. Despite surgical advances in treatment, patients with parastomal varices have a high risk of morbidity (13%), mortality (6.3%), and recurrence (11% after 3 years) [4]. Given the significant number of affected patients, further research is needed to investigate appropriate medical or surgical approaches for managing parastomal varices bleeding.

References

[1] V. H. Chong, K. K. Tan, and F. Sharif, "Successful treatment of parastomal varices bleeding with percutaneous *N*-butyl-2-cyanoacrylate glue injection," *Surgical Laparoscopy, Endoscopy & Percutaneous Techniques*, vol. 18, no. 5, pp. 520–522, 2008.

[2] M. O. Pennick and D. Y. Artioukh, "Management of parastomal varices: who re-bleeds and who does not? A systematic review of the literature," *Techniques in Coloproctology*, vol. 17, no. 2, pp. 163–170, 2012.

[3] M. McGee and P. Cataldo, "Intestinal stomas," in *The ASCRS Text Book of Colon and Rectal Surgery*, S. Steele, T. Hull, and T. Read, Eds., pp. 971–1013, Springer, New York, NY, USA, Third edition, 2016.

[4] S. Tsujinaka, K.-Y. Tan, Y. Miyakura et al., "Current management of intestinal stomas and their complications," *Journal of the Anus, Rectum and Colon*, vol. 4, no. 1, pp. 25–33, 2020.

[5] D. Krishnamurty, J. Blatnik, and M. Mutch, "Stoma complications," *Clinics in Colon and Rectal Surgery*, vol. 30, no. 03, pp. 193–200, 2017.

[6] W. Osborne, J. North, and J. Williams, "Using a risk assessment tool for parastomal hernia prevention," *British Journal of Nursing*, vol. 27, no. 5, pp. 15–19, 2018.

[7] W. E. Saad, N. E. Saad, and J. Koizumi, "Stomal varices: management with decompression TIPS and transvenous obliteration or sclerosis," *Techniques in Vascular and Interventional Radiology*, vol. 16, no. 2, pp. 126–134, 2013.

[8] K. Tran-Harding, M. Winkler, and D. Raissi, "Bleeding stomal varices in portal hypertension," *Radiology Case Reports*, vol. 13, no. 2, pp. 356–360, 2018.

[9] L. Lian, X.-R. Wu, X.-S. He et al., "Extraperitoneal vs. intraperitoneal route for permanent colostomy: a meta-analysis of 1,071 patients," *International Journal of Colorectal Disease*, vol. 27, no. 1, pp. 59–64, 2012.

8

Diffuse Large B Cell Lymphoma with Cutaneous and Gastrointestinal Involvement

Aye-Mya-Mya Kyaw,[1] Than-Than Aye,[1] and Lin-Lin Htun[2]

[1]*Gastroenterology Department, Thingangyun General Hospital, Yangon, Myanmar*
[2]*Pathology Department, Thingangyun General Hospital, Yangon, Myanmar*

Correspondence should be addressed to Aye-Mya-Mya Kyaw; ammk.intmed@gmail.com

Academic Editor: Yoshihiro Moriwaki

Diffuse large B cell lymphoma (DLBCL) is the histological subtype of non-Hodgkin's lymphoma, representing approximately 30%. The most common primary extranodal sites of DLBCL are the gastrointestinal (GI) tract, the head and neck, and the skin/soft tissue. We report a case of DLBCL with cutaneous involvement presenting with skin nodules and GI manifestations such as obstructive jaundice and upper GI bleeding. Malignant cystic pancreatic tumor occupying the head and body with invasion to lower end of common bile duct and periampullary region causing biliary obstruction and mesenteric lymphadenopathy were found in abdominal computed tomography and endoscopic ultrasonography. There was also a large gastric ulcer (Forrest IIa) at the greater curvature of body of the stomach. Histopathological results of the skin and stomach were consistent with diffuse large B cell lymphoma; gastric biopsy being negative for leucocyte common antigen. The patient was considered to have disseminated DLBCL. The aim of the present case report was to present the clinical, radiological, and histological characteristics of the patient, which may aid physicians in diagnosing involvement of multiple extranodal sites in DLBCL.

1. Introduction

Gastrointestinal tract (GIT) is the most common extranodal site for non-Hodgkin's lymphoma (NHL), constituting about 10%–15% of all NHL. Diffuse large B cell lymphoma (DLBCL) is the most common histological subtype, representing approximately 30% of NHLs. The most common primary extranodal sites of DLBCL are the gastrointestinal tract, the head and neck, and the skin/soft tissue [1]. Here, we report a case of DLBCL presenting with both gastrointestinal and dermatological manifestations.

2. Case Report

A 39-year-old lady from a remote area was referred from dermatological unit for the large ulcerative skin lesion over the abdomen and trunk associated with progressive obstructive jaundice and significant weight loss over 1 month. Because of cholangitis with sepsis at that moment, she was decided to treat GI pathology first. On reviewing her history, since 2015, she has had progressive infiltrative skin lesions on her left lower chest (Figure 1(a)), right upper chest, and left lumber region for which indigenous medicine has been taking prior to medical consultation.

The physical examination revealed jaundice, abdominal tenderness, and multiple skin lesions on the chest and left loin region (Figure 1(b)). All the skin lesions had no bleeding or tenderness. Lymphadenopathy, organomegaly, or ascites was not detected.

The liver function test revealed high bilirubin and alkaline phosphatase. There was also hypochromic microcystic anaemia (hemoglobin, 10 g/dl; mean corpuscular volume (MCV), 76.6 fl). Lactate dehydrogenase (LDH) was 770 U/L, and tumor markers such as CA 19-9 and alpha-fetoprotein were normal. There is no abnormal finding in chest X-ray (CXR, PA view).

In abdominal computed tomography (CT), there was malignant cystic pancreatic tumor ($6.3 \times 4.7 \times 3.8$ cm) occupying the head and body with invasion to lower end of

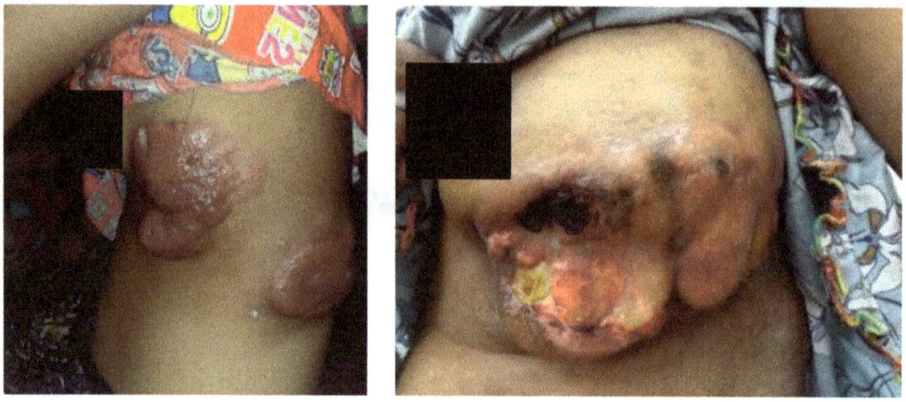

(a) (b)

FIGURE 1: (a). Cutaneous manifestations at 2015: skin nodules on the left lower chest and loin region. (b) One of the cutaneous manifestations at the time of admission: large ulcer with some necrotic tissue (11 × 6 cm in size) at left lower chest wall.

common bile duct (CBD) and periampullary region causing biliary obstruction and mesenteric lymphadenopathy (Figures 2(a) and 2(b)). There was no abnormal finding in the liver and spleen.

Endoscopic ultrasound (EUS) showed a large inhomogenous hypoechoic mass (4 × 3.6 cm in diameter) in pancreatic head region with dilatation of proximal CBD and both intrahepatic ducts (IHD) (Figures 3(a) and 3(b)). EUS-guided fine needle aspiration cytology (FNAC) from pancreatic head mass found large atypical cells with hypochromatic nuclei and few papillae with stratification and irregular chromatin (positive for malignancy). However, EUS-guided fine needle aspiration biopsy (FNAB) came back as the tissue was not adequate for analysis. Straight plastic biliary stent was placed for cholangitis with long CBD stricture (5.1 cm in length).

On the other hand, immunohistochemical (IHC) staining of the skin biopsy revealed strongly positive CD20, high Ki67 (Figure 4), but negative expression for CD3, CD45, CD30, AE1/3, CD10, Bcl-6, Bcl-2, and MUM-1. Findings were consistent with diffuse large B cell lymphoma.

On the first day of post-ERCP, the patient had hypovolaemic shock with gastrointestinal bleeding. In EGD, there was a large gastric ulcer (Forrest IIa) at the greater curvature of body of the stomach (Figure 5(a)), which would have been missed in ERCP. Combined adrenalin injection and heater probe coagulation were applied. Histopathological result of gastric ulcer initially came out as poorly differentiated adenocarcinoma or lymphoma in H&E staining (Figure 5(b)). Histochemical staining of both leucocyte common antigen (LCA) and epithelial membrane antigen (EMA) were negative in this case (Figures 5(c) and 5(d)). However, due to different anatomical sites involvement and getting the IHC result of skin biopsy just before it, the suspection of lymphoma behoved us to exclude the possibility of LCA-negative lymphoma. The subsequent IHC panel revealed diffusely positive for CD20 in these atypical cells (Figure 5(e)).

After stabilizing the general condition of the patient for a few weeks, second EUS procedure was repeated with the intention to take adequate FNA biopsy from pancreatic mass. At that time, because there was extrinsic compression of the first part of duodenum and an infiltrative lesion along second part of the duodenum, the EUS linear scope was not able to pass through luminal narrowing. Because of the cost issue, we did not proceed to IHC stainings on duodenal tissue but assumed to be the same pathology.

The final diagnosis was disseminated diffuse large B cell lymphoma (DLBCL) with cutaneous and gastrointestinal involvement. Unfortunately, the patient expired just before receiving chemotherapy in the oncology ward.

3. Discussion

Most DLBCLs originate in lymph nodes, but ≤40% initially present in extranodal sites [2]. Like most other NHLs, there is a male predominance with approximately 55% of cases occurring in men [3]. Sixty percentage of patients will present with advanced stage DLBCL (usually stage III or IV disease), while 40% have a more localized disease [4, 5]. The patient in this report had cutaneous manifestation since 5 years ago. At the time of admission, she presented with obstructive jaundice due to CBD stricture with pancreatic involvement and gastrointestinal bleeding due to gastric involvement.

Depending on the site of involvement, there are 2 distinct subsets: primary cutaneous DLBCL which initially presents on the skin and DLBCL accompanied by secondary spread to the skin [6]. The presence of multiple skin lesions and time of evolution at presentation were associated with poorer prognosis in secondary cutaneous DLBCL [7]. In this patient, we assumed that her cutaneous manifestation was initial presentation of disseminated DLBCL. Because of delay in seeking medical advice, we could not exclude whether gastrointestinal involvement preceded subcutaneous nodules appearance or not.

Gastrointestinal bleeding is the presenting symptom in 20–30% of gastric DLBCL cases. Lymphoma can be recognized as ulceration, diffuse infiltration, or a polypoid mass during an endoscopic examination. *Helicobacter pylori*

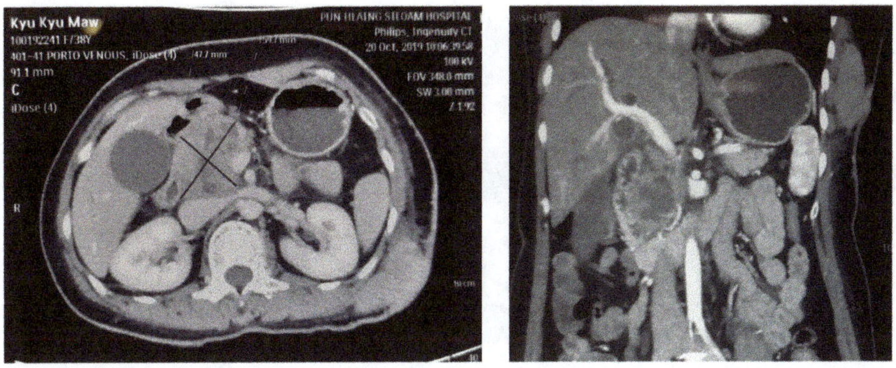

(a) (b)

Figure 2: (a), (b) CT revealed malignant cystic pancreatic tumor occupying head and body with invasion to lower end of CBD and periampullary region causing biliary obstruction.

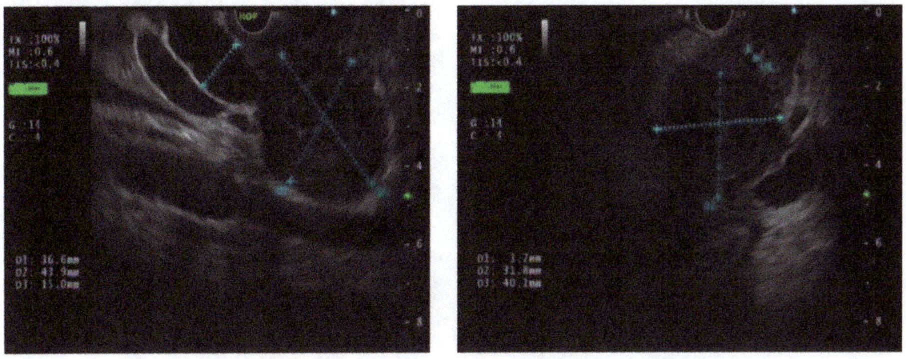

(a) (b)

Figure 3: (a), (b) EUS showing a large inhomogenous hypoechoic mass (4 × 3.6 cm in diameter) in pancreatic head region with dilatation of CBD (1.4 cm) and both IHDs. Main pancreatic duct (MPD) is mildly dilated (3.4 mm) in head region.

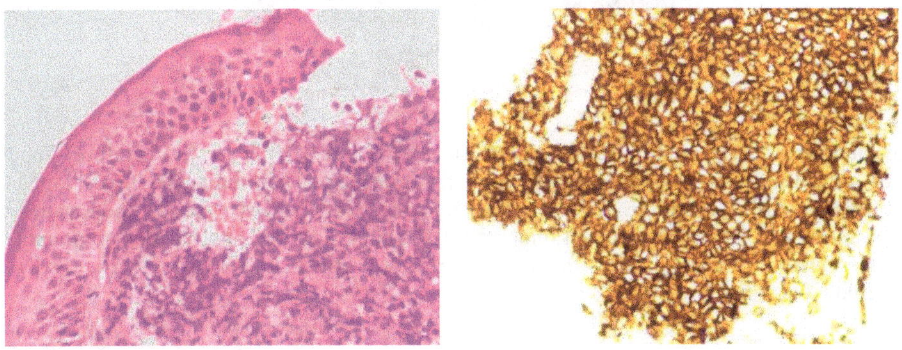

(a) (b)

Figure 4: IHC analysis of skin biopsy. (a) The subcutaneous tissue infiltrated by diffuse sheet of atypical large lymphoid cells with vesicular nuclei, prominent nucleoli, and moderate cytoplasm (hematoxylin and eosin (H&E staining, x20). (b) Strongly membranous positive CD 20 in lesional lymphoid cells (IHC-CD20, x40).

association can be found in 63% of high-grade lymphoma and 88% of low-grade lymphoma [8]. Endoscopy finding of our patient revealed a large ulcer (Forrest IIa) at the greater curvature of body of stomach.

In pancreatic lymphoma, abdominal pain is the most common presenting symptom (83%), followed by abdominal mass (58%), weight loss (50%), jaundice (37%), acute pancreatitis (12%), small bowel obstruction (12%), and diarrhea (12%) [9]. Our patient presented with biliary obstruction due to pancreatic lesion. Theoretically, obstructive jaundice is less frequent than in pancreatic adenocarcinoma [9].

To differentiate pancreatic lymphoma from adenocarcinoma in imagings, Merkle et al. reported that findings of a

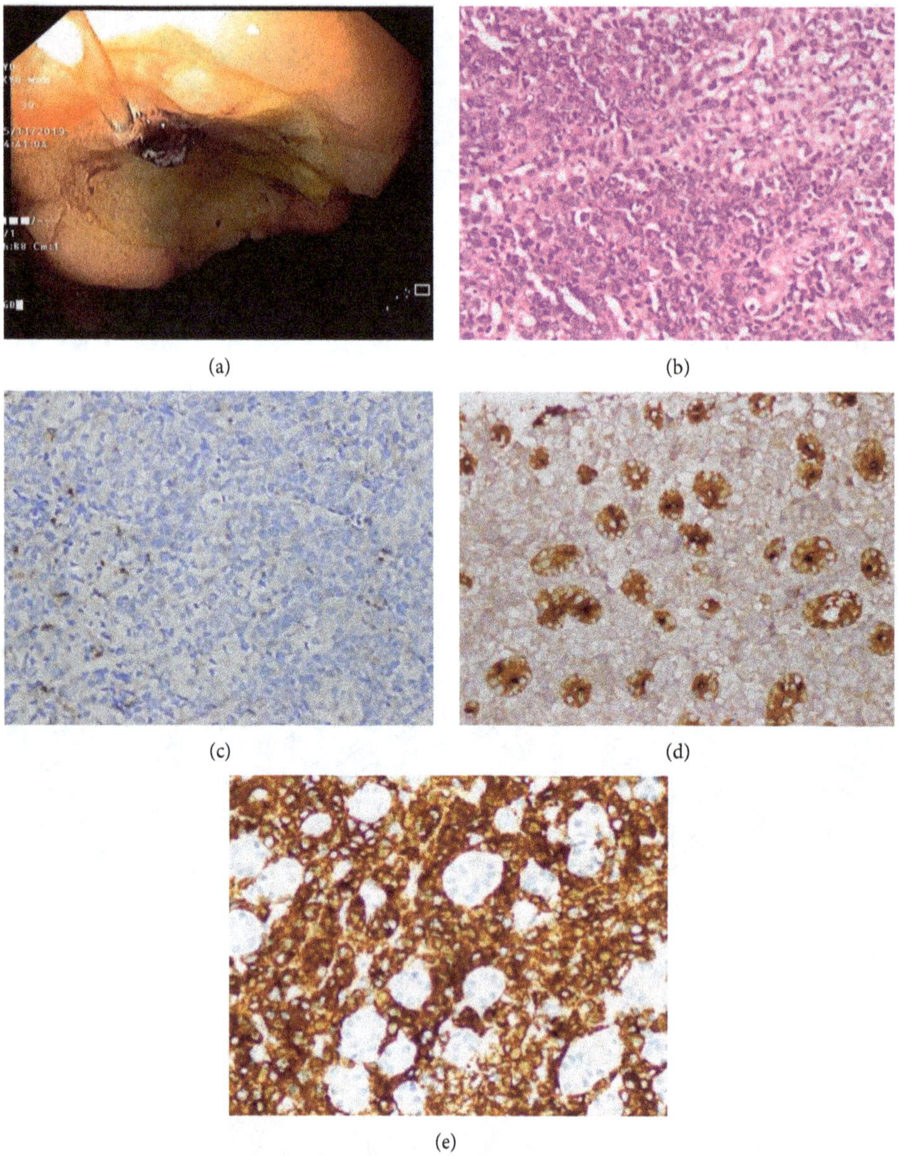

Figure 5: Gastroscopic biopsies and IHC staining. (a) A large gastric ulcer (Forrest IIa) at greater curvature of body of the stomach. (b) Diffuse sheets of atypical large lymphoid cells having vesicular nuclei, prominent nucleoli, and moderate eosinophilic cytoplasm. They are spilling into gastric epithelial cells (IEL, intraepithelial lymphoid cells). Mitoses are occasionally seen (H and E staining; magnification, x40). (c) LCA (leucocyte common antigen, CD 45) negative in tumor cells (IHC x40). (d) EMA (epithelial membrane antigen) negative in tumor cells and positive only in residual gastric glands (IHC x40). (e) CD 20 strongly positive in lesional large lymphoid cells and negative in gastric epithelial cells (IHC staining; magnification, x100).

bulky localized tumor in the pancreatic head without significant dilatation of the main pancreatic duct, invasive tumor growth not respecting anatomic boundaries, and the absence of calcifications and necrosis within the tumor mass, all seen more commonly in lymphoma [9, 10]. Enlarged lymph nodes below the renal vein also rules out pancreatic cancer and favors a diagnosis of pancreatic lymphoma [11]. Ultrasound or CT-guided fine needle biopsy of the pancreatic mass can also help to distinguish pancreatic lymphoma from pancreatic adenocarcinoma [12]. Unfortunately, in this patient, the tissue of FNB was not adequate for interpretation.

Staining for pan-B cell markers such as CD20 and CD79a should be performed for the diagnosis, and a much broader set of stains may be needed in cases with atypical morphological features [13]. The distinction between poorly differentiated adenocarcinoma and gastric lymphoma in endoscopic biopsies is sometimes difficult owing to the morphologic similarities that these neoplasias can share and the small amount of tissue obtained by this technique. An additional factor that may contribute to this confusion is the presence of artifactual lymphocytes resembling signet-ring cells [14]. Therefore, Arista-Nasr et al. suggested that the diagnosis of gastric lymphoma must be excluded using histochemical and immunohistochemical studies if a poorly differentiated neoplasm consistent with signet-ring adenocarcinoma is found in an endoscopic biopsy with artificial changes [14].

In our patient, IHC staining of gastric biopsy was LCA-negative, CD 20-positive DLBCL. Rare cases of LCA-negative large B cell lymphomas previously reported have an extranodal presentation, urinary bladder [15], thyroid gland [16], and cerebellum [17], and have been reclassified as plasmablastic lymphoma or ALK-positive large B cell lymphoma in literature. Loss of LCA expression on lymphoma cells usually suggests that neoplastic transformation has occurred during the differentiation pathway to plasma cells just before its CD20 expression [16].

In conclusion, we reported a rare case of diffuse large B cell lymphoma with cutaneous and gastrointestinal involvement. Pancreatic head mass was also assumed to be lymphoma, although we could not confirm the diagnosis. Histopathological diagnosis with histochemical and IHC studies are important in distinguishing lymphoma from adenocarcinoma. Although most cases of DLBCL respond well to chemotherapy, our patient could not undergo adequate treatment for her disease because of poor performance status and large burden of disease since the time of presentation, leading to her death.

Authors' Contributions

All authors have contributed in writing and reviewing the manuscript.

Acknowledgments

The authors thank their colleagues of Gastroenterology Department and Associate Professor Dr. Aye Aye Win from the Pathology Department, Thingangyun General Hospital, for their assistance in investigations and treatment of this case.

References

[1] D. Yang, W.-P. Zhang, J.-M. Yang, M.-X. He, C. Cheng, and J. Chen, "Secondary skin involvement in gastric diffuse large B-cell lymphoma treated with chidamide," *Medicine*, vol. 97, no. 49, 2018.

[2] U. Vitolo, J. F. Seymour, M. Martelli et al., "Extranodal diffuse large B-cell lymphoma (DLBCL) and primary mediastinal B-cell lymphoma: ESMO clinical practice guidelines for diagnosis, treatment and follow-up," *Annals of Oncology, Official Journal of the European Society for Medical Oncology*, vol. 27, no. Supplement 5, pp. v91–v102, 2016.

[3] L. M. Morton, S. S. Wang, S. S. Devesa, P. Hartge, D. D. Weisenburger, and M. S. Linet, "Lymphoma incidence patterns by WHO subtype in the United States, 1992-2001," *Blood*, vol. 107, no. 1, pp. 265–276, 2006.

[4] J. O. Armitage and D. D. Weisenburger, "New approach to classifying non-Hodgkin's Lymphomas: clinical features of the major histologic subtypes. non-Hodgkin's Lymphoma classification project," *Journal of Clinical Oncology Official Journal of the European Society for Medical Oncology*, vol. 16, no. 8, pp. 2780–2795, 1998.

[5] "A clinical evaluation of the international lymphoma study group classification of non-Hodgkin's lymphoma. The non-Hodgkin's lymphoma classification project," *Blood*, vol. 89, no. 11, pp. 3909–3918, 1997.

[6] W. J. Lee, K. H. Won, C. H. Won et al., "Secondary cutaneous diffuse large B-cell lymphoma has a higher international prognostic index score and worse prognosis than diffuse large B-cell lymphoma, leg type," *Acta Dermato-Venereologica*, vol. 96, no. 2, pp. 245–250, 2016.

[7] J. B. Ferrão, J. V. Barreira, S. Marote, and A. Parmanande, "Diffuse large B cell lymphoma: cutaneous presentation," *BMJ Case Reports*, vol. 11, no. 1, Article ID e226839, 2018.

[8] M. W. Saif, S. Khubchandani, and M. Walczak, "Secondary pancreatic involvement by a diffuse large B-cell lymphoma presenting as acute pancreatitis," *World Journal of Gastroenterology*, vol. 13, no. 36, pp. 4909–4911, 2007.

[9] E. M. Merkle, G. N. Bender, and H.-J. Brambs, "Imaging findings in pancreatic lymphoma," *AJR. American Journal of Roentgenology*, vol. 174, no. 3, pp. 671–675, 2000.

[10] D. Anand, C. Lall, P. Bhosale, D. Ganeshan, and A. Qayyum, "Current update on primary pancreatic lymphoma," *Abdominal Radiology (New York)*, vol. 41, no. 2, pp. 347–355, 2016.

[11] N. L. Kelekis and R. C. Semelka, "MRI of pancreatic tumors," *European Radiology*, vol. 7, no. 6, pp. 875–886, 1997.

[12] D. V. Gopal, E. A. Johnson, P. R. Pfau, M. E. Benson, N. Guda, and T. J. Frick, "Differentiating primary pancreatic lymphoma from adenocarcinoma using endoscopic ultrasound characteristics and flow cytometry: a case-control study," *Endoscopic Ultrasound*, vol. 3, no. 4, pp. 221–225, 2014.

[13] U. A. Pirzada, K. Kumar, H. Tariq, M. Niazi, and J. Makker, "Case of gastric diffuse large B-cell lymphoma," *Case Reports in Oncology*, vol. 12, no. 1, pp. 39–46, 2019.

[14] J. Arista-Nasr, P. Romero-Lagarza, and R. Pichardo Bahena, "Artifactual signet-ring-like cells in endoscopic biopsy of gastric lymphoma," *Archives of Pathology and Laboratory Medicine*, vol. 121, no. 6, pp. 623–625, 1997.

[15] S. Pasricha, N. Singh, G. Gupta, A. Sharma, and M. Anurag, "LCA-negative DLBCL: a potential diagnostic pitfall," *Indian Journal of Hematology and Blood Transfusion*, vol. 33, no. Suppl 1, pp. S1–S126, Guwahati, India, 2017.

[16] T. Inaba, H. Nishimura, J. Saito et al., "A Case of CD45-negative diffuse large B-cell lymphoma in thyroid gland," *Laboratory Hematology, Official Journal of the European Society for Medical Oncology*, vol. 14, no. 2, pp. 12–14, 2008.

[17] B. Jha, I. Mohapatra, S. Gajendra, and R. Sachdev, "CD45-negative primary diffuse large B-cell lymphoma of the cerebellum," *Neurology India*, vol. 63, no. 2, pp. 276–279, 2015.

9

Benign Recurrent Intrahepatic Cholestasis (BRIC): An African Case Report

Adil Salyani, Linda Barasa, Allan Rajula, and Sayed K. Ali

Department of Medicine, Aga Khan University Hospital, Nairobi, Kenya

Correspondence should be addressed to Sayed K. Ali; sayed.karar@aku.edu

Academic Editor: Chia-Tung Shun

Benign recurrent intrahepatic cholestasis (BRIC) is a rare disorder characterised by recurrent episodes of cholestatic jaundice. First described in 1959, BRIC has been reported in patients all over the world including of African descent. Here, we describe a case of a 21-year-old male with recurring episodes of cholestatic jaundice where we diagnosed BRIC and terminated an episode with rifampicin. To our knowledge, this is the first case report of BRIC diagnosed in Africa.

1. Introduction

Benign recurrent intrahepatic cholestasis (BRIC) is a rare, autosomal recessive disorder characterised by recurrent, self-limited episodes of cholestasis manifested by pruritus, anorexia, fatigue, steatorrhea, and jaundice [1, 2]. The index episode usually occurs in the first two decades of life [2,3]. Episodes can be spontaneous or triggered by infections or pregnancy and can last from weeks to months [2,4,5]. Diagnosis is based on a compatible clinical presentation, laboratory parameters and histology with exclusion of other causes of cholestasis [2] and confirmed by genetic testing [1]. Treatment is supportive often aimed at relief of symptoms, shortening of episodes, and prevention of complications [6].

2. Case

A 21-year-old male of Somali descent presented to our institution in December 2018. He complained of pruritus for a month and jaundice for two weeks. The pruritus was severe, generalised, and worse at night. He also reported fatigue, loss of appetite, dyspepsia, bloating, and right upper quadrant discomfort associated with nonbilious vomiting. His urine was dark and his stools loose, fatty, and pale. There was recent easy bruising of the skin, but no mucous membrane bleeding. He had lost 6 kilograms of weight since onset of symptoms. He denied fever, arthralgia, myalgia, or rash. He had no recent drug ingestion, risk factors for acquisition of viral hepatitis, food or drug allergies, and did not smoke tobacco, consume alcohol, use injectionor inhaled drugs.

He was the second-last born of 21 siblings and half siblings and was unemployed. He reported no family history of cholestasis or liver disease. Several of his sisters were parous with gestations uncomplicated by jaundice or pruritus.

On further questioning, he reported four similar prior episodes over 7 years of varying severities lasting between two to eight weeks with intervening symptom-free periods (Table 1). These episodes were unprovoked except for two occasions triggered by cutaneous infections. The episodes followed a stereotyped pattern; the onset marked by loss of appetite and severe generalised pruritus closely followed by intense fatigue, bloating, right upper quadrant discomfort, loose fatty stools, and dark urine. Scleral icterus characteristically developed two weeks later. Termination also followed a typical pattern with sudden reduction, then resolution of pruritus, a ravenous increase in appetite with resolution of fatigue and other symptoms. Scleral icterus was the last to resolve after a delay of two weeks. These episodes were punctuated by a weight loss of 5-6 kilograms that was regained back to baseline on recovery.

On examination, we found a lean young male with scleral icterus and excoriation marks on his body. He was alert and oriented in time, place, and person. There were no

Table 1: Previous attacks.

Attack	Month, year	Age at onset	Trigger (s)	Duration	Severity	Period to next attack
1	2014	14	None	2 weeks	Mild	2 years
2	June, 2016	16	Skin abscesses	7 weeks	Severe	7 months
3	April, 2017	17	None	8 weeks	Severe	6 months
4	December, 2017	18	Skin abscesses	5 weeks	Moderate	11 months

stigmata of chronic liver disease. Abdominal examination revealed mild right upper quadrant tenderness with a negative Murphy's sign, a normal liver span, and no clinically detectable ascites. The rest of the examination was unremarkable.

His liver function tests revealed a cholestatic picture with markedly elevated total bilirubin, predominantly direct. Alkaline phosphatase was elevated to four times the upper limit of normal, but gamma glutamyl transferase was normal, as were the transaminases. Prothrombin time was prolonged with an INR of 1.98. Serology for hepatitis A, B, and C and HIV 1&2 was negative. These results, along with those from testing performed during the previous episodes where he did not receive a diagnosis are charted in Table 2.

An abdominal ultrasound and magnetic resonance cholangiopancreatography (MRCP) both revealed a normal liver with normal biliary and pancreatic ducts. The patient declined a liver biopsy due to financial constraints at that time. He was prescribed ursodeoxycholic acid, which he did not take. The episode resolved spontaneously after seven weeks, and follow-up liver function tests were subsequently normal.

In June 2019, he presented 2 weeks into his sixth episode. Laboratory testing again revealed a cholestatic picture with peak total bilirubin 408 umol/l, direct bilirubin 326 umol/l, alkaline phosphatase 688 U/L, GGT 7 U/L, and normal transaminases. This time underwent a liver biopsy that revealed preserved liver architecture without inflammation, steatosis, or fibrosis with intrahepatic cholestasis predominantly in the centrilobular zone (Figure 1).

Based on clinical, laboratory, and histologic findings, he was diagnosed with BRIC as per the criteria proposed by Luketic and Shiffman (Table 3). He was initiated on rifampicin 150 mg twice daily for a duration of two weeks with rapid resolution of symptoms and improvement in biochemical parameters.

3. Discussion

BRIC, first described in 1959 in two English patients, [7] has since been reported to occur worldwide [2] including 4 patients of African descent in a 1989 case series from France and Belgium [3] and recently in a North African teenager in Switzerland [8]. While reports continue to emerge from other parts of the world [8–11], there have been no reports of cases diagnosed within Africa. This may be due to the rarity of the condition compounded by a lack of awareness of among clinicians.

Inheritance follows an autosomal recessive pattern with mutations in both alleles of ATP8B1 (BRIC1) or ABCB11 (BRIC2) [1]. Both mutations cause cholestasis by impairing the function of the bile salt export pump (BSEP), which actively transports bile into canaliculi. ATP8B1 gene codes for familial intrahepatic cholestasis type 1 transporter (FIC1), a flippase involved in translocation of phospholipids across the plasma membrane. Deficiency of FIC1 decreases plasma membrane stability, impairing the function of transmembrane transporters including the BSEP, which is encoded by ABCB11. Unlike the BSEP that is only expressed in the canalicular membrane of hepatocytes, FIC1 is also expressed in the small intestine and pancreas. This explains why extrahepatic manifestations of BRIC1 such as diarrhoea and pancreatitis are absent in BRIC2 [9].

Despite a genetic basis, most cases are sporadic. The first episode usually occurs in the first two decades of life. Episodes can last from weeks to months and can be of varying severity. In between episodes, patients remain totally devoid of symptoms for periods ranging from months to years [2, 3]. Triggers include stress, pregnancy, and airway and gastrointestinal infections [2, 4, 10, 11]. Episodes triggered by cutaneous infections seen in our patient have not been described previously.

Pruritus and jaundice are the cardinal symptoms. Other symptoms include malaise, right upper quadrant pain, anorexia, nausea, vomiting, steatorrhea, and weight loss [2]. Prolonged episodes can lead to coagulopathy and haemorrhagic tendencies due to vitamin K malabsorption [12]. Termination of the episodes is heralded by abrupt resolution in anorexia and pruritus followed by gradual resolution in jaundice. The symptoms vary from patient to patient but remain consistent in the same individual across episodes [2].

Laboratory findings during episodes reveal an elevated total bilirubin, which is predominantly direct. Alkaline phosphatase is always elevated, sometimes markedly. Transaminases are normal or mildly elevated but can also be markedly elevated [3, 13]. Early ALT rise that eventually resolves has also been described, a trend seen in our patient during his second episode [4]. The hallmark of BRIC and the other familial causes of intrahepatic cholestasis is that the GGT is normal or only mildly elevated in comparison with the other causes of intrahepatic cholestasis [2]. GGT release is associated with damage to cholangiocytes caused by elevated toxic bile salts in bile. Impaired function of the BSEP markedly reduces the concentration of bile salts in bile, thereby explaining the low levels of GGT seen in these conditions [1].

Liver biopsies performed during episodes reveal centrilobular cholestasis with bile deposition in canaliculi, hepatocytes, and Kupffer's cells. Hepatocyte degeneration, necrosis, and portal and parenchymal inflammation may be seen. These changes resolve completely between episodes [2, 10].

Table 2: Laboratory results.

Investigation	Reference range	26/06/16 attack 2	09/07/16 attack 2	13/07/16 attack 2	07/01/18, 20/01/18 attack 4	04/12/18 attack 5
White cell count (×109/L)	4–10	7.04				
Neutrophils (%)	45–75	65				
Lymphocytes (%)	25–40	26				
Monocytes (%)	2–10	7				
Eosinophils (%)	1–6	2				
Basophils (%)	0–2	0				
Red cell count (×1012/L)	4.5–6.5	5.46				
Haematocrit (%)	40–54	50.6				
Haemoglobin (g/dL)	13–18	16.4				
Platelets (×109/L)	150–400	369				
International normalised ratio (INR)						**1.98**
Total bilirubin (umol/L)	0–21	**134.7**	**229.1**	**293.7**		**393**
Direct bilirubin (umol/L)	0–3.4	**108.4**	**204.9**	**249.3**		**337**
Alkaline phosphatase (U/L)	52–171	**288.5**	**313.0**	**370.0**		**692**
Gamma glutamyl transferase (U/L)	2–42	18.1	8.0	9.0		12
Aspartate aminotransferase (U/L)	0–50	**186.5**	**60.7**	46.1		48
Alanine aminotransferase (U/L)	0–50	**400.4**	**62.4**	43.7		32
Total protein (g/L)	60–85					**91**
Albumin (g/L)	35–55					46
Hepatitis B surface antigen	Negative	Negative				Negative
Hepatitis A IgM antibody	Negative	Negative		Negative		Negative
Hepatitis A total antibody	Negative			**Positive**		
Hepatitis C antibody	Negative		Negative			Negative
Antinuclear antibody					Negative	
Antimitochondrial antibody					Negative	
Anti-LKM A[±]					Negative	
Liver antibodies*					Negative	

[±]Antiliver kidney microsome type 1 antibody. *ASMA, AMA-M2, M2-3E, SP-100, PML, gp210, LKM-1, LC-1, SLA/LP, and Ro-52.

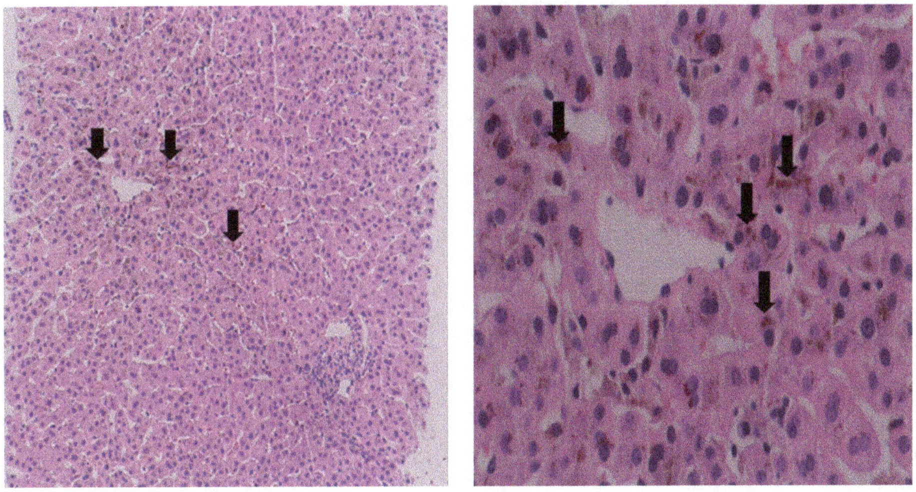

(a) (b)

Figure 1: Liver histology. (a) Liver architecture is preserved. No inflammation, steatosis, or fibrosis seen (haematoxylin and eosin (H&E) × 100). Intrahepatic cholestasis predominantly in the centrilobular zone is identified (black arrows). (b) Intrahepatic cholestasis (black arrows) better demonstrated at a higher magnification (H&E × 400). Central vein at the middle.

Table 3: Diagnostic criteria.

Diagnostic criteria for BRIC (LUKETIC and SHIFFMAN, 2004)
At least two attacks of jaundice separated by a symptom-free interval lasting several months to years
Laboratory values consistent with intrahepatic cholestasis
GGT either normal or only minimally elevated
Severe pruritus secondary to cholestasis
Liver histology demonstrating centrilobular cholestasis
Normal intra- and extrahepatic bile ducts by cholangiography
Absence of factors known to be associated with cholestasis (i.e., drugs and pregnancy)

Diagnosis is based on the criteria proposed by Luketic and Shiffman [2] (Table 3) with genetic testing for mutations used as a confirmation [4].

Treatment is mainly supportive, aimed at relieving symptoms, shortening the episodes, and preventing complications. High dose fat-soluble vitamins should be supplemented to prevent deficiency during prolonged episodes. Bile acid sequestrants such as cholestyramine, opioid antagonists, and ursodeoxycholic acid may reduce pruritus but not the duration of episodes [2, 14]. Rifampicin, plasmapheresis, and endoscopic nasobiliary drainage have all been shown to relieve symptoms and shorten episodes [4, 15].

Rifampicin is safe and effective in reducing pruritus associated with chronic cholestasis [16]. The mechanism of action is related to its enzyme-inducing effects. It activates transcription of CYP3A4, hence stimulating 6α-hydroxylation of bile salts, which can be excreted at the basolateral membrane by ABCC4 transporter. It also induces UGT1A1 and ABCC2, which conjugate and excrete bilirubin [17]. In episodes of BRIC, rifampicin therapy leads to reduced symptoms, improved biochemical parameters, and termination of episodes and hence is considered first-line therapy [4, 10, 18–20].

Our case, the first reported diagnosis of BRIC in Africa, highlights the challenges faced in African countries in diagnosing such rare diseases, including lack of specialists and availability and affordability of diagnostic tests, ultimately resulting in patients receiving delayed, wrong, or no diagnosis. It also adds to the literature on safety and effectiveness of rifampicin in therapy of BRIC episodes.

References

[1] E. Sticova, M. Jirsa, and J. Pawlowska, "New insights in genetic cholestasis: from molecular mechanisms to clinical implications," *Canadian Journal of Gastroenterology & Hepatology*, vol. 2018, Article ID 2313675, 12 pages, 2018.

[2] V. A. Luketic and M. L. Shiffman, "Benign recurrent intrahepatic cholestasis," *Clinics in Liver Disease*, vol. 8, no. 1, pp. 133–149, 2004.

[3] R. Brenard, A. P. Geubel, and J. P. Benhamou, "Benign recurrent intrahepatic cholestasis," *Journal of Clinical Gastroenterology*, vol. 11, no. 5, pp. 546–551, 1989.

[4] G. Folvik, O. Hilde, and G. O. Helge, "Benign recurrent intrahepatic cholestasis: review and long-term follow-up of five cases," *Scandinavian Journal of Gastroenterology*, vol. 47, no. 4, pp. 482–488, 2012.

[5] A. G. F. De Pagter, G. P. Van Berge Henegouwen, J. A. ten Bokkel Huinink, and K.-H. Brandt, "Familial benign recurrent intrahepatic cholestasis," *Gastroenterology*, vol. 71, no. 2, pp. 202–207, 1976.

[6] W. L. Van Der Woerd, R. H. Houwen, and S. F. Van De Graaf, "Current and future therapies for inherited cholestatic liver diseases," *World Journal of Gastroenterology*, vol. 23, no. 5, pp. 763–775, 2017.

[7] W. H. J. Summerskill and J. M. Walshe, "Benign recurrent intrahepatic "obstructive" jaundice," *The Lancet*, vol. 274, no. 7105, pp. 686–690, 1959.

[8] P. Schreiner, B. Stieger, V. McLin et al., "A rare cause of a cholestatic jaundice in a north African teenager," *Liver In-*

ternational: Official Journal of the International Association for the Study of the Liver, vol. 39, no. 11, pp. 2036–2041, 2019.

[9] W. L. van der Woerd, S. W. C. van Mil, J. M. Stapelbroek, L. W. J. Klomp, S. F. J. van de Graaf, and R. H. J. Houwen, "Familial cholestasis: progressive familial intrahepatic cholestasis, benign recurrent intrahepatic cholestasis and intrahepatic cholestasis of pregnancy," *Best Practice & Research Clinical Gastroenterology*, vol. 24, no. 5, pp. 541–553, 2010.

[10] F. Ermis, K. Oncu, M. Ozel et al., "Benign recurrent intrahepatic cholestasis: late initial diagnosis in adulthood," *Annals of Hepatology*, vol. 9, no. 2, pp. 207–210, 2010.

[11] A. Norouzi, S. Ghajarieh Sepanlou, S. Tavassoli, and R. Malekzadeh, "Clinical challenge in hepatology," *Middle East Journal of Digestive Diseases*, vol. 3, no. 3, pp. 138–148, 2011.

[12] W. H. J. Summerskill, "The syndrome of benign recurrent cholestasis," *The American Journal of Medicine*, vol. 38, no. 2, pp. 298–305, 1965.

[13] M. Nakamuta, S. Sakamoto, Y. Miyata, M. Sato, and H. Nawata, "Benign recurrent intrahepatic cholestasis: a long-term follow-up," *Hepato-gastroenterology*, vol. 41, no. 41, pp. 287–289, 1994.

[14] L. European Association for the Study of the, "EASL clinical practice guidelines: management of cholestatic liver diseases," *Journal of Hepatology*, vol. 51, no. 2, pp. 237–267, 2009.

[15] T. Yakar, M. Demir, H. S. Gokturk et al., "Nasobiliary drainage for benign recurrent intrahepatic cholestasis in patients refractory to standard therapy," *Clinical and Investigative Medicine Medecine Clinique Et Experimentale*, vol. 39, no. 6, p. 27522, 2016.

[16] S. Khurana and P. Singh, "Rifampin is safe for treatment of pruritus due to chronic cholestasis: a meta-analysis of prospective randomized-controlled trials," *Liver International*, vol. 26, no. 8, pp. 943–948, 2006.

[17] J. M. Stapelbroek, K. J. van Erpecum, L. W. J. Klomp, and R. H. J. Houwen, "Liver disease associated with canalicular transport defects: current and future therapies," *Journal of Hepatology*, vol. 52, no. 2, pp. 258–271, 2010.

[18] E. Cançado, R. M. Cubero Leitão, F. J. Carrilho, and A. A. Laudanna, "Unexpected clinical remission of cholestasis after rifampicin therapy in patients with normal or slightly increased levels of γ-glutamyl transpeptidase," *The American Journal of Gastroenterology*, vol. 93, no. 9, pp. 1510–1517, 1998.

[19] T. Mizuochi, A. Kimura, A. Tanaka et al., "Characterization of urinary bile acids in a pediatric BRIC-1 patient: effect of rifampicin treatment," *Clinica Chimica Acta; International Journal of Clinical Chemistry*, vol. 413, no. 15-16, pp. 1301–1304, 2012.

[20] T. Kumagi and E. J. Heathcote, "Successfully treated intractable pruritus with rifampin in a case of benign recurrent intrahepatic cholestasis," *Clinical Journal of Gastroenterology*, vol. 1, no. 4, pp. 160–163, 2008.

CMV-Related Gastric Ulcer and Gastroduodenitis in an Immunocompetent Patient: A Case Report and Literature Review

Andrawus Beany [1,2] and Tova Rainis [1,2]

[1] *Division of Gastroenterology, Bnai Zion Medical Center, Haifa, Israel*
[2] *The Ruth and Bruce Rappaport Faculty of Medicine, Technion, Haifa, Israel*

Correspondence should be addressed to Andrawus Beany; andrewbeany@gmail.com

Academic Editor: Chia-Tung Shun

Background. Cytomegalovirus (CMV)- related gastroduodenal infection is rare in immunocompetent hosts, and although it is considered a self-limiting condition in most cases, there is scarce literature to assert its management. *Case Presentation.* We report a case of a 66-year-old immunocompetent male patient diagnosed with a giant gastric ulcer caused by CMV infection. The ulcer manifested as refractory vomiting and melena. Rapid and full resolution was observed on proton-pump inhibitor (PPI) monotherapy. *Conclusion.* Gastric CMV infection might mimic an advanced gastric tumor in individuals with an intact immune system. The condition is rare, and the diagnosis is challenging and oftentimes overlooked. However, a rapid resolution has been documented in all cases, even without antiviral therapy.

1. Background

Cytomegalovirus (CMV), a DNA virus and a member of the Herpesviridae family, is related to one of the most prevalent infectious diseases. The seroprevalence rates, as an evidence of prior infection with CMV, range between 40 to 100 percent of the adult population [1] and increase with age [2].

The spectrum of diseases caused by the virus in humans is diverse, and most cases are asymptomatic or experience an indolent course with nonspecific symptoms [3]. Acute CMV infection may manifest as infectious mononucleosis, or, less commonly, as a systemic disease with significant morbidity [4]. Single organ involvement; colitis, encephalitis, and myocarditis among others; or multisystemic disorders have been reported [5], mainly in patients with immunosuppression. Immunocompetent hosts, however, usually have a mild and self-limiting disease. Viral reactivation is common among critically ill immunocompetent patients [6] and immunocompromised individuals [7] and is associated with severe morbidity and high mortality rate.

In this paper, we report a case of a rare manifestation of gastrointestinal CMV infection in an immunocompetent patient, followed by a review of the literature.

2. Case Presentation

A 66-year-old male with a 3-week history of nausea and vomiting was admitted. He also reported a one-month history of weakness, night sweats, anorexia, and diarrhea.

Lab work performed prior to admission was notable for CMV-specific IgM and IgG antibodies and an elevated C-reactive protein (CRP). A left lower lobe consolidation was demonstrated in a chest X-ray. He was started on oral cefuroxime and roxithromycin for a diagnosis of lobar pneumonia. However, he continued to suffer from nausea and vomiting.

His past medical history included hypertension, treated with angiotensin converting enzyme inhibitor (ACE-I) and hydrochlorothiazide. The patient denied personal history of smoking, alcohol abuse, and the use of aspirin or nonsteroidal anti-inflammatory drugs (NSAIDs).

His vital signs were normal, and physical exam on admission was only notable for scant petechial skin eruption.

In-hospital complete blood count (CBC) and chemistry were only notable for mild leukocytosis, without reactive lymphocytosis, and a slightly elevated CRP.

Further infectious workup was performed, including blood and urine cultures, serology for *Brucella*, hepatitis B and C viruses, human-immunodeficiency virus, *Coxiella burnetii*, and leptospira, and stool *Clostridium difficile* toxin assay. Results returned negative in due course; however, the polymerase chain reaction (PCR) for CMV-DNA in the serum was positive (1,278 IU/ml).

During the second day of admission, the patient reported tarry stools and a CBC showed a 2 gr/dl decrease in hemoglobin.

An esophagogastroduodenoscopy (EGD) revealed a large, irregularly shaped, deep ulcer in the gastric antrum, involving the angular incisure and the prepyloric region, with a deformation and narrowing of the pylorus (Figure 1). A few adjacent erosions were also seen. Biopsies were obtained from the stomach and duodenum. Colonoscopy was only notable for diverticulosis.

Abdominal computed tomography scans revealed diffuse antral-wall thickening with mild mesenteric lymphadenopathy (Figure 2).

Staining of the gastric biopsy specimens with hematoxylin and eosin (H&E) revealed severe chronic active gastritis with ulceration and scattered large cells with inclusion bodies, characteristic of CMV infection (Figure 3(a)). Immunohistochemistry (IHC) using monoclonal CMV antibodies was also positive (Figure 3(b)). Staining for *Helicobacter pylori* bacilli was negative. Duodenal mucosa staining yielded duodenitis and scattered large cells with inclusion bodies (Figure 3(c)).

The patient was commenced on oral esomeprazole 40 mg. On this regimen, his gastrointestinal (GI) and systemic symptoms rapidly and fully resolved.

Follow-up EGD, carried 50 days after the initiation of treatment, was only notable for a residual antral scar (Figure 4). Histology from obtained biopsies revealed gastric mucosa with mild chronic inflammation and normal duodenal mucosa. The patient completed the prescribed therapy for three months with no significant adverse or unanticipated events.

Follow-up 5 years later was carried out by examining his medical inpatient and outpatient records and by contacting him via phone. The patient was healthy, with no evidence of immunosuppressive state.

3. Discussion and Conclusions

While CMV infection in immunocompromised patients is associated with substantial morbidity and high mortality rate, immunocompetent individuals are usually asymptomatic [3].

The colitis [8] and esophagitis [9] are the most common GI manifestation areas of a CMV infection. It is uncommon in immunocompetent individuals, and most cases were reported in scenarios of critical illness or immunosuppression such as organ transplantation, long-term renal hemodialysis, HIV infection, hematological and solid malignancies, and immunosuppressive chemotherapies and radiotherapies, among others.

Gastroduodenal CMV infection is uncommon and rarely reported in immunocompetent hosts. A prospective study of 38 immunocompetent patients with gastroduodenal ulcerations failed to show CMV involvement, even as a superinfection within areas of previous peptic or NSAIDs-related mucosal injury [10].

We searched PubMed for case reports up to April 2021 using the following keywords: (cytomegalovirus) AND (gastric ulcer OR gastritis) AND (immunocompetent). Of the 25 search results, articles published in English on CMV gastric disease in immunocompetent patients older than 18 years were included. We found 7 cases eligible for inclusion, as summarized in Table 1. Similar to the patient we report, all patients were male; one was elderly and diabetic, and most of the remaining were in their late twenties and early thirties with no underlying disease.

CMV infection of the upper GI tract in immunocompetent hosts has been reported to cause multiple shallow gastric erosions and ulcers similar to *Helicobacter pylori*- and NSAIDs-related ulcers [15]. Giant obstructive ulcers, mimicking advanced gastric carcinoma or primary gastric lymphoma, were mostly reported in patients with AIDS [18, 19] and renal transplant recipients [20]. Differently, we describe a case of an immunocompetent patient presenting with an ulcer mimicking an advanced gastric malignancy.

The pathogenesis of CMV-related ulceration is ill-defined. Cytomegalic vasculitis, in which CMV infection induces ischemic injury in the involved endothelial cells, has been proposed as a possible mechanism of ulceration [21, 22].

Reported gastric CMV infections were mostly accompanied with systemic inflammatory symptoms, mainly low-grade fever and fatigue. Epigastric pain was also a predominant symptom, described in five of the seven included case reports [11, 13–15]. Our patient presented without fever or abdominal pain, and Vergara et al. describe a case where gastric ulcer was the sole manifestation of CMV infection in an otherwise asymptomatic healthy host [23]. Of note, febrile and symptomatic patients with acute infectious diseases rarely undergo invasive procedures. Thus, underdiagnosis may partly explain the few documented cases of CMV-related gastroduodenal ulcerations.

The diagnosis of gastric CMV ulcers is challenging due to their rarity and the absence of distinct morphological characteristics. If CMV infection is suspected, it is important to obtain biopsies from the ulcer base and examine the biopsy specimens for inclusion bodies using H&E staining and IHC. The latter method has a better sensitivity [13]. The different available diagnostic methods are not always in concordance. In our literature review, one case was reported where IHC was positive in the absence of inclusion bodies

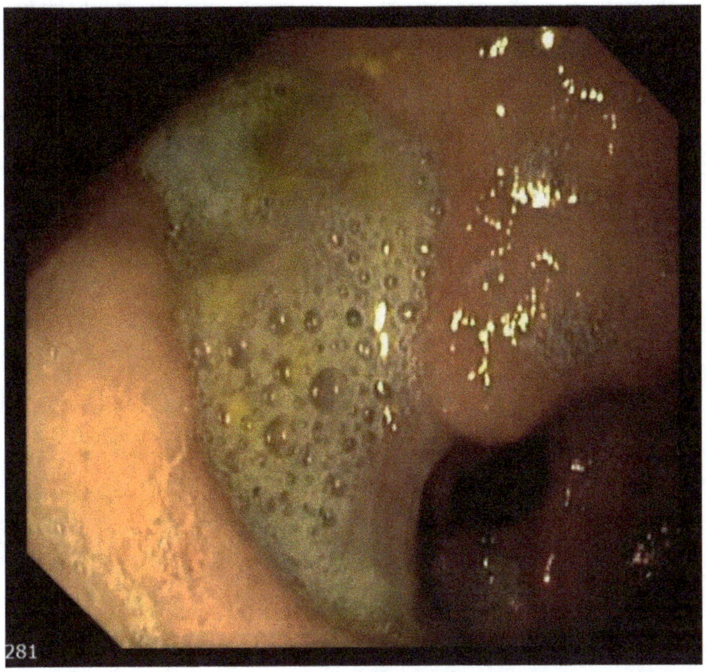

FIGURE 1: Endoscopy showing the gastric ulcer.

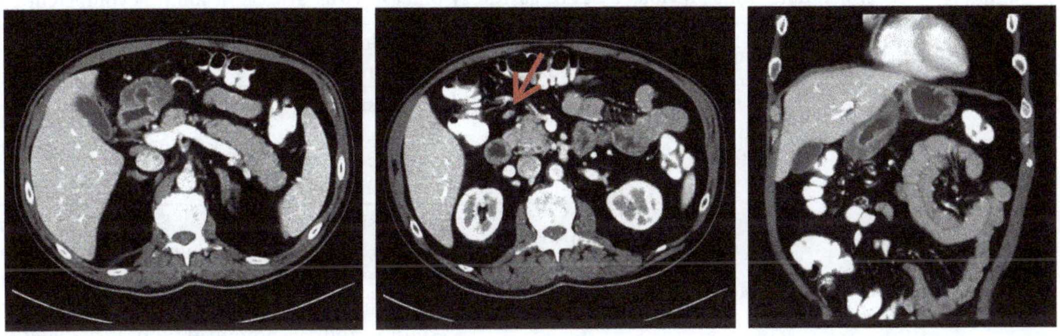

FIGURE 2: Computed tomography showing antral-wall thickening and mesenteric lymphadenopathy (arrow).

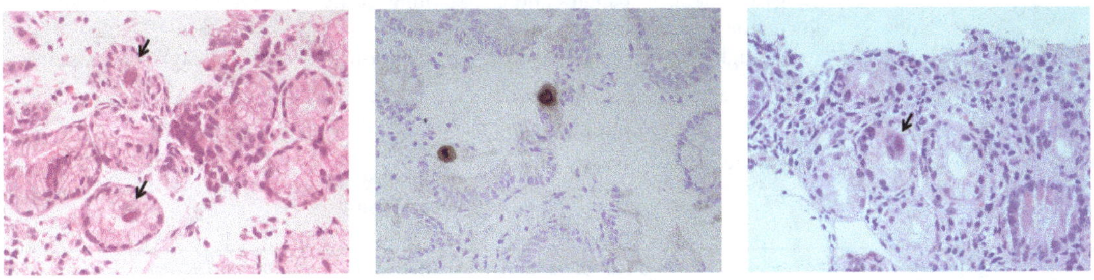

(a) (b) (c)

FIGURE 3: The patient's histological findings. (a) H&E staining showing chronic gastritis and scattered large cells with intranuclear and intracytoplasmatic inclusion bodies (arrows); (b) positive IHC in a representative duodenal specimen; (c) H&E staining showing duodenitis and large cells with inclusion bodies (arrow).

[13]. Quantitative PCR technique can help establish the diagnosis when histopathologic testing is inconclusive or negative [14]. Occasionally, repeated endoscopy and careful observation of deep biopsies are conducive to establish the diagnosis [16].

It is unclear whether CMV is the primary etiology of the gastric lesion or colonizes it post factum as an innocent bystander. Halme and colleagues showed that CMV-positive cells were found in duodenal biopsy specimens obtained from 19% of immunocompetent patients who underwent

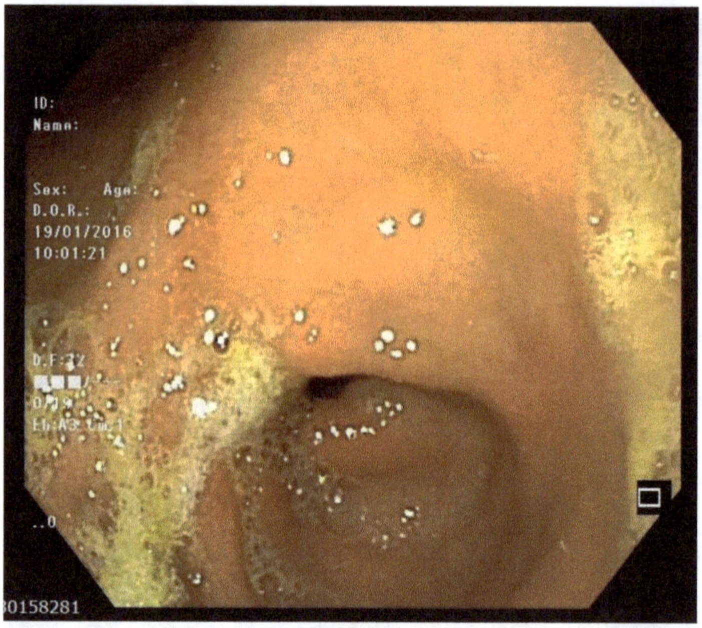

Figure 4: Follow-up endoscopy showing a residual scar.

Table 1: Summary of published data from previous cases of gastric cytomegalovirus disease in immunocompetent patients.

Ref.	Age/ gender	Comorbidities	Symptoms	Endoscopic findings	Histologic findings	Treatment	Follow-up endoscopy
Crespo et al. [11]	31/ male	None	Epigastric pain, fever	Superficial erosions of the gastric antrum	Inclusion bodies and positive IHC staining	IV ganciclovir 5 mg/kg twice daily for 7 days	Full resolution, time of repeated endoscopy is not mentioned
Fyock et al. [12]	83/ male	DM	Melena	Gastritis with multiple small antral, duodenal, and colonic ulcers	Inclusion bodies and positive IHC staining, culture, and PCR	21-day course of oral ganciclovir followed by IV administration	Partial healing of the duodenal ulcers after the antiviral therapy; full resolution 4 years later with the persistence of CMV
Ebisutani et al. [13]	33/ male	None	Epigastric pain, low-grade fever, cough	Multiple gastric papules and a large irregularly shaped shallow ulcer	Positive IHC staining in the absence of inclusion bodies	Oral PPI (rabeprazole, 20 mg/day)	Small gastric ulcer on day 40; a residual ulcer scar on day 68
Matsui et al. [14]	29/ male	N/A	Epigastric pain, fever	Multiple shallow gastric ulcers and mucosal erosions	Positive PCR for CMV-DNA in the absence of inclusion bodies	Oral PPI	Full resolution 2 months later
Himoto et al. [15]	31/ male	None	Epigastric pain, fever	Multiple shallow gastric ulcers and mucosal edema	Inclusion bodies and positive IHC staining	Oral PPI (lansoprazole, 30 mg/day)	Full resolution 2 months later
Xiong et al. [16]	44/ male	None	Epigastric pain, abdominal distention	Multiple erosions in the gastric antrum and thickening of the stomach wall	Inclusion bodies and positive IHC staining, negative PCR for CMV-DNA	IV ganciclovir for 3 months	Full resolution 3 months later

Table 1: Continued.

Ref.	Age/ gender	Comorbidities	Symptoms	Endoscopic findings	Histologic findings	Treatment	Follow-up endoscopy
Yamamoto et al. [17]†	35/ male	None	Infectious mononucleosis syndrome	Thickened and eroded mucosa throughout the stomach	Positive IHC staining in the absence of inclusion bodies	None	Improvement, time of repeated endoscopy is not mentioned

†CMV-EBV coinfection.

upper GI endoscopies for dyspeptic symptoms. No gastric CMV infection was found, and the histopathological findings in the CMV-positive mucosa were nonspecific and mild [24]. In the present case, we could not document any other potential causative agent and the inclusion bodies had disappeared in the specimens obtained from the healing lesion. Hence, from these findings and the active CMV infection documented by blood PCR, we concluded that CMV infection was the etiology of the gastric ulceration in our patient.

CMV-associated ulcers in the GI tracts of immunocompetent hosts often resolve rapidly on oral proton-pump inhibitors (PPIs). Antiviral therapy may be a reasonable second-line therapy in PPI refractory cases [11, 12]. The decision to use antivirals can be complex and challenging. Fyock and colleagues suggest an algorithm to determine whether or not to use antivirals based on several risk factors extrapolated from a meta-analysis of cases with CMV colitis in immunocompetent hosts [12, 25]. Male patients older than 55 years, pregnant women, or patients with comorbidities (diabetes, chronic kidney disease, or malignancies) may benefit from antiviral therapy [12]. However, our 66-year-old patient demonstrated complete endoscopic and histologic resolution within 2 months on PPIs monotherapy.

As in our case, the time to ulcer resolution was 10 weeks in most cases, similar to that of *Helicobacter pylori*-related ulcers [13].

In conclusion, in this case report, we describe a case of gastric CMV infection mimicking an advanced gastric tumor in an immunocompetent patient. Literature review yielded scarce reports on CMV-related gastric ulcers in patients with an intact immune system. Review of previous cases reveals the condition to be self-limiting and rapidly resolving. The diagnosis may be challenging and requires raised awareness of the clinician, due to the sometimes unrevealing nature of the standard biopsy and staining and the overall rarity of the condition. Whether its discovery should lead to a search for an immunocompromised state remains unknown and will require further data collection and a larger case series in the future.

Abbreviations

ACE-I: Angiotensin converting enzyme inhibitor
CBC: Complete blood count
CMV: Cytomegalovirus
CRP: C-reactive protein
EGD: Esophagogastroduodenoscopy
GI: Gastrointestinal
H&E: Hematoxylin and eosin
IHC: Immunohistochemistry
NSAIDs: Nonsteroidal anti-inflammatory drugs
PCR: Polymerase chain reaction
PPI: Proton-pump inhibitors.

Authors' Contributions

AB and TR were directly responsible for the patient and managed the whole clinical case. AB was a major contributor in writing of the manuscript, and both authors read and approved the final manuscript.

References

[1] U. Krech, "Complement-fixing antibodies against cytomegalovirus in different parts of the world," *Bulletin of the World Health Organization*, vol. 49, no. 1, pp. 103–106, 1973.

[2] S. L. Bate, S. C. Dollard, and M. J. Cannon, "Cytomegalovirus seroprevalence in the United States: the national health and nutrition examination surveys, 1988-2004," *Clinical Infectious Diseases*, vol. 50, no. 11, pp. 1439–1447, 2010.

[3] J. I. Cohen and G. R. Corey, "Cytomegalovirus infection in the normal host," *Medicine*, vol. 64, no. 2, pp. 100–114, 1985.

[4] C. A. Horwitz, W. Henle, G. Henle et al., "Clinical and laboratory evaluation of cytomegalovirus-induced mononucleosis in previously healthy individuals," *Medicine*, vol. 65, no. 2, pp. 124–134, 1986.

[5] M. Eddleston, S. Peacock, M. Juniper, and D. A. Warrell, "Severe cytomegalovirus infection in immunocompetent patients," *Clinical Infectious Diseases*, vol. 24, no. 1, pp. 52–56, 1997.

[6] A. P. Limaye, "Cytomegalovirus reactivation in critically ill immunocompetent patients," *Journal of the American Medical Association*, vol. 300, no. 4, pp. 413–422, 2008.

[7] R. R. Razonable and A. Humar, "Cytomegalovirus in solid organ transplantation," *American Journal of Transplantation*, vol. 13, no. s4, pp. 93–106, 2013.

[8] D. S. Siegal, N. Hamid, and B. A. Cunha, "Cytomegalovirus colitis mimicking ischemic colitis in an immunocompetent host," *Heart & Lung: The Journal of Critical care*, vol. 34, no. 4, pp. 291–294, 2005.

[9] A. Venkataramani, A. J. Schlueter, T. J. Spech, and E. Greenberg, "Cytomegalovirus esophagitis in an immunocompetent host," *Gastrointestinal Endoscopy*, vol. 40, no. 3, pp. 392-393, 1994.

[10] R. N. Murray, A. Parker, S. C. Kadakia, E. Ayala, and E. M. Martinez, "Cytomegalovirus in upper gastrointestinal ulcers," *Journal of Clinical Gastroenterology*, vol. 19, no. 3, pp. 198–201, 1994.

[11] P. Crespo, N. Dias, N. Marques, and J. Saraiva da Cunha, "Gastritis as a manifestation of primary CMV infection in an immunocompetent host," *BMJ Case Reports*, vol. 2015, p. bcr2014206991, 2015.

[12] C. Fyock, M. Gaitanis, J. Gao, M. Resnick, and S. Shah, "Gastrointestinal CMV in an elderly, immunocompetent patient," *Rhode Island Medical Journal*, vol. 97, pp. 53–56, 2014.

[13] C. Ebisutani, A. Kawamura, N. Shibata et al., "Gastric ulcer associated with cytomegalovirus in an immunocompetent patient: method for diagnosis," *Case Reports in Gastroenterology*, vol. 6, no. 2, pp. 365–368, 2012.

[14] Y. Matsui, N. Sugino, H. Kaneko, M. Watanabe, Y. Miura, and M. Tsudo, "CMV quantitative PCR in the diagnosis of CMV-associated AGML in an immunocompetent host," *Internal Medicine*, vol. 49, no. 12, pp. 1265–1267, 2010.

[15] T. Himoto, F. Goda, H. Okuyama et al., "Cytomegalovirus-associated acute gastric mucosal lesion in an immunocompetent host," *Internal Medicine*, vol. 48, no. 17, pp. 1521–1524, 2009.

[16] X. Xiong, F. Liu, W. Zhao et al., "Cytomegalovirus infective gastritis in an immunocompetent host misdiagnosed as malignancy on upper gastrointestinal endoscopy: a case report and review of literature," *Human Pathology*, vol. 92, pp. 107–112, 2019.

[17] S. Yamamoto and Y. Sakai, "Acute gastritis caused by concurrent infection with Epstein-Barr virus and cytomegalovirus in an immunocompetent adult," *Clinical Journal of Gastroenterology*, vol. 12, no. 3, pp. 274–278, 2019.

[18] N. A. Andreollo, "Obstructive gastric pseudotumor caused by cytomegalovirus in an AIDS patient: a case report and review of surgical treatment," *American Journal of Case Reports*, vol. 16, pp. 536–541, 2015.

[19] J. Pérez-Pereyra, D. Morales, R. Díaz, M. Yoza, and O. Frisancho, "Giant gastric ulcer by cytomegalovirus in infection VIH/SIDA," *Revista de Gastroenterología del Perú*, vol. 28, no. 4, pp. 379–382, 2008.

[20] C.-J. Lin, C.-F. Pan, C.-J. Wu, H.-H. Chen, C.-R. Kao, and C.-C. Lee, "A giant gastric ulcer mimicking carcinoma in a renal transplant recipient with CMV infection," *Southern Medical Journal*, vol. 101, no. 3, p. 327, 2008.

[21] S. Patra, S. C. Samal, A. Chacko, V. I. Mathan, and M. M. Mathan, "Cytomegalovirus infection of the human gastrointestinal tract," *Journal of Gastroenterology and Hepatology*, vol. 14, no. 10, pp. 973–976, 1999.

[22] D. A. Campbell, J. R. A. Piercey, T. K. Shnitka, G. Goldsand, R. D. O. Devine, and W. M. Weinstein, "Cytomegalovirus-associated gastric ulcer," *Gastroenterology*, vol. 72, no. 3, pp. 533–535, 1977.

[23] M. Vergara, J. Herrero, I. de Torres, J. R. Armengol, E. Saperas, and J. R. Malagelada, "Gastric ulcers as the only manifestation of infection by cytomegalovirus in immunocompetent patients," *Journal of Gastroenterology and Hepatology*, vol. 21, no. 7, pp. 332–334, 1998.

[24] L. Halme, J. Arola, K. Höckerstedt, and I. Lautenschlager, "Human herpesvirus 6 infection of the gastroduodenal mucosa," *Clinical Infectious Diseases*, vol. 46, no. 3, pp. 434–439, 2008.

[25] P. Galiatsatos, I. Shrier, E. Lamoureux, and A. Szilagyi, "Meta-analysis of outcome of cytomegalovirus colitis in immunocompetent hosts," *Digestive Diseases and Sciences*, vol. 50, no. 4, pp. 609–616, 2005.

11

Intussusception in the Setting of an Ulcerative Colitis Flare

Varag Abed, Alexis Faber, Cristina Jageka, Ryan Goleniak, and Raef Fadel

Henry Ford Health System, 2799 W Grand Blvd, Detroit, MI 48202, USA

Correspondence should be addressed to Varag Abed; varagabed@yahoo.com

Academic Editor: Hirotada Akiho

Intussusception is an extraordinary cause of acute abdomen in adults and has been defined as the telescoping of a bowel segment into the lumen of an adjacent segment. A 43-year-old female presented to our hospital's emergency department (ED) with 10+ episodes of bloody diarrhea per day, left-sided abdominal pain, and the inability to tolerate oral intake for one month. She was initially diagnosed with ulcerative colitis (UC) ten years ago and is currently on mesalamine oral and enema therapy. She presented to our gastroenterology clinic two weeks after the beginning of her flare and was started on prednisone 40 mg daily. This did not improve her symptoms, and she presented to the ED two weeks later. She underwent a computed tomography (CT) abdomen/pelvis which revealed intussusception in the left hemiabdomen with no definite lead point measuring 5.6 cm in the craniocaudal dimension with pneumatosis and no evidence of bowel obstruction. There were no other significant laboratory abnormalities. Acute care surgery was consulted and suggested obtaining a CT enterography for further evaluation which showed spontaneous resolution of intussusception with no evidence of pneumatosis, portal venous gas, or intraperitoneal free air. She reports that following oral contrast intake, she "felt movement and relaxation" in her abdomen with substantial pain relief. Infectious workup was negative, and therapy was initiated with intravenous steroids. In conclusion, intussusception has been very rarely reported in patients with UC with the most common treatment being surgical resection. However, conservative management in the absence of bowel obstruction can be attempted.

1. Introduction

Intussusception is a very rare cause of acute abdomen in adults and has been defined as the telescoping of a bowel segment into the lumen of an adjacent segment [1, 2]. In patients with ulcerative colitis (UC), only seven cases of concurrent intussusception have been reported in the literature [2–8]. Abdominal pain is usually the presenting sign with most patients requiring surgical resection [9]. In this case report, we describe a patient with an active UC flare who developed symptomatic abdominal pain and intussusception that resolved following oral contrast administration at a university teaching hospital.

2. Case Report

A 43-year-old female presented to our hospital's emergency department (ED) with 10+ episodes of bloody diarrhea per day, left-sided abdominal pain, and the inability to tolerate oral intake for one month. She was initially diagnosed with ulcerative colitis ten years ago and is currently on mesalamine oral and enema therapy. Most recent colonoscopy was done in 2020 and revealed extensive colitis of the transverse, descending, and sigmoid colon with active proctitis. She usually has two to three flares a year where she manages them by herself through diet modification and lifestyle changes (liquid diet and small meals with lean proteins), but this time her symptoms continued worsening causing her to come to the hospital. She presented to our gastroenterology (GI) clinic two weeks after the beginning of this current flare and was started on prednisone 40 mg daily. They recommended discontinuing the mesalamine enema due to excess diarrhea, which she did, but she inadvertently also stopped taking her oral mesalamine. The prednisone did not improve her symptoms, as she was still having 10+ bloody bowel movements per day and severe left-sided abdominal pain described as a constant throbbing sensation with swelling and warmth overlying the skin. She presented to our ED two

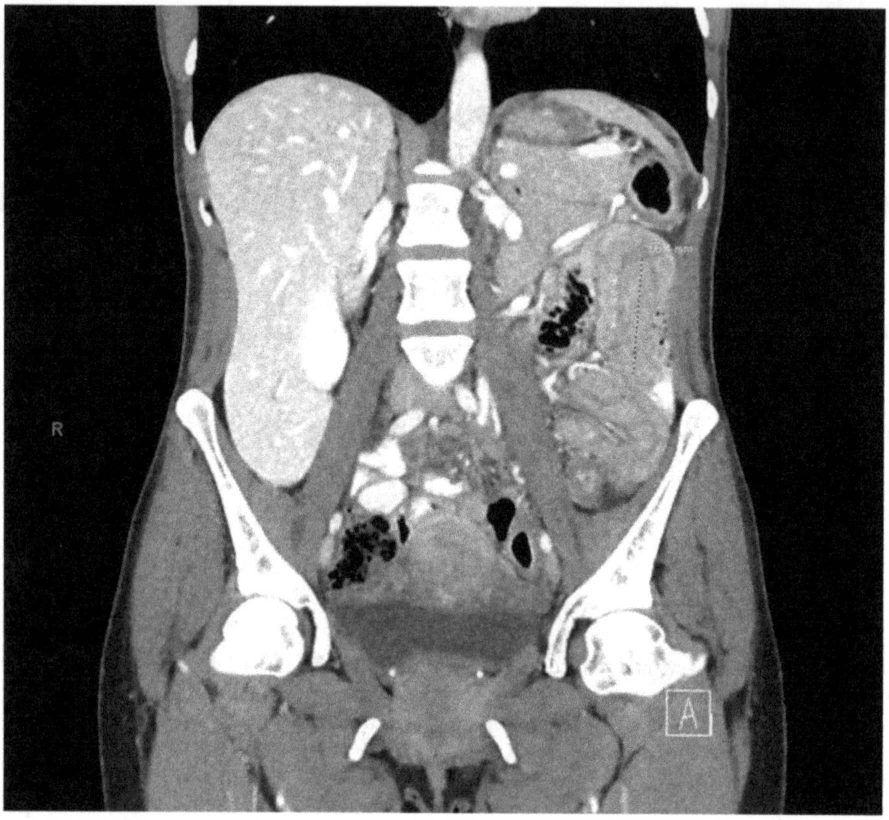

Figure 1: CT scan showing intussusception in the left hemiabdomen.

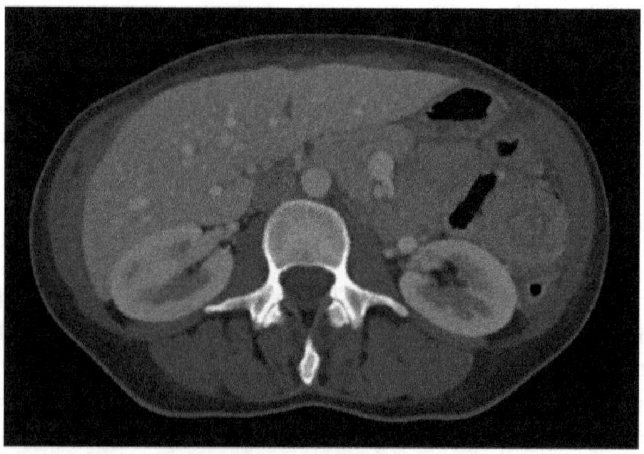

Figure 2: CT scan showing the "Target Sign."

weeks later and was found to have an elevated c-reactive protein of 4.4 mg/dL, erythrocyte sedimentation rate of 51 mm/Hr, blood pressure of 164/101 mmHg, pulse of 107 with a soft, nondistended, tender abdomen, and dry mucous membranes. A Truelove and Witts severity index scoring was utilized, resulting in a severe classification. Also, the Montreal classification for inflammatory bowel disease scoring was rated as E3 S3. She underwent a computed tomography (CT) abdomen/pelvis which revealed intussusception in the left hemiabdomen with no definite lead point measuring 5.6 cm in the craniocaudal dimension with pneumatosis and no evidence of bowel obstruction. Diffuse colorectal wall thickening, mucosal hyperenhancement, and fat stranding were also seen suggesting proctocolitis (Figures 1 and 2). There were no other significant laboratory abnormalities. Acute care surgery was consulted and suggested obtaining a CT enterography for further evaluation, which showed spontaneous resolution of intussusception with no evidence of pneumatosis, portal venous gas, or intraperitoneal free air. She reports that following oral contrast (Breeza) intake, she "felt movement and relaxation" in her abdomen with substantial pain relief. She was subsequently transferred to the medicine floor with a GI consultation for management of her UC flare. Infectious workup was negative, and therapy was initiated with intravenous steroids. Her hospital stay was uneventful as she was discharged five days later on an oral prednisone taper with GI follow-up.

3. Discussion

To the best of our knowledge, there have only been seven cases of patients with UC complicated with intussusception in the literature (Table 1). In the adult population, neoplastic lead points are the most common cause of intussusception [10], but surprisingly, none of the previous reported cases have been found to have an underlying neoplasm. Tanabe et al. [2] hypothesized that this could be due to the frequent colonoscopies patients with UC receive. The most common cause has been inflammatory polyps with four of the previous seven case reports citing them as the underlying etiology, and the most common treatment was surgical resection in five of the seven previous cases (Table 1).

Table 1: Reported cases of concurrent intussusception and ulcerative colitis.

Author	Year	Age	Gender	Location	Etiology	Symptoms	Treatment
Tanabe et al. [2]	2020	18	Male	Transverse colon	Inflammatory polyps	None	Surgical resection
Burchard and Thomay [3]	2018	39	Female	Appendix	Appendicitis	Abdominal pain	Surgical resection
Coghlan et al. [4]	2010	35	Female	Transverse colon	CMV infection	Abdominal pain	Conservative medical approach
Davey et al. [5]	2020	42	Male	Hepatic flexure	Appendicitis	Abdominal pain	Surgical resection
Esaki et al. [6]	2009	27	Male	Hepatic flexure	Inflammatory polyps	Abdominal pain	Enema reduction
Forde et al. [7]	1978	22	Male	Transverse colon	Inflammatory polyps	Abdominal pain	Surgical resection
Maldonado et al. [8]	2004	27	Male	Splenic flexure	Inflammatory polyps	Abdominal pain	Surgical resection
Current case	2022	43	Female	Left hemiabdomen	Unknown	Abdominal pain	Oral contrast reduction

Table adapted from Tanabe et al. [2].

CT scan has been regarded as the modality of choice for diagnosing intussusception [11]. Due to the clinical progression of our patient, we believe intussusception was the likely cause of her UC flare which was found on initial CT. Most studies of intussusception have been performed on children, as they are much more likely to receive the diagnosis than adults. Nonsurgical conservative management for intussusception consists of barium, water-soluble contrast media, water, electrolyte solutions, or air [12]. Our patient had resolution of her intussusception with the oral contrast used for CT enterography, which to our knowledge has not been reported in the literature. However, we cannot definitively determine this to be the reason as the intussusception could have been transient which resolved spontaneously [13]. Notwithstanding, resolution of intussusception has been seen previously after oral gastrografin ingestion [14].

In conclusion, intussusception has been previously reported with patients with UC with the most common treatment being surgical resection. However, based on our findings, conservative management with oral contrast could be attempted before surgical resection in adults in the absence of bowel obstruction.

References

[1] M. Sertkaya, A. Emre, E. Mehmet Pircanoglu, F. Mehmet Yazar, and M. Tepe, "A rare cause of acute abdomen: diagnosis and management of adult colonic intussusception," *Euroasian Journal of Hepato-Gastroenterology*, vol. 6, no. 2, pp. 179–182, 2016.

[2] T. Tanabe, S. Furukawa, T. Masuda, K. Morimoto, T. Yamana, and R. Sahara, "Asymptomatic colonic intussusception in ulcerative colitis: a case report," *Journal of Surgical Case Reports*, vol. 2020, no. 7, 2020.

[3] P. R. Burchard and A. A. Thomay, "Appendiceal intussusception in the setting of ulcerative colitis," *Journal of Surgical Case Reports*, vol. 2018, no. 4, 2018.

[4] E. Coghlan, A. Nadales, L. Laferrere, M. Terres, and J. P. Perotti, "Colocolic intussusception in a patient with ulcerative colitis," *Inflammatory Bowel Diseases*, vol. 16, no. 7, pp. 1085–1087, 2010.

[5] M. G. Davey, E. T. Conlon, G. Forde, V. M. Byrnes, and P. A. Carroll, "Adult intussusception secondary to an appendiceal tumour in a patient with ulcerative colitis: a case report," *Surg Case Rep*, vol. 6, no. 1, p. 234, 2020.

[6] M. Esaki, T. Matsumoto, Y. Fuyuno et al., "Giant inflammatory polyposis of the cecum with repeated intussusception in ulcerative colitis: report of a case," *American Journal of Gastroenterology*, vol. 104, no. 11, pp. 2873-2874, 2009.

[7] K. A. Forde, R. P. Gold, S. Holck, M. D. Goldberg, and P. S. Kaim, "Giant pseudopolyposis in colitis with colonic intussusception," *Gastroenterology*, vol. 75, no. 6, pp. 1142–1146, 1978.

[8] T. S. Maldonado, B. Firoozi, D. Stone, and K. Hiotis, "Colocolonic intussusception of a giant pseudopolyp in a patient with ulcerative colitis: a case report and review of the literature," *Inflammatory Bowel Diseases*, vol. 10, no. 1, pp. 41–44, 2004.

[9] P. A. Ongom, C. K. Opio, and S. C. Kijjambu, "Presentation, aetiology and treatment of adult intussusception in a tertiary Sub-Saharan hospital: a 10-year retrospective study," *BMC Gastroenterology*, vol. 14, no. 1, p. 86, 2014.

[10] T. Lu and Y. M. Chng, "Adult intussusception," *The Permanente Journal*, vol. 19, no. 1, pp. 79–81, 2015.

[11] B. Y. Huang and D. M. Warshauer, "Adult intussusception," *Radiologic Clinics of North America*, vol. 41, no. 6, pp. 1137–1151, 2003.

[12] G. Del-Pozo, J. C. Albillos, D. Tejedor et al., "Intussusception in children: current concepts in diagnosis and enema reduction," *RadioGraphics*, vol. 19, no. 2, pp. 299–319, 1999.

[13] H. Aref, A. Nawawi, A. Altaf, and M. Aljiffry, "Transient small bowel intussusception in an adult: case report with intraoperative video and literature review," *BMC Surgery*, vol. 15, no. 1, 2015.

[14] M. Romano, E. Tartaglia, F. Amodio, A. Gragnaniello, S. Bortone, and M. Fabozzi, "Treatment of postoperative jejunal intussusception in adult with oral gastrografin after laparoscopic low rectal resection. A case report," *International Journal of Surgery Case Reports*, vol. 74, pp. 120–123, 2020.

12

Stevens–Johnson Syndrome and Herpes Simplex Type 1 Infection during Adalimumab Therapy for Crohn's Disease

Jenny Roselli,[1] Tommaso Innocenti,[1] Erica Nicola Lynch,[1] Laura Parisio,[1] Pasquale Apolito,[1] Tommaso Mello,[1] Giuseppe Macrì,[2] Monica Milla,[2] Maria Rosa Biagini,[1] Mirko Tarocchi,[1] Stefano Milani,[1] and Andrea Galli[1]

[1]*Department of Biomedical, Experimental and Clinical Sciences, University of Florence, Florence, Italy*
[2]*Azienda Ospedaliero-Universitaria Careggi, Florence, Italy*

Correspondence should be addressed to Tommaso Innocenti; tommaso.innocenti@unifi.it

Academic Editor: Daniel C. Damin

Stevens–Johnson syndrome (SJS) is a severe mucocutaneous adverse drug reaction with a relatively high mortality rate. SJS is described during herpes simplex virus type 1 (HSV1) infection and, rarely, even during adalimumab therapy. We report the case of a patient with Crohn's disease who developed SJS during an HSV1 infection and a contemporaneous anti-TNFα therapy with adalimumab. Remission was achieved with suspension of adalimumab and high doses of intravenous steroids and antivirals. Patients with HSV1 infection and on adalimumab therapy have a combined risk of SJS and should be monitored closely.

1. Introduction

Stevens–Johnson syndrome (SJS) is a severe mucocutaneous adverse reaction, characterized by necrosis of skin and mucosa upper layers, with consequent formation of vesicles, bullae, and ulcers. In SJS, skin detachment involves less than 10% of the body surface area [1]. Common initial clinical manifestations of SJS are malaise, fatigue, persistent high fever, skin tenderness, and pain. In SJS, the primary immunological barrier of the skin is disrupted and there is an increased risk of infections [2, 3]. SJS is considered a severe drug reaction, as drugs are its most common trigger [4, 5]. It is a medical condition that usually requires hospitalization and that has a mortality rate of 1–5% [6].

We describe the case of an IBD patient who developed SJS during a herpes simplex type 1 infection and a contemporary anti-TNF alpha therapy with adalimumab.

2. Case Report

A 44-year-old female patient was diagnosed with ileocolonic steno-penetrating Crohn's disease in 2006. She also suffered from dermatological manifestations of the disease (erythema nodosum and psoriasiform dermatitis). Initially, the patient was treated with systemic steroids and mesalamine and achieved a good clinical response. Subsequently, mesalamine was interrupted due to drug intolerance. In 2007, the disease flared up, so the patient underwent an ileocolonic resection. No postoperative treatment was initiated. The patient was first referred to our Inflammatory Bowel Disease Center (AOU Careggi, Florence) in 2015 because of a disease relapse. In order to assess disease activity, a colonoscopy, abdomen CT scan, and digestive MRI scan were carried out, which revealed a 8–10-cm long preanastomotic stricture. Thus, in October 2015, the patient started treatment with adalimumab. After three months of therapy, the patient was admitted to our hospital with malaise, high fever, pain, pruritus, and skin and mucosa detachment of <5% of body surface area (mouth, periorbital region, palms, and soles) with positive Nikolsky sign; (Figures 1 and 2) she also presented with vesicular lesions of the nostrils and nasolabial fold. The patient underwent a vesicle swab, which demonstrated the presence of HSV1 DNA. The patient was evaluated by our consultant Dermatologist and was diagnosed

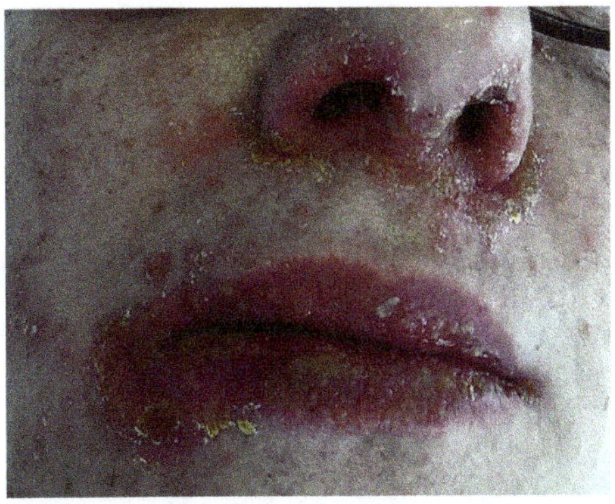

Figure 1: Perioral desquamative lesions.

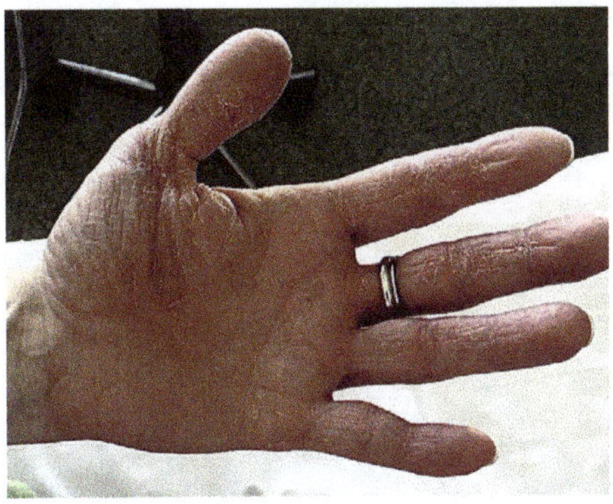

Figure 2: Palmar desquamative lesions.

with herpes simplex type 1 infection complicated by bacterial superinfection with impetigo and SJS. Isolation precautions were used because of the patient's high risk of acquiring infection. The patient was treated with fluids, antivirals, and high doses of intravenous steroids until she achieved complete remission. This event could either have been a consequence of the herpes simplex type 1 infection, or an adverse reaction to adalimumab, therefore, in this eventuality, the treatment was discontinued. Nevertheless, we decided to start treatment with infliximab in December 2017, after consulting our Immunologist who confirmed the absence of contraindications to the treatment with a different anti-TNF alpha drug. She is currently still being treated with infliximab and regularly attends follow-up visits at our Outpatient Department. She has not developed any adverse events to the drug.

3. Discussion

Skin reactions to adalimumab are frequent and extremely varied. The most common dermatologic adverse event to adalimumab is injection-site erythema and pruritus, which resolve spontaneously and occur less frequently with time. Conversely, eczema and psoriasiform lesions can be so severe as to cause treatment interruption [7].

In the literature, only two other cases of SJS during adalimumab therapy are described: Mounach et al. presented the case of a 53-year-old patient who was treated with adalimumab for rheumatoid arthritis [8], while Salama and Lawrance described the case of a 29-year-old patient with ileocolonic steno-penetrating Crohn's disease, with dermatological and rheumatological extraintestinal manifestations [9].

In both these cases, the clinical manifestations were pathognomonic, with peripheral rash, abdominal skin detachment, and oral cavity mucositis, so that biopsy was not necessary for diagnosis. In both these cases, as well as in our, SJS resolved with the suspension of adalimumab and with the administration of high doses of intravenous steroids; the patients were then switched to infliximab therapy without complications [8, 9].

On the other hand, herpes simplex type 1 infection is also a well-known cause of SJS and one of the most frequent triggers of erythema multiforme [10, 11]. In 1992, Detjen et al. described a case of SJS in a 36-year-old man with recurrent HSV-related oropharyngitis; even in this case, as in ours, the patient was treated with antivirals and steroids, achieving complete resolution of signs and symptoms [12].

4. Conclusions

SJS is a severe medical condition, described during HSV type 1 infection and, rarely, even during adalimumab therapy.

Patients in treatment with biologic drugs, such as adalimumab, are more susceptible to recurrent reactivation of HSV type 1 infection. As a result, they have a combined risk of SJS. Patients who are treated with adalimumab should be monitored closely, especially in case of simultaneous therapy with other drugs, and should be advised to seek immediate medical care if alarming symptoms appear.

References

[1] E.-J. Kim, H. Lim, S. Y. Park et al., "Rapid onset of Stevens-Johnson syndrome and toxic epidermal necrolysis after ingestion of acetaminophen," *Asia Pacific Allergy*, vol. 4, no. 1, pp. 68–72, 2014.

[2] R. P. Dodiuk-Gad, W.-H. Chung, L. Valeyrie-Allanore, and N. H. Shear, "Stevens-Johnson syndrome and toxic epidermal necrolysis: an update," *American Journal of Clinical Dermatology*, vol. 16, no. 6, pp. 475–493, 2015.

[3] F. A. Pereira, A. V. Mudgil, and D. M. Rosmarin, "Toxic epidermal necrolysis," *Journal of the American Academy of Dermatology*, vol. 56, no. 2, pp. 181–200, 2007.

[4] S. Anne, S. Kosanam, and L. N. Prasanthi, "Steven Johnson syndrome and toxic epidermal necrolysis: a review," *International Journal of Pharmaceutical Research*, vol. 4, pp. 158–165, 2014.

[5] L. E. French, "Toxic epidermal necrolysis and Stevens Johnson syndrome: our current understanding," *Allergology International*, vol. 55, no. 1, pp. 9–16, 2006.

[6] T. Harr and L. E. French, "Toxic epidermal necrolysis and Stevens-Johnson syndrome," *Orphanet Journal of Rare Diseases*, vol. 5, no. 1, p. 39, 2010.

[7] C. Hillemand and R. Leong, "Gastrointestinal: cutaneous reaction associated with loss of response to adalimumab," *Journal of Gastroenterology and Hepatology*, vol. 28, no. 7, p. 1073, 2013.

[8] A. Mounach, A. Rezqi, A. Nouijai et al., "Stevens-Johnson syndrome complicating adalimumab therapy in rheumatoid arthritis disease," *Rheumatology International*, vol. 33, no. 5, pp. 1351–1353, 2013.

[9] M. Salama and I. C. Lawrance, "Stevens-Johnson syndrome complicating adalimumab therapy in Crohn's disease," *World Journal of Gastroenterology*, vol. 15, no. 35, pp. 4449–4452, 2009.

[10] W. B. Shelly, "Herpes simplex virus as a cause of erythema multiforme," *JAMA*, vol. 201, pp. 153–156, 1967.

[11] P. W. Orton, J. C. Huff, M. G. Tonnesen, and W. L. Weston, "Detection of a herpes simplex viral antigen in skin lesions of erythema multiforme," *Annals of Internal Medicine*, vol. 101, no. 1, pp. 48–50, 1984.

[12] P. F. Detjen, R. Patterson, G. A. Noskin, J. P. Phair, and S. O. Loyd, "Herpes simplex virus associated with recurrent Stevens-Johnson syndrome," *Archives of Internal Medicine*, vol. 152, no. 7, pp. 1513–1516, 1992.

13

Helicobacter suis-Associated Gastritis Mimicking Conventional *H. pylori*-Associated Atrophic Gastritis

Masaya Iwamuro,[1] Somay Yamagata Murayama,[2] Masahiko Nakamura,[3] Kenta Hamada,[1] Takehiro Tanaka,[4] and Hiroyuki Okada[1]

[1]*Department of Gastroenterology and Hepatology, Okayama University Graduate School of Medicine, Dentistry and Pharmaceutical Sciences, Okayama 700-8558, Japan*
[2]*Department of Fungal Infection, National Institute of Infectious Diseases, Tokyo 162-8340, Japan*
[3]*Omura Satoshi Memorial Institute, Kitasato University, Tokyo 108-8641, Japan*
[4]*Department of Pathology, Okayama University Graduate School of Medicine, Dentistry and Pharmaceutical Sciences, Okayama 700-8558, Japan*

Correspondence should be addressed to Masaya Iwamuro; pr145h2k@okayama-u.ac.jp

Academic Editor: Hirotada Akiho

A 45-year-old Japanese man underwent esophagogastroduodenoscopy, which revealed spotty redness at the gastric fornix, mucosal swelling, diffuse redness in the corpus, and mucosal atrophy in the gastric angle and antrum. Histological examination showed rod-shaped bacteria that appeared larger than *Helicobacter pylori*. The patient tested positive for rapid urease test, and serum anti-*H. pylori* IgG antibody test results were negative. Further examination of the bacteria revealed that *H. suis* antibody test was positive, and the presence of *H. suis* was confirmed using *H. suis*-specific real-time PCR. *H. suis* was successfully eradicated after triple therapy with vonoprazan, amoxicillin, and clarithromycin. This case reinforces the notion that non-*H. pylori* Helicobacter species such as *H. suis* and *H. heilmannii* may be involved in the pathogenesis of active gastritis in patients who test negative for *H. pylori* antibodies.

1. Introduction

Since its discovery in 1982, *Helicobacter pylori* has been widely recognized as a pathogenic organism that causes gastritis, peptic ulcer disease, and gastric cancer [1]. In addition to *H. pylori*, various spiral-shaped organisms have been identified in humans and other animals. Helicobacter species other than *H. pylori* are known as non-*Helicobacter pylori* Helicobacter, which include *H. suis*, *H. heilmannii*, *H. bizzozeroni*, *H. salomonis*, and *H. felis*. Among these, *H. suis* is the primary human pathogenic organism [2].

Although *H. suis* infection in the human stomach causes gastritis, the clinicopathological features of *H. suis*-associated gastritis have long been uninvestigated because its isolation and cultivation are technically difficult [3]. Herein, we report the case of a patient with *H. suis*-associated gastritis, who showed endoscopic features similar to those of conventional *H. pylori*-associated atrophic gastritis.

2. Case Presentation

A 45-year-old Japanese male underwent upper gastrointestinal series and was diagnosed with chronic gastritis. Subsequently, the patient underwent esophagogastroduodenoscopy, which revealed spotty redness at the gastric fornix (Figure 1(a)), mucosal swelling, diffuse redness in the corpus (Figure 1(b)), and mucosal atrophy at the gastric angle (Figure 1(c)) and antrum (Figure 1(d)). Regular arrangement of collecting venules was scarcely identified throughout the stomach. Thus, atrophic gastritis and current infection of *H. pylori* were suspected. However, the serum

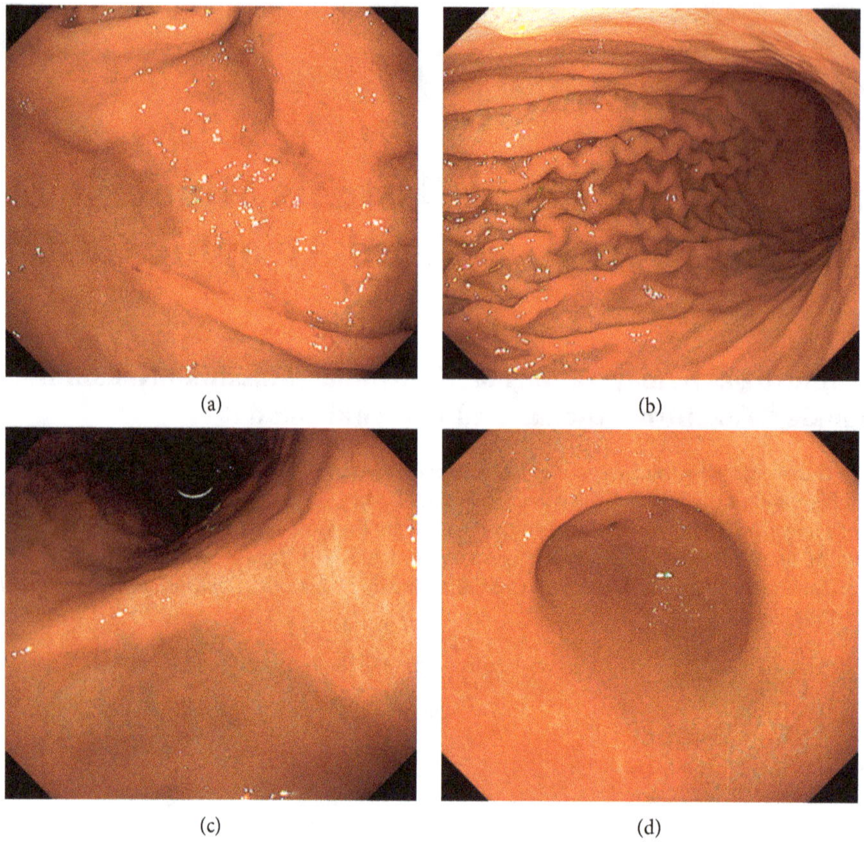

Figure 1: Esophagogastroduodenoscopy images. Endoscopy reveals spotty redness at the gastric fornix (a), mucosal swelling with diffuse redness in the corpus (b), and mucosal atrophy in the gastric angle (c) and antrum (d).

anti-*H. pylori* IgG antibody test results were negative. Histological examination revealed rod-shaped bacteria that appeared larger than *H. pylori* (Figure 2, arrows). Infection of non-*H. pylori* Helicobacter species, such as *H. suis* and *H. heilmannii*, was then suspected, and the patient was referred to our hospital for further investigation.

The patient had no history of other diseases and was not taking any medication. Physical examination revealed no abnormalities and no evidence of hepatosplenomegaly or peripheral lymphadenopathy. All laboratory findings, including lactate dehydrogenase and soluble interleukin-2 receptor levels, were within the normal ranges. Repeat esophagogastroduodenoscopy and biopsy showed rod-shaped bacteria that seemed larger than *H. pylori*. The patient tested positive in the rapid urease test. The serum anti-*H. pylori* IgG antibody test was negative, whereas the in-house ELISA test for the *H. suis* antibody was positive. The presence of *H. suis* was further confirmed using *H. suis*-specific real-time polymerase chain reaction (PCR) targeting ureA and outer membrane protein genes (Figure 3) [4, 5]. *H. pylori* was negative on PCR test. Consequently, the patient was diagnosed with *H. suis*-associated gastritis. *H. suis* was successfully eradicated after triple therapy with vonoprazan, amoxicillin, and clarithromycin. Esophagogastroduodenoscopy performed two months after eradication therapy showed that spotty redness remained at the gastric fornix (Figure 4(a)), while mucosal swelling and diffuse redness in the corpus disappeared (Figure 4(b)).

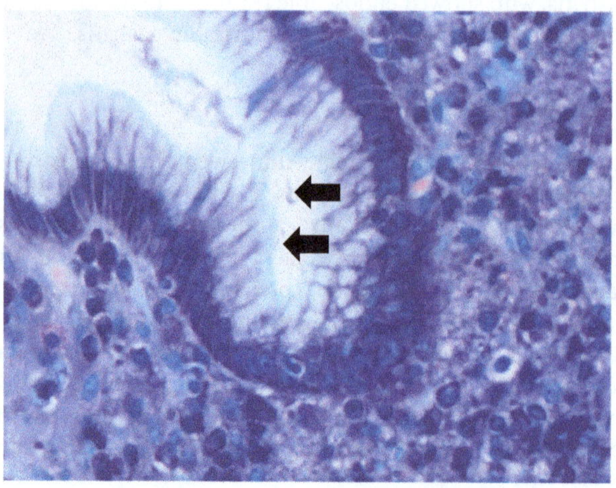

Figure 2: Histological image. Giemsa stain shows rod-shaped bacteria appearing larger than *H. pylori* (arrows), suggesting a non-*Helicobacter pylori* Helicobacter infection.

3. Discussion

H. suis is a zoonotic pathogen that colonizes the gastric mucosa of 60–95% of pigs at the slaughter age. *H. suis* primarily infects the fundic and pyloric gland zones of the porcine stomach, leading to gastritis, gastric ulcers, and

ureA, *H. suis* Sequence (5'-3')	omp, *H. suis* Sequence (5'-3')
CACCACCCCGGGGAAGTGATCTTG	GATGGGCGCTTCTGGTTTA
CTACATCAATCAAATGCACGGTTTTTTCTTCG	CTGGTAATGCATCATTAGAAGCAAA
	56-FAM/TGTACACAC/ZEN/CAAACAGATGAGCCGT/3IABkFQ

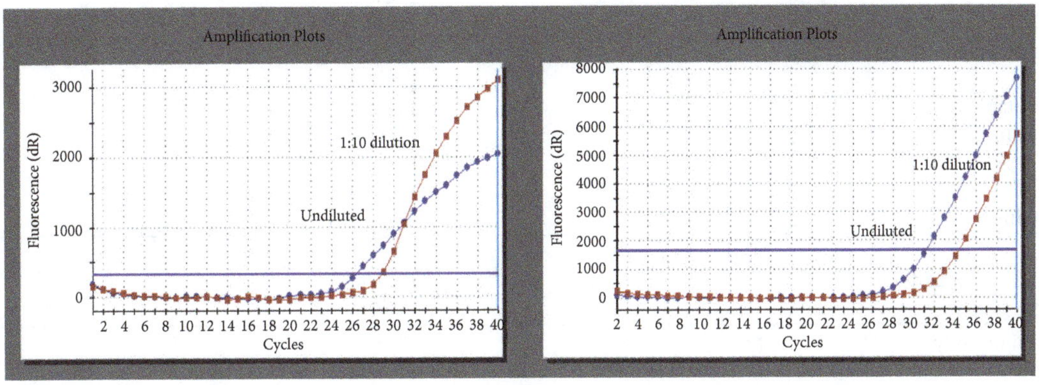

FIGURE 3: PCR analysis. The presence of *H. suis* is confirmed using *H. suis*-specific real-time PCR, targeting ureA and outer membrane protein genes.

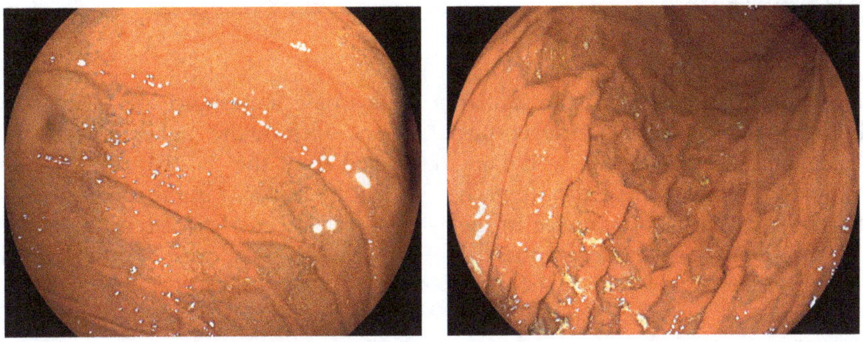

(a) (b)

FIGURE 4: Esophagogastroduodenoscopy images two months after the eradication therapy. Spotty redness still exists at the gastric fornix (a), while mucosal swelling and diffuse redness are not observed in the corpus (b).

decreased daily weight gain [6]. Since the first human case of *H. suis*-associated erosive gastritis was reported in 1994 [7], *H. suis* infection in humans has been described in only a small number of cases. This is mainly because it is difficult to isolate and cultivate the pathogen. Rimbara et al. reported that *H. suis* is not viable at neutral pH. Thus, endoscopic biopsy specimens containing *H. suis* require a low-pH medium for transport and successful isolation [3]. In the present patient, an in-house enzyme-linked immunosorbent assay for the detection of human IgG antibodies to *H. suis* was positive. In addition, we extracted the DNA from the gastric biopsy specimens and performed nested PCR using the specific primers for *H. suis* [8], which was also positive. Consequently, the patient was diagnosed with *H. suis*-associated gastritis.

Although *H. suis* has urease activity, its activity is generally lower than that of *H. pylori* [9]. Therefore, the urea breath test and rapid urease test, which are commonly used to detect urease activity in *H. pylori*, often yield negative results for *H. suis* [3, 10]. However, the patient tested positive in the rapid urease test. Since both serum *H. pylori* antibody and PCR assays for *H. pylori* were negative, co-infection with *H. suis* and *H. pylori* was unlikely. Consequently, the urease activity of *H. suis* detected in the present patient may have been comparable to that of *H. pylori*. Another explanation is that the bacterial density of *H. suis* was greater than that of other patients with *H. suis* infections.

The typical endoscopic features of non-*Helicobacter pylori* Helicobacter-associated gastric lesions include spotty redness, crack-like mucosa, nodular gastritis-like appearance, and white marbled appearance. Erosions, ulcers, and even extranodal marginal zone lymphoma of the mucosa-associated lymphoid tissue can be found in the stomach, in association with non-*Helicobacter pylori* Helicobacter infection [11, 12]. Tsukadaira et al. investigated 50 patients with non-*Helicobacter pylori* Helicobacter infections in the stomach, including 26 cases of *H. suis* and two cases of *H. heilmannii*/*H. ailurogastricus* [13]. The authors reported that the crack-like mucosa was observed in 45 out of 50 patients (90.0%), which was defined as a mesh-like morphology composed of faded, depressed, and varying width lines on coarse and slightly reddish mucosa extending from the gastric antrum to the angle. Nodular gastritis was noted

TABLE 1: Endoscopic features according to the Kyoto classification of gastritis.

	Typical case of active infection with *H. pylori*	Present patient
Entire stomach		
Atrophy	Present	Present
Diffuse redness	Present	Present
Foveolar-hyperplastic polyp	Present	Absent
Xanthoma	Present	Absent
Intestinal metaplasia	Present	Absent
Mucosal swelling	Present	Present
Patchy redness	Present	Absent
Depressive erosion	Present	Absent
Map-like redness	Absent	Absent
Gastric body		
Enlarged and tortuous folds	Present	Present
Sticky mucus	Present	Absent
Gastric fornix and body		
Spotty redness	Present	Present
Fundic gland polyp	Absent	Absent
Lower gastric body to antrum		
Nodularity	Present	Absent
Regular arrangement of collecting venules	Absent	Absent

in 11 out of 50 patients (22.0%). All the patients had a regular arrangement of collecting venules in the gastric corpus (100%). Shiratori et al. reported two patients with non-*Helicobacter pylori* Helicobacter infection of the stomach [14]. Both patients had a white marble appearance in the lesser curvature of the gastric angle and antrum, and the authors speculated that the white marble appearance is a potential characteristic finding of non-*Helicobacter pylori* Helicobacter infection gastritis.

Table 1 shows the endoscopic features of the stomach that are characteristic of patients with current *H. pylori* infection according to the Kyoto classification of gastritis [15]. They include atrophy, diffuse redness, foveolar-hyperplastic polyps, xanthomas, intestinal metaplasia, mucosal swelling, patchy redness, depressive erosions, enlarged and tortuous folds, sticky mucus, spotty redness, and nodularity. In contrast, fundic gland polyps and the regular arrangement of collecting venules are absent or reduced in the stomachs of patients with current *H. pylori* infection, as opposed to those of people without the infection. Map-like redness is a representative endoscopic feature observed in the stomachs of patients in whom *H. pylori* infection has been previously eradicated.

The esophagogastroduodenoscopy performed in the present patient revealed that the crack-like mucosa and white marble appearance were absent, and a regular arrangement of collecting venules was scarcely identified throughout the stomach. Instead, spotty redness at the gastric fornix, mucosal swelling, diffuse redness in the corpus, and mucosal atrophy in the gastric angle were observed (Table 1). In a previous report, the spotty redness in the corpus was found in 4 out of 50 patients (8.0%), and mucosal swelling was observed in only 1 out of 50 patients (2.0%) [13]. The endoscopic features of our patient were indistinguishable from those of conventional *H. pylori*-induced gastritis. Although the exact cause of the infrequent endoscopic appearance of *H. suis*-associated gastritis remains unclear, the higher urease activity, which was presumed from the positive results of the rapid urease test, might be involved in the unique endoscopic features of the present patient. However, as this report describes only one patient, this issue must be investigated.

4. Conclusions

This case reinforces the notion that non-*H. pylori* Helicobacter species, such as *H. suis*, may be involved in the pathogenesis of active gastritis in patients who tested negative for *H. pylori* antibodies. It is also noteworthy that *H. suis*-associated gastritis may present with endoscopic features indistinguishable from those of *H. pylori* infection.

References

[1] E. Bessède and F. Mégraud, "Microbiota and gastric cancer," *Seminars in Cancer Biology*, 2022, In press.

[2] M. Padra, B. Adamczyk, B. Flahou et al., "Helicobacter suis infection alters glycosylation and decreases the pathogen growth inhibiting effect and binding avidity of gastric mucins," *Mucosal Immunology*, vol. 12, no. 3, pp. 784–794, 2019.

[3] E. Rimbara, M. Suzuki, H. Matsui et al., "Isolation and characterization of Helicobacter suis from human stomach," *Proceedings of the National Academy of Sciences of the United States of America*, vol. 118, no. 13, Article ID e2026337118, 2021.

[4] J. Liu, L. He, F. Haesebrouck et al., "Prevalence of coinfection with gastric non-Helicobacter pylori Helicobacter (NHPH) species in Helicobacter pylori-infected patients suffering from gastric disease in Beijing, China," *Helicobacter*, vol. 20, no. 4, pp. 284–290, 2015.

[5] H. Takigawa, S. Masaki, T. Naito et al., "Helicobacter suis infection is associated with nodular gastritis-like appearance of gastric mucosa-associated lymphoid tissue lymphoma," *Cancer Medicine*, vol. 8, no. 9, pp. 4370–4379, 2019.

[6] E. De Bruyne, B. Flahou, K. Chiers et al., "An experimental Helicobacter suis infection causes gastritis and reduced daily weight gain in pigs," *Veterinary Microbiology*, vol. 160, no. 3-4, pp. 449–454, 2012.

[7] M. Tanaka, A. Saitoh, T. Narita et al., "Gastrospirillum hominis-associated gastritis: the first reported case in Japan," *Journal of Gastroenterology*, vol. 29, no. 2, pp. 199–202, 1994.

[8] H. Matsui, T. Takahashi, S. Y. Murayama et al., "Development of new PCR primers by comparative genomics for the detection of Helicobacter suis in gastric biopsy specimens," *Helicobacter*, vol. 19, no. 4, pp. 260–271, 2014.

[9] D. De Groote, R. Ducatelle, L. J. van Doorn, K. Tilmant, A. Verschuuren, and F. Haesebrouck, "Detection of 'Candidatus Helicobacter suis' in gastric samples of pigs by PCR: comparison with other invasive diagnostic techniques," *Journal of Clinical Microbiology*, vol. 38, no. 3, pp. 1131–1135, 2000.

[10] S. Goji, Y. Tamura, M. Sasaki et al., "Helicobacter suis-infected nodular gastritis and a review of diagnostic sensitivity for Helicobacter heilmannii-like organisms," *Case Reports in Gastroenterology*, vol. 9, no. 2, pp. 179–187, 2015.

[11] H. Kadota, R. Yuge, R. Miyamoto et al., "Investigation of endoscopic findings in nine cases of Helicobacter suis-infected gastritis complicated by gastric mucosa-associated lymphoid tissue lymphoma," *Helicobacter*, vol. 27, no. 3, Article ID e12887, 2022.

[12] S. Nakagawa, T. Shimoyama, M. Nakamura et al., "The resolution of Helicobacter suis-associated gastric lesions after eradication therapy," *Internal Medicine*, vol. 57, no. 2, pp. 203–207, 2018.

[13] T. Tsukadaira, S. Hayashi, H. Ota et al., "Prevalence, clinical features, and esophagogastroduodenoscopy (EGD) findings of non-Helicobacter pylori Helicobacter infection: a study of 50 cases at a single facility in Japan," *Helicobacter*, vol. 26, no. 4, Article ID e12811, 2021.

[14] S. Shiratori, K. Mabe, S. Yoshii et al., "Two cases of chronic gastritis with non-Helicobacter pylori Helicobacter infection," *Internal Medicine*, vol. 55, no. 14, pp. 1865–1869, 2016.

[15] M. Hojo, A. Nagahara, T. Kudo et al., "Endoscopic findings of *Helicobacter pylori* gastritis in children and young adults based on the Kyoto classification of gastritis and age-associated changes," *JGH Open*, vol. 5, no. 10, pp. 1197–1202, 2021.

14

Zinc Acetate Dihydrate Tablet-Associated Gastritis Occurring in a Post-Hematopoietic Stem Cell Transplant Recipient

Masaya Iwamuro,[1] Takehiro Tanaka,[2] Akifumi Matsumura,[3] Seiji Kawano,[1] Yoshiro Kawahara,[4] and Hiroyuki Okada[1]

[1]*Department of Gastroenterology and Hepatology, Okayama University Graduate School of Medicine, Dentistry and Pharmaceutical Sciences, Okayama 700-8558, Japan*
[2]*Department of Pathology, Okayama University Graduate School of Medicine, Dentistry and Pharmaceutical Sciences, Okayama 700-8558, Japan*
[3]*Department of Hematology and Oncology, Okayama University Graduate School of Medicine, Dentistry and Pharmaceutical Sciences, Okayama 700-8558, Japan*
[4]*Department of Practical Gastrointestinal Endoscopy, Okayama University Hospital, Okayama 700-8558, Japan*

Correspondence should be addressed to Masaya Iwamuro; pr145h2k@okayama-u.ac.jp

Academic Editor: Olga I. Giouleme

A 65-year-old Japanese woman underwent umbilical cord blood transplantation for acute myeloid leukemia. Zinc acetate dihydrate tablets were administered for hypozincemia after transplantation, and vomiting and appetite loss occurred soon thereafter. Esophagogastroduodenoscopy revealed mucosal redness, erosion, white coat adhesion, and ulcers. Although graft-versus-host disease, intestinal transplant-associated microangiopathy, and cytomegalovirus infection were considered as possible causes, we diagnosed the patient with zinc acetate dihydrate tablet-associated gastric mucosal alterations based on the endoscopic features. This case reinforces the notion that medication-associated gastric lesions should be suspected in patients taking zinc acetate dihydrate tablets.

1. Introduction

Zinc is one of the most important trace elements in the body. A shortage of zinc may result from insufficient zinc intake, malabsorption, increased zinc demand, and increased excretion. Low-birth-weight infants, pregnant women, and the elderly are prone to zinc deficiency. Chronic liver disease, short bowel syndrome, diabetes, chronic renal disease, long-term use of chelating agents, parenteral nutrition, and tube feeding with insufficient zinc supplementation may also cause zinc deficiency [1–6]. Zinc deficiency leads to taste disorders, dermatitis, hair loss, anemia, stomatitis, male sexual dysfunction, increased susceptibility to infections, and osteoporosis. Zinc acetate dihydrate is prescribed as a supplement for patients with zinc deficiency.

Zinc acetate dihydrate is generally safe and well tolerated. Meanwhile, erosions and ulcers have recently been reported in the stomach of patients taking zinc acetate dihydrate [7, 8]. Herein, we describe a case of a patient who developed gastric ulcers after hematopoietic stem cell transplantation. Although various diseases, such as graft-versus-host disease, transplant-associated microangiopathy, and cytomegalovirus gastritis, had been considered as possible causes, the patient was finally diagnosed with zinc acetate dihydrate tablet-induced gastric mucosal damage.

2. Case Report

A 65-year-old Japanese woman was diagnosed with *FMS-like tyrosine kinase 3*-internal tandem duplication mutation-positive acute myeloid leukemia. Treatment with idarubicin and cytarabine was initiated but was ineffective. The patient was treated with gilteritinib. Because her acute myeloid leukemia did not respond to gilteritinib, she underwent umbilical cord blood transplantation after one cycle of treatment with gilteritinib, 5-azacytidine, and venetoclax. The patient complained of dysgeusia after transplantation and blood tests revealed decreased serum zinc levels (66 μg/dL; reference range, 80–130 μg/dL), which was considered to be a possible cause of dysgeusia. Thus, zinc acetate dihydrate tablets were administered for hypozincemia 35 days after transplantation. Vomiting and appetite loss occurred on the day of zinc acetate dihydrate tablet administration. The patient was referred to the department of gastroenterology for investigation of gastrointestinal symptoms. She had been taking amlodipine, lansoprazole, ursodeoxycholic acid, ambroxol, brotizolam, acyclovir, letermovir, *Clostridium butyricum* preparation, and mycophenolate mofetil, in addition to zinc acetate dihydrate tablets.

Esophagogastroduodenoscopy performed 41 days after transplantation revealed multiple reddish spots in the gastric body (Figure 1(a)) and shallow ulcers with white coat adhesion in the gastric fornix (Figure 1(b)). Zinc acetate dihydrate tablets were discontinued because we suspected that they were associated with the gastric lesions. As the patient was a hematopoietic stem cell transplant recipient under immunosuppressive treatment, involvement of graft-versus-host disease, intestinal transplant-associated microangiopathy, and cytomegalovirus infection were also considered as differential diagnoses of gastric mucosal damage. However, these findings were ruled out by pathological analysis. A biopsy of one ulcer showed focal inflammation, erosion, and degenerative epithelium (Figure 2), which were consistent with the pathological features specific to zinc acetate dihydrate tablet-associated gastric lesions. Esophagogastroduodenoscopy performed 6 days after cessation of zinc acetate dihydrate tablet intake showed improvement in gastric lesions (Figure 3).

3. Discussion

Medications containing the active ingredient zinc commercially available in Japan include polaprezinc and zinc acetate [9]. Polaprezinc has been used for the treatment of gastric ulcers, whereas zinc acetate is prescribed to patients with Wilson's disease or hypozincemia [10]. Although dietary zinc intake is recommended as an initial treatment for hypozincemia, zinc acetate dihydrate is used when dietary therapy is insufficient. In patients with Wilson's disease, chelating agents excrete copper in the body into the urine, whereas zinc acetate dihydrate inhibits the absorption of copper from food and excretes copper into feces. Ingested zinc induces the production of metallothionein in intestinal mucosal epithelial cells, which is the major endogenous copper-binding protein [11]. Patients with Wilson's disease need to avoid copper-rich foods, such as organ meat and shellfish. However, dietary restrictions are usually insufficient to control Wilson's disease on their own. Thus, zinc acetate dihydrate is prescribed in combination with chelating drugs, such as penicillamine and trientine, which have different mechanisms of action, aiming to relax strict dietary restrictions. Zinc acetate dihydrate may also be used as a prophylactic agent in asymptomatic patients with Wilson's disease [12, 13].

Adverse events associated with zinc acetate dihydrate include copper deficiency and increased levels of blood amylase, lipase, and alkaline phosphatase. Gastrointestinal symptoms, such as epigastric discomfort, nausea, vomiting, abdominal pain, diarrhea, and constipation, may occur [14]. In addition, gastric mucosal injury has recently been reported to be associated with zinc acetate dihydrate tablet intake. Kitagawa et al. reported that in three cases of Wilson's disease treated with zinc acetate, lustrous white erosions surrounded by erythematous mucosa were observed in the greater curvature of the gastric corpus [8]. We retrospectively analyzed 47 patients who underwent upper gastrointestinal endoscopy while taking oral zinc acetate dihydrate [7]. Gastric mucosal injury was identified in 29 patients (61.7%), including mucosal redness (93.1%), erosion (90.0%), white coat adhesion (86.2%), and ulcers (31.0%). The most frequently involved area was the middle third of the stomach (96.6%), followed by the upper third (65.5%) and lower third (46.4%). Therefore, ulcers and erosions with white coat and redness of the surrounding mucosa, which were observed in the present case, are typical endoscopic features of zinc acetate dihydrate-associated gastric lesions.

The mechanism of zinc acetate dihydrate-associated gastric lesions has not yet been elucidated. Kitagawa et al. reported that orcein-positive granules were observed in the fundic glands and interstitium of the stomach in three cases of Wilson's disease, suggesting cytotoxicity induced by copper deposition [8]. Although we performed energy-dispersive X-ray analysis of the biopsy specimen from another patient with hypozincemia, no copper or zinc was detected [15]. Possible factors other than copper deposition include the corrosive action of high concentrations of zinc. For instance, oral intake of iron causes bleeding, erosion, and necrosis when in contact with the gastrointestinal mucosa for a long period [16]. Polaprezinc, a complex of zinc and L-carnosine, contains 17 mg of zinc per tablet, giving a daily zinc intake of 34 mg. Regarding zinc acetate dihydrate, 50–150 and 150–250 mg of zinc are administered per day for hypozincemia and Wilson's disease, respectively. Therefore, higher concentrations of zinc, compared with polaprezinc, may damage the gastric mucosa.

Generally, hematopoietic stem cell transplant recipients may develop gastrointestinal lesions due to various causes, such as graft-versus-host disease, transplant-associated microangiopathy, and cytomegalovirus infection [17]. Because each disease requires different treatments, prompt diagnosis of the underlying cause is essential. Although biopsy and pathological analysis are inevitable, this case reinforces that the recognition of representative endoscopic features of zinc acetate dihydrate tablet-associated gastric mucosal alterations enabling appropriate diagnosis and management without delay, particularly when various potential causes can be considered.

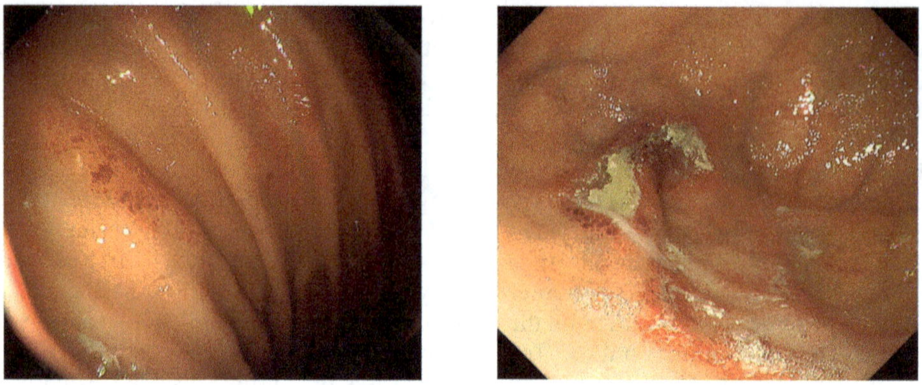

(a) (b)

Figure 1: Endoscopic images. (a) Esophagogastroduodenoscopy reveals multiple reddish spots in the gastric body. (b) Shallow ulcers with white coat adhesion in the gastric fornix.

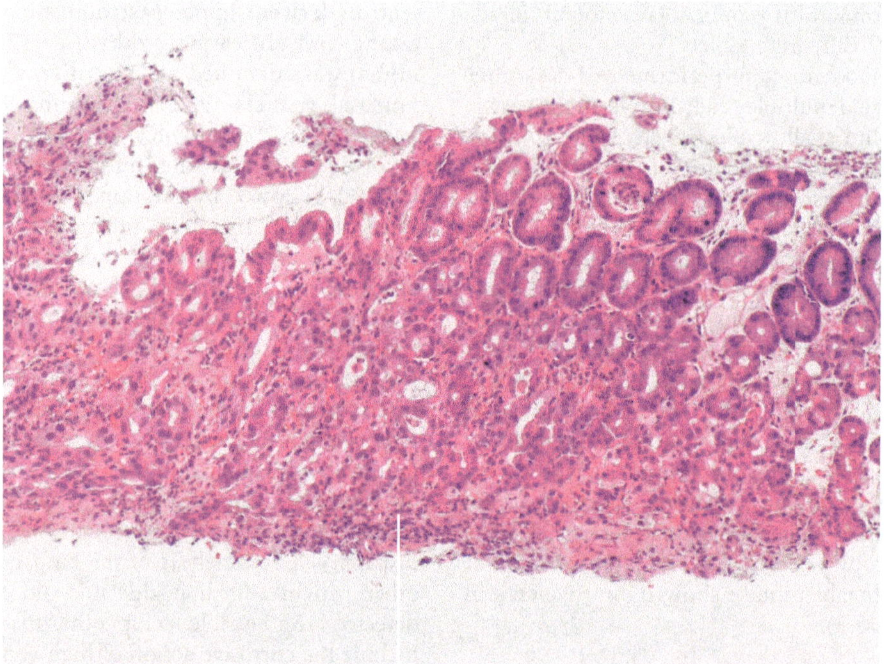

Figure 2: A pathology image. A biopsy from the gastric ulcer shows focal inflammation, erosion, and degenerative epithelium. These features are consistent with pathological features specific to zinc acetate dihydrate tablet-associated gastric lesions.

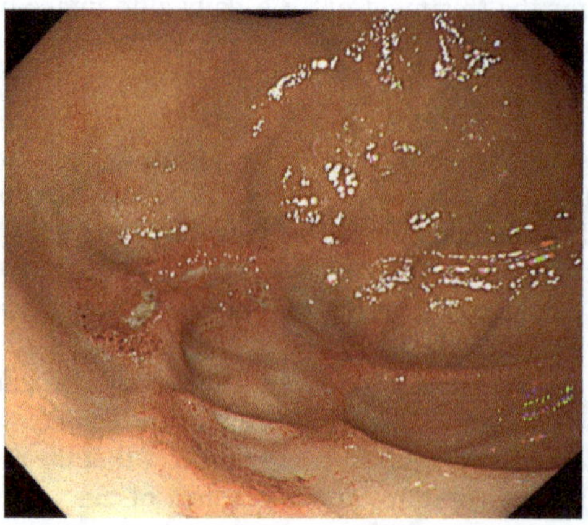

Figure 3: An endoscopy image performed 6 days after cessation of zinc acetate dihydrate tablet intake. Esophagogastroduodenoscopy shows improvement in gastric lesions.

4. Conclusions

We experienced a case of zinc acetate dihydrate tablet-associated gastric lesions, which presented with typical features of mucosal redness, erosion, white coat adhesion, and ulcers. Medication-associated gastric lesions should be suspected in patients taking zinc acetate dihydrate tablets.

References

[1] R. Sun, J. Wang, J. Feng, and B. Cao, "Zinc in cognitive impairment and aging," *Biomolecules*, vol. 12, no. 7, p. 1000, 2022.

[2] Y. Wan and B. Zhang, "The impact of zinc and zinc homeostasis on the intestinal mucosal barrier and intestinal diseases," *Biomolecules*, vol. 12, no. 7, p. 900, 2022.

[3] A. Abdollahi, A. Ghahramani, and N. Ghahramani, "Zinc and kidney disease: a review," *Iranian Journal of Kidney Diseases*, vol. 16, no. 2, pp. 79–87, 2022.

[4] H. Hata, Y. Ota, K. Uesaka et al., "Oral adverse events due to zinc deficiency after pancreaticoduodenectomy requiring continuous intravenous zinc supplementation: a case report and literature review," *BMC Oral Health*, vol. 22, no. 1, p. 52, 2022.

[5] K. Grüngreiff, T. Gottstein, and D. Reinhold, "Zinc deficiency-an independent risk factor in the pathogenesis of haemorrhagic stroke?" *Nutrients*, vol. 12, no. 11, p. 3548, 2020.

[6] H. Kodama, M. Tanaka, Y. Naito, K. Katayama, and M. Moriyama, "Japan's practical guidelines for zinc deficiency with a particular focus on taste disorders, inflammatory bowel disease, and liver cirrhosis," *International Journal of Molecular Sciences*, vol. 21, no. 8, p. 2941, 2020.

[7] M. Iwamuro, T. Tanaka, S. Kuraoka et al., "Zinc acetate dihydrate tablet-associated gastric lesions," *Internal Medicine*, vol. 61, no. 13, pp. 8625-21-1938, 2022.

[8] D. Kitagawa, M. Ominami, K. Taira et al., "Lustrous white erosions surrounded by an erythematous mucosa: a novel endoscopic finding of gastric lesions in patients with Wilson disease," *Internal Medicine*, vol. 61, no. 12, pp. 8076-21-1841, 2022.

[9] T. Okamoto, S. Hatakeyama, K. Togashi et al., "Pre-dialysis serum creatinine as an independent predictor of responsiveness to zinc supplementation among patients on hemodialysis," *Clinical and Experimental Nephrology*, vol. 24, no. 10, pp. 955–962, 2020.

[10] D. Sato, T. Gohda, M. Kihara et al., "Effect of zinc acetate dihydrate (NobelzinR) treatment on anemia and taste disorders in patients with chronic kidney disease with hypozincemia," *Acta Medica Okayama*, vol. 72, no. 5, pp. 535–538, 2018.

[11] L. Chen, L. Ma, Q. Bai et al., "Heavy metal-induced metallothionein expression is regulated by specific protein phosphatase 2A complexes," *Journal of Biological Chemistry*, vol. 289, no. 32, pp. 22413–22426, 2014.

[12] M. A. Camarata, A. Ala, and M. L. Schilsky, "Zinc maintenance therapy for Wilson disease: a comparison between zinc acetate and alternative zinc preparations," *Hepatology Communications*, vol. 3, no. 8, pp. 1151–1158, 2019.

[13] R. Santiago, F. Gottrand, D. Debray et al., "Zinc therapy for Wilson disease in children in French pediatric centers," *Journal of Pediatric Gastroenterology and Nutrition*, vol. 61, no. 6, pp. 613–618, 2015.

[14] Wilzin, "25-mg hard capsules and wilzin 50-mg hard capsules, package leaflet," 2019, https://www.medicines.org.uk/emc/files/pil.6244.pdf.

[15] M. Iwamuro, Y. Kono, T. Tanaka et al., "Zinc acetate-associated gastric lesions: a case report," *Nihon Shokakibyo Gakkai Zasshi*, vol. 119, pp. 853–857. in press, 2022.

[16] T. Sunkara, M. E. Caughey, S. Nigar, R. Olivo, and V. Gaduputi, "Iron pill gastritis: an under diagnosed condition with potentially serious outcomes," *Gastroenterology Research*, vol. 10, no. 2, pp. 138–140, 2017.

[17] J. H. Lee, G. Y. Lim, S. A. Im, N. G. Chung, and S. T. Hahn, "Gastrointestinal complications following hematopoietic stem cell transplantation in children," *Korean Journal of Radiology*, vol. 9, no. 5, pp. 449–457, 2008.

15

Sevelamer Carbonate Crystal-Induced Colitis

T. Lai, [1] **A. Frugoli**, [2] **B. Barrows**, [3] **and M. Salehpour** [4]

[1] *Community Memorial Health System, Graduate Medical Education, Ventura, CA, USA*
[2] *Community Memorial Health System, Graduate Medical Education, Department of Internal Medicine, Pacific Inpatient Physicians, Ventura, CA, USA*
[3] *Community Memorial Hospital, Department of Pathology, Ventura, CA, USA*
[4] *Community Memorial Hospital, Department of General Surgery, Ventura, CA, USA*

Correspondence should be addressed to T. Lai; thaihnglai@gmail.com

Academic Editor: Olga I. Giouleme

Hyperphosphatemia is a common and well-described complication of end-stage renal disease. Despite strict dietary constraints and compliance, phosphate binders such as calcium acetate and/or sevelamer carbonate are also needed to treat secondary hyperparathyroidism. This case vignette describes an underrecognized adverse effect of a phosphate binder, sevelamer carbonate, inducing colitis in a 47-year-old male with insulin-dependent diabetes complicated by end-stage renal disease. He presented for recurrent abdominal pain with associated nausea and was found to have multiple circumferential lesions on computed tomography including distal ascending, transverse, and proximal descending colon. Colonoscopy demonstrated nearly obstructing lesions worrisome for colonic ischemia or inflammatory bowel disease. Pathological review of histology demonstrated ragged colonic mucosa with ulcerative debris and nonpolarizing crystalline material at the sites of ulceration, morphologically consistent with the phosphate binder, sevelamer carbonate. Sevelamer carbonate was discontinued, and the patient was transitioned to calcium carbonate with strict dietary restrictions. His symptoms improved with the cessation of sevelamer, and he was subsequently discharged home. He eventually underwent renal transplant without redevelopment of symptoms. Recognition of this underreported complication of sevelamer carbonate, phosphate binder, is of utmost importance in directing appropriate therapy with cessation of this medication in the setting of gastrointestinal complaints or more specifically enteritis and colitis. Clinicians providing care to end-stage renal patients taking either sevelamer and/or sodium polystyrene sulfonate should have increased awareness of the possible gastrointestinal side effects.

1. Introduction

End-stage renal disease (ESRD) is associated with multiple metabolic and electrolyte derangements. Hormonal and electrolyte imbalance of calcium, phosphorus, and PTH can result in short-term complications such as calciphylaxis and long-term sequelae such as renal osteodystrophy, increased cardiovascular events, and all-cause mortality [1–3]. As a result, many patients have strict dietary constraints, and despite compliance, phosphate binders such as calcium acetate and/or sevelamer carbonate are also needed to treat secondary hyperparathyroidism [1, 2]. Of the two more commonly used, sevelamer carbonate is a calcium-free phosphate binder that is composed of a nonabsorbable resin and has been considered one of the preferred agents by NKF KDOQI guidelines [4, 5]. It has many common gastrointestinal side effects including nausea, vomiting, constipation, and abdominal pain that limit patient compliance [2, 6]. These symptoms previously had no specific etiology, but recently, sevelamer carbonate is receiving recognition as a possible cause of mucosal injury [6–8]. The exact mechanism of injury remains elusive, but in the last 5 years, Swanson et al. described that variable degrees of mucosal injury throughout the gastrointestinal tract from "gum to bum" are believed to be associated with sevelamer use. These include acute and chronic inflammation, ulceration, and features of ischemia with mucosal necrosis from samples obtained via endoscopy/colonoscopy [7].

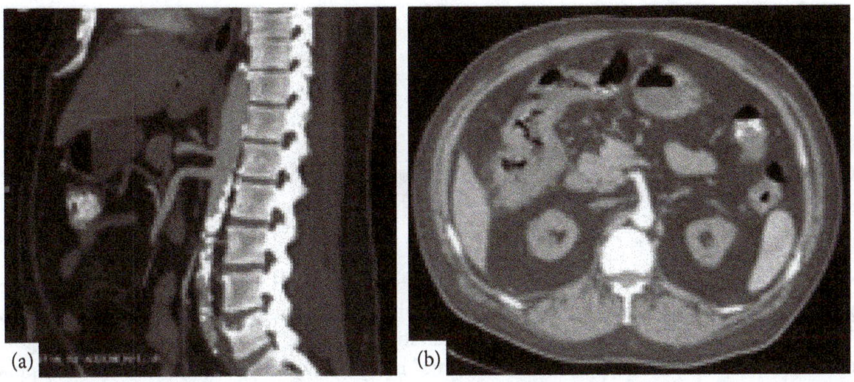

FIGURE 1: Computed tomography angiogram with contrast of the abdomen and pelvis demonstrating atherosclerotic disease of the abdominal aorta without involvement of major arterial supply of the intestine (a) and pericolic fat stranding with wall thickening of the right hepatic flexure (b).

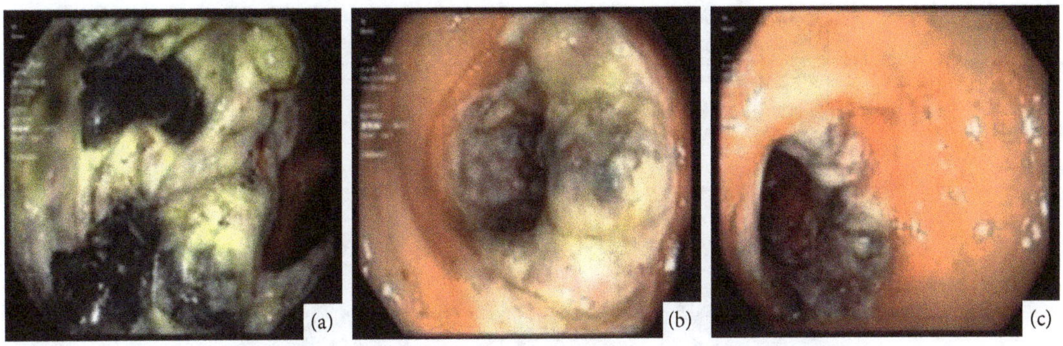

FIGURE 2: Images from colonoscopy demonstrating multiple lesions including obstructing circumferential lesion in the ascending colon (a, b) and circumferential but nonobstructing lesion in the transverse colon (c).

2. Clinical Case

A 47-year-old male with hypertension and insulin-dependent diabetes complicated by end-stage renal disease presented with a 2-day history of crampy abdominal pain. It was associated with nausea and anorexia but without additional gastrointestinal symptoms such as diarrhea or hematochezia. He had a similar episode 1 month prior with workup including computed tomography imaging followed by colonoscopy, notable for numerous circumferential lesions.

Biopsy histology was suspicious for colonic ischemia, and there were no histologic features of inflammatory bowel disease. It was suspected this constellation of symptoms could have developed as sequelae to hypotension during hemodialysis while on antihypertensive medications. His antihypertensive medications were discontinued, and he was provided supportive care with nonoperative management. He had resolution of his pain and was able to tolerate diet and was discharged home. He returned one month later for recurrence of abdominal pain and nausea. He was empirically started on antimicrobials and underwent repeat imaging with the computed tomography mesenteric angiogram that demonstrated only moderate features of atherosclerotic disease with patent celiac, superior mesenteric artery (SMA), and inferior mesenteric artery (IMA) (Figure 1(a)). Additional findings included features of colitis with pericolic fat stranding in the distal ascending, transverse, and proximal descending colon (Figure 1(b)). He underwent repeat colonoscopy showing similar findings (3 regions of circumferential ulceration in the ascending/hepatic flexure, splenic flexure, and descending colon) (Figures 2(a)–2(c)). Biopsy histology demonstrated ragged colonic mucosa with ulcerative debris and nonpolarizing crystalline material at the sites of ulceration (Figures 3–5). Clinical workup for additional causes including cardioembolic events and vasculitis was completed and found to be nondiagnostic. Histology from the current and prior colon biopsy specimens demonstrated crystalline material morphologically consistent with the phosphate binder sevelamer carbonate. Sevelamer carbonate was discontinued, and the patient was transitioned to calcium carbonate with strict dietary restrictions. His symptoms improved with the cessation of sevelamer, and he was subsequently discharged home. He eventually underwent renal transplant without redevelopment of symptoms.

3. Discussion

This vignette illustrates a rare and likely underrecognized adverse effect of therapy with sevelamer carbonate in the treatment of hyperphosphatemia in patients with end-stage renal disease. Review of the literature shows a limited number of reported cases (estimate of about 50 cases) and

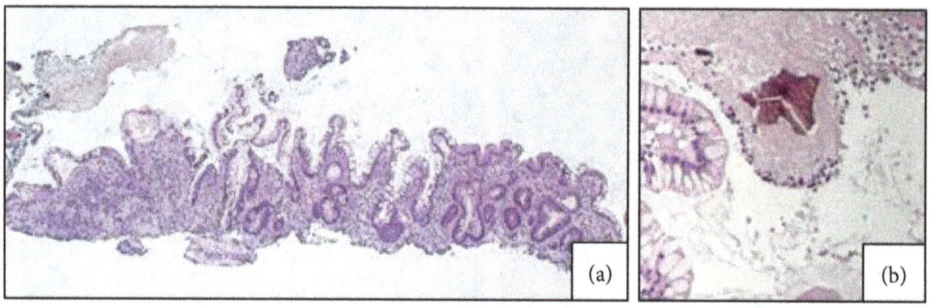

FIGURE 3: (a) Ragged colonic mucosa from the circumferential lesions biopsied during colonoscopy. (b) A high power view of a sevelamer crystal on hematoxylin and eosin-stained (H&E) slide with characteristic "fish scale" morphology and yellow/gold color. Both sevelamer (Figure 3(b)) and sodium polystyrene sulfonate have similar "fish scale" morphology and are nonpolarizable by polarized light microscopy. The primary morphologic difference between these two crystal types can be seen on standard H&E-stained slides. Sevelamer crystals can be distinguished by yellow/gold color when compared with sodium polystyrene sulfonate crystals, which show dark violet staining.

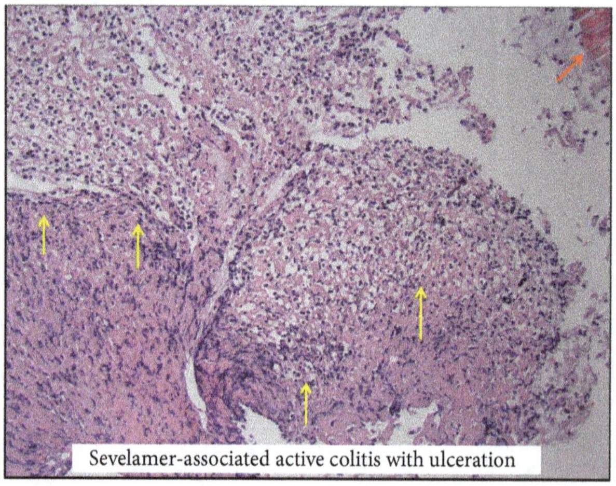

FIGURE 4: Image from histology demonstrating ulcerated colonic mucosa with adherent fibrinous exudate (yellow arrows) in the presence of sevelamer crystals (red arrow) seen in the top right corner.

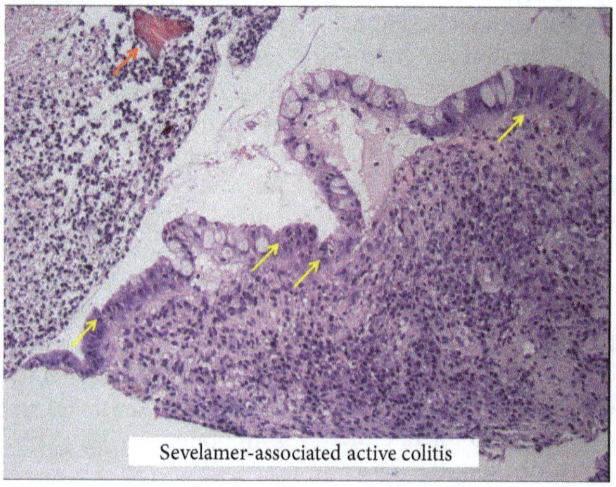

FIGURE 5: Image from histology demonstrating active colitis (yellow arrows) again in the presence of sevelamer crystals (red arrow) as previously seen, top left corner.

illustrates the immense range of presenting symptoms and possible pathology identified. This condition is likely more common, but underrecognized as there are many reasons for patients with end-stage renal disease to have gastrointestinal complaints. Additionally, the relative rarity of complications with severity to prompt further evaluation is complicated by nonspecific colonoscopic findings and potentially subtle histopathologic features, which may not include crystals dependent on biopsy sampling. It is also possible that the pathology is missed as a result of misidentification or failure to identify crystals from resin-based medications like sevelamer and sodium polystyrene sulfonate [9–13].

Although not previously described, there are clinical circumstances when patients with ESRD may chronically be taking more than one medication associated with mucosal injury. This creates a diagnostic dilemma, in which the diagnosis may solely rely on the histopathologic review of tissue and identification by crystal morphology. As previously discussed by Gonzales et al. in their review and comparison of classic features of medication resins, sevelamer carbonate morphology was described as flaky (commonly described as "fish scales"), rectangular in shape, with hues of pink (central) with peripheral transition to yellow/orange pigment by H&E staining [9].

Recognition of this underreported complication of sevelamer carbonate, phosphate binder, is of utmost importance in directing appropriate therapy with cessation of this medication in the setting of gastrointestinal complaints or more specifically enteritis and colitis. Clinicians providing care to end-stage renal patients taking either sevelamer and/or sodium polystyrene sulfonate should have increased awareness of the possible gastrointestinal side effects.

References

[1] S. Chan, K. Au, R. S. Francis, D. W. Mudge, D. W. Johnson, and P. I. Pillans, "Phosphate binders in patients with chronic kidney disease," *Australian Prescriber*, vol. 40, no. 1, pp. 9–14, 2017.

[2] A. M. Shaman and S. R. Kowalski, "Hyperphosphatemia management in patients with chronic kidney disease," *Saudi Pharmaceutical Journal*, vol. 24, no. 4, pp. 494–505, 2016.

[3] H. Eddington, R. Hoefield, S. Sinha et al., "Serum phosphate and mortality in patients with chronic kidney disease," *Clinical Journal of the American Society of Nephrology*, vol. 5, no. 12, pp. 2251–2257, 2010.

[4] J. Grinfeld, A. Inaba, and A. J. Hutchison, "Update and critical appraisal of sevelamer in the management of chronic renal failure," *Open Access Journal of Urology*, vol. 2, pp. 161–170, 2010.

[5] National Kidney Foundation, "KDOQI clinical practice guidelines for bone metabolism and disease in chronic kidney disease," *American Journal of Kidney Diseases*, vol. 42, no. 4, 2003.

[6] C. Yuste, E. Mérida, E. Hernández et al., "Gastrointestinal complications induced by sevelamer crystals," *Clinical Kidney Journal*, vol. 10, no. 4, pp. 539–544, 2017.

[7] B. J. Swanson, B. N. Limketkai, T.-C. Liu et al., "Sevelamer crystals in the gastrointestinal tract (GIT)," *The American Journal of Surgical Pathology*, vol. 37, no. 11, pp. 1686–1693, 2013.

[8] J. Magee, M. Robles, and P. Dunaway, "Sevelamer-induced gastrointestinal injury presenting as gastroenteritis," *Case Reports in Gastroenterology*, vol. 12, no. 1, pp. 41–45, 2018.

[9] R. S. Gonzalez, S. M. Lagana, O. Szeto, and C. A. Arnold, "Challenges in diagnosing medication resins in surgical pathology specimens: a crystal-clear review guide," *Archives of Pathology & Laboratory Medicine*, vol. 141, no. 9, pp. 1276–1282, 2017.

[10] M. Desai, A. Reiprich, N. Khov, Z. Yang, A. Mathew, and J. Levenick, "Crystal-associated colitis with ulceration leading to hematochezia and abdominal pain," *Case Reports in Gastroenterology*, vol. 10, no. 2, pp. 332–337, 2016.

[11] C. E. McGowan, S. Saha, G. Chu, M. B. Resnick, and S. F. Moss, "Intestinal necrosis due to sodium polystyrene sulfonate (kayexalate) in sorbitol," *Southern Medical Journal*, vol. 102, no. 5, pp. 493–497, 2009.

[12] C. Okwara, C. Choi, and J. Y. Park, "Sevelamer-induced colitis presenting as a pseudotumor," *Clinical Gastroenterology and Hepatology*, vol. 13, no. 7, pp. A39–A40, 2015.

[13] National Kidney Foundation, "Sevelamer induced diffuse crystal colitis: a case report of a rarely reported side effect," *American Journal of Kidney Diseases*, vol. 69, no. 4, p. A31, 2017.

16

Colouterine and Jejunouterine Fistula Secondary to Chronic Diverticulitis

Ilias Galanis, Georgios Floros, Christophoros Theodoropoulos, Myriam Metaxa, Panagiotis Theodoropoulos, Panagiotis Tsintavis, Dimitrios Bartziotas, Georgios Giannos, Georgios Stylianidis, and Georgios Papadopoulos

Department of Surgery, Evaggelismos General Hospital, Athens, Greece

Correspondence should be addressed to Ilias Galanis; iliasg100@gmail.com

Academic Editor: Hirotada Akiho

Fistulae between the colon or the small intestine and the uterus are extremely rare as the uterus is a thick, muscular organ. Here, we present the case of a 74-year-old female presenting to our surgical department because of fecal vaginal discharge for the past few months, which proved to be caused by a combined colouterine and jejunouterine fistula due to chronic diverticulitis. Total abdominal hysterectomy with bilateral oophorectomy with en bloc resection of part of the jejunum and the sigmoid colon and primary anastomoses were performed. This case represents an unusual type of diverticulitis complication and aims to point out the diagnostic and therapeutic issues of such a rare medical condition.

1. Introduction

Diverticulosis is one of the most common colonic pathologies. It affects, mostly, those who are living in developed countries, and its incidence is well known to increase with age. However, the incidence of diverticular disease has, recently, been increasing in Third-World countries [1]. Diverticulitis is the result of infection and inflammation of diverticula. The complications of diverticulitis are stricture, bleeding, perforation, fistula formation, and death [2]. Fistulisation is defined as a communication between two surfaces getting in contact [3]. Fistulae constitute up to 20% of complications. The formation of the fistula results from a local inflammatory process which decompresses by perforating into an adjacent tissue. The most common type of fistulae due to diverticulitis is colovesical fistulae, with colovaginal fistulae being the second most common. Colouterine, as well as jejunouterine, fistulae are very rare because the uterus is a very thick and muscular organ, preventing any benign or malignant disease from invading it [4]. Except for diverticulitis, malignant disease, spontaneous rupture of a gravid uterus, and obstetric trauma such as curettage and radiation therapy may result in a fistula between the intestine and the uterus [5]. A colouterine fistula was, first, described by Lejemtel in 1909, and the first report of the colouterine fistula related to diverticulitis was given by Noecker in 1929 [1]. Since then, only very few cases have been reported in the literature, indicating the rarity of this condition.

2. Case

A 74-year-old female was referred to our department of surgery with malodorous fecal vaginal discharge that had lasted several weeks. Medical history included multiple episodes of acute diverticulitis and dementia. She had no abdominal pain or fever. Upon admission, her laboratory tests were within the normal range. Pelvic examination revealed an atrophied vagina and malodorous yellowish vaginal discharge. A colovaginal fistula, secondary to diverticular disease, was suspected as it is the most common type of fistula between the gastrointestinal and female reproductive system. Cultures of the vaginal discharge were sent. Nil per os, total parenteral nutrition, and intravenous antibiotic therapy with ciprofloxacin and metronidazole were applied to the patient until a definitive diagnosis would be made. An abdominal computed tomography (CT) showed multiple diverticula and findings indicative of chronic diverticulitis, such as thickening of the wall of the sigmoid colon and pericolic fat stranding (Figures 1 and 2). A colonoscopy was performed, revealing diverticula of the sigmoid colon. Magnetic resonance imaging (MRI) revealed a fistula between the sigmoid colon and the uterine fundus and air bubbles in the uterine cavity and the vagina (Figure 3). Surgical management was decided. Intraoperative findings included a colouterine fistula side to side to a jejunouterine fistula as well (Figure 4). Inflammatory adhesions of the sigmoid colon and the jejunum to the wall of the uterus, as a result of the repeated episodes of diverticulitis, were found, explaining the presence of the fistulae, as well as adhesive lesions between the urinary bladder and uterus. Taking in mind the age of the patient and the intraoperative findings, we performed a total abdominal hysterectomy with bilateral oophorectomy and en bloc resection of the defective part of the sigmoid colon and jejunum (Figures 5 and 6). Primary jejunojejunal and colocolonic anastomoses were performed. During surgery, a bladder injury was recognized and repaired immediately. Postoperatively, the patient had a fever because of an urinary tract infection which was treated with antibiotics. Rest of the postoperative course was uneventful, and the patient was discharged on the 21st postoperative day.

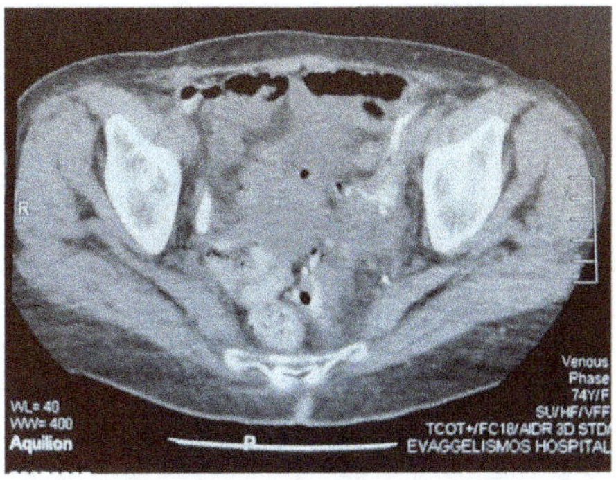

FIGURE 1: CT scan showing findings of chronic diverticulitis.

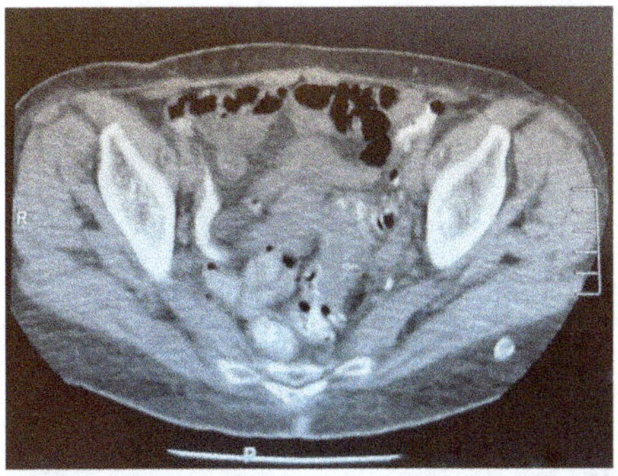

FIGURE 2: CT scan showing findings of chronic diverticulitis.

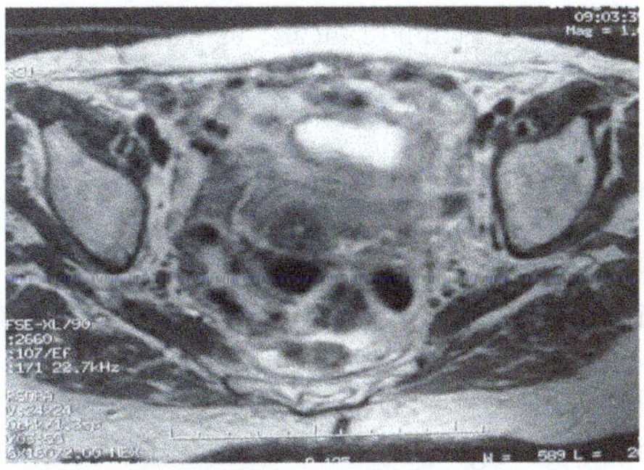

FIGURE 3: MRI revealing the colouterine fistula.

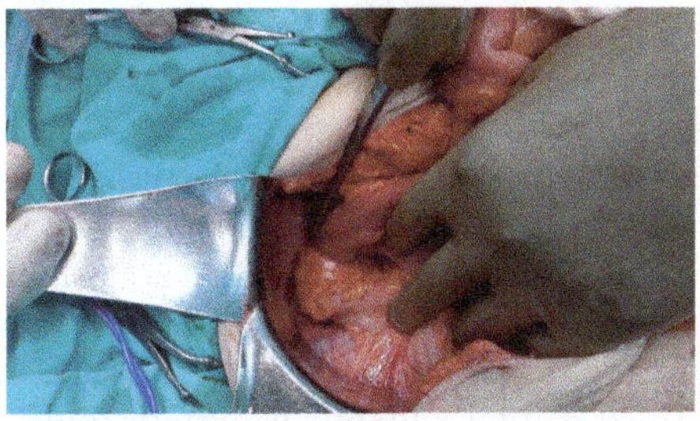

FIGURE 4: Colouterine and jejunouterine fistulae discovered intraoperatively.

3. Discussion

Fistula creation between the gastrointestinal tract and the uterus is rare. The fistula is usually found between the fundus of the uterus and loops of the sigmoid colon or small bowel [6]. In cases of diverticulitis, the inflammatory adherence of the bowel wall to the uterus may result in fistula formation, especially in older people whose uterine wall becomes thinner and mucosa atrophic. Clinical manifestations of a colouterine or a jejunouterine fistula may vary, but typical symptoms include malodorous fecal or purulent vaginal discharge for weeks or months. Fever and recurrent abdominal pain may, also, be present, in case of diverticulitis, but they may be absent in case of a chronic inflammation, as in our case. A palpable abdominal mass may be reported, especially if an abscess has been described [7].

Many imaging modalities have been suggested for establishing the diagnosis of a colouterine or jejunouterine fistula. Vaginal or cervical cultures will determine the source of vaginal discharge and will be useful for selecting the appropriate antibiotic therapy. The imaging modality for diverticular fistulae has been contrast radiology, either rectally or vaginally. Computed tomography (CT) may reveal evidence of diverticulitis and communication between the uterus and the colon, but it may fail to demonstrate the fistulous tract. A multidetector computed tomography (MDCT) has been used to provide better visualisation of the fistula, but it is associated with great radiation. Magnetic resonance imaging (MRI) is a more accurate diagnostic tool, able to identify fistulae, and demonstrate the degree of pericolic inflammation, especially in T1-weighted images. In our case, MRI was the effective modality for diagnosis as it was the only imaging technique indicating the colouterine fistula. The charcoal test depends on demonstrating the passage of orally administered activated charcoal from the

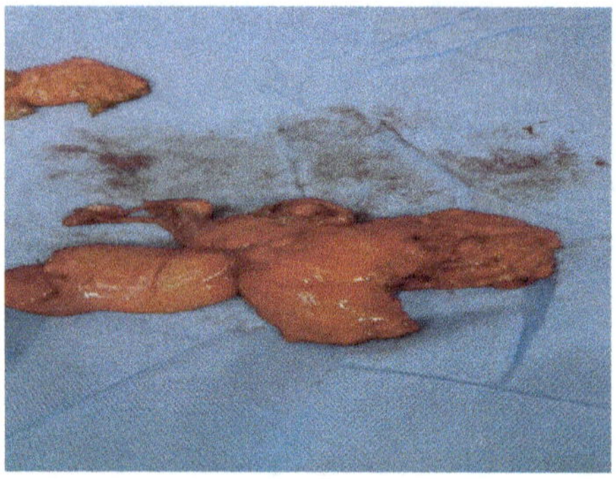

Figure 5: En bloc resection of the uterus with part of the sigmoid colon and jejunum.

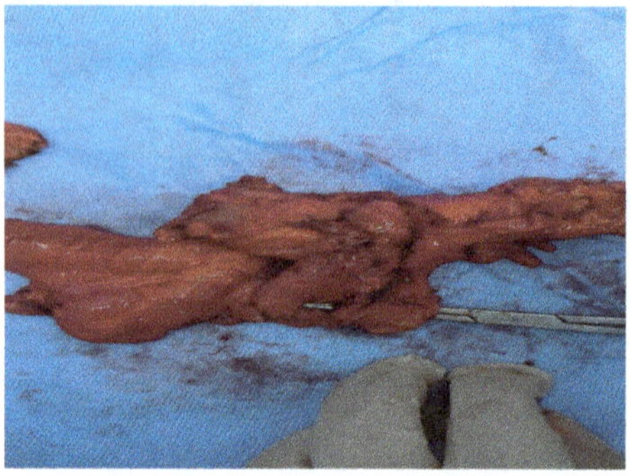

Figure 6: En bloc resection of the uterus with part of the sigmoid colon and jejunum.

cervical os at pelvic examination on the next day. A colonoscopy may be useful in the diagnosis of diverticulosis, but it is not very helpful in the detection of fistulae. Finally, endovaginal ultrasonography and sonohysterography using a contrast medium could be used to visualise both the fistula tract and the uterine wall and colon [1, 8].

Surgical management is the treatment of choice, in most cases. Many surgical approaches have been suggested. Hartmann procedure with hysterectomy, transverse colostomy followed by hysterectomy and closure of the fistula without bowel resection, and an en bloc resection of the uterus and the colon or small bowel are several examples [9]. Hysterectomy may be necessary if malignancy is suspected, but it is not mandatory in case of benign disease [7]. When there is severe local inflammation, a two-stage procedure with reanastomosis at a later time is preferable. In our case, because of the age of the patient and the fact that there was no acute infection, we performed a total abdominal hysterectomy with bilateral oophorectomy and en bloc resection of the sigmoid colon and part of the jejunum and primary anastomoses of the intestines. Laparoscopic approach may, also, be used [2]. Conservative treatment has been suggested with antibiotics and drainage of any abscesses, but it is used, mainly, in patients with major contradictions for surgery [1]. Prognosis for patients with fistulae secondary to diverticulitis is excellent after surgical treatment [9].

4. Conclusion

Fistulae between the uterus and the bowel are very rare complications of diverticulitis. They should be suspected in case of malodorous discharge from the vagina so that the appropriate diagnostic tests may be conducted and the best therapeutic options may be applied. Accurate diagnosis is the key to prompt treatment of this very rare condition.

Disclosure

This case report was performed as part of the employment of the authors by Evaggelismos General Hospital.

References

[1] A. Mohamed, Y. A. Suhaibani, F. Emran, and S. Al Shami, "Colo-uterine fistula, a rare Complication of diverticular Disease of the colon, case Report and literature review," *The Internet Journal of Surgery*, vol. 25, no. 1, 2009.

[2] R. Naval, S. Naval, A. Padmawar, and R. Patankar, "Total laparoscopic management of colouterine fistula," *Journal of Datta Meghe Institute of Medical Sciences University*, vol. 11, no. 4, p. 460, 2016.

[3] G. Zanghì, V. Leanza, R. Vecchio et al., "Neoplastic sigmoid-uterine fistula. An exceptional complication of large intestine cancer," *G Chir*, vol. 38, no. 1, pp. 37–40, 2017.

[4] R. Aggarwal, V. Indiran, and P. Maduraimuthu, "Different etiologies of an unusual disease: colouterine fistula - report of two cases," *Indian Journal of Radiology and Imaging*, vol. 28, no. 1, pp. 37–40, 2018.

[5] S. Jain, S. Jain, S. Jain, V. Jain, and M. Jain, "Sigmoidouterine fistula: anal menstruation as a rare presentation," *Obstetrics & Gynecology: An International Journal*, vol. 2014, Article ID 306195, 7 pages, 2014.

[6] M. E. C. McFarlane, J. M. Plummer, T. Remy et al., "Jejunouterine fistula: a case report," *Gynecological Surgery*, vol. 5, no. 2, p. 173, 2008.

[7] L. Sentilhes, O. Foulatier, E. Verspyck et al., "Colouterine fistula complicating diverticulitis: a case report and review of the literature," *European Journal of Obstetrics & Gynecology and Reproductive Biology*, vol. 110, no. 1, pp. 107–110, 2003.

[8] L. H. Banu, A. Siddiqua, and S. Siddique, "Colouterine fistula," *Journal of Bangladesh College of Physicians and Surgeons*, vol. 35, no. 1, pp. 31–33, 2017.

[9] P. W. Choi, "Colouterine fistula caused by diverticulitis of the sigmoid colon," *Journal of the Korean Society of Coloproctology*, vol. 28, no. 6, pp. 321–324, 2012.

17

Late-Onset Posttransplant Lymphoproliferative Disorder Results in Jejunal Stricture Managed with Endoscopic Dilation

Steven Park,[1] John Miller,[2] Janice Cheong,[2] Asad Ullah,[2] Lawrence Saubermann,[2] and Arthur Decross[2]

[1]*Department of Internal Medicine, University of Rochester Medical Center, Rochester, NY, USA*
[2]*Division of Gastroenterology & Hepatology, University of Rochester Medical Center, Rochester, NY, USA*

Correspondence should be addressed to Steven Park; steven_park@urmc.rochester.edu

Academic Editor: Yoshihiro Moriwaki

Background. Late-onset posttransplant lymphoproliferative disorder (PTLD) after orthotopic heart transplantation is rare. *Case Presentation.* We present a rare diagnosis of small bowel stricture caused by healed lymphomatous ulcers in a patient with orthotopic heart transplantation and PTLD diagnosed 25 years after initial transplantation. We also demonstrate successful endoscopic balloon dilations that improved the patient's obstructive symptoms. *Conclusion.* It is important to consider stricture from healed lymphomatous ulcers in posttransplant patients presenting with obstructive symptoms.

1. Background

Late-onset posttransplant lymphoproliferative disorder (PTLD) after orthotopic heart transplantation is rare. We present a rare diagnosis of small bowel stricture caused by healed lymphomatous ulcers in a patient with orthotopic heart transplantation and PTLD diagnosed 25 years after initial transplantation. We also demonstrate successful endoscopic balloon dilations that improved the patient's obstructive symptoms.

2. Case Presentation

A 31-year-old female with a past medical history of two orthotopic heart transplants (at age six for viral cardiomyopathy and at age thirteen for graft vasculopathy) complicated by posttransplant lymphoproliferative disorder (PTLD) (monomorphic with germinal center B-cell type; EBV-negative) presented to our hospital with two weeks of postprandial emesis. Nausea and emesis occurred two to four hours after meals and consisted of nonbloody, nonbilious emesis. Bloodwork was notable for hemoglobin of 8 g/dL (11.2–15.7 g/dL). 6 days prior to admission, she had received third cycle of triweekly chemotherapy with cyclophosphamide, doxorubicin, vincristine, and prednisone (CHOP).

Upper endoscopy performed 1 month prior to admission to evaluate for a source of anemia demonstrated scattered, large, nonbleeding, clean-based ulcers in the proximal jejunum and a segment of circumferential ulceration. Biopsies of the jejunal ulcers confirmed involvement by patient's known monomorphic-type PTLD (germinal center B-cell type; EBV-negative). To evaluate for gastric outlet obstruction (GOO) suggested by CT scan in the setting of nausea and emesis, we performed an upper endoscopy. This endoscopy revealed a wide-open pylorus without GOO, and no endoscopic abnormality was seen through the fourth portion of the duodenum. Duodenal biopsies were negative for cytomegalovirus, adenovirus, and herpes simplex. Congo red stains were negative for amyloid, and morphologic evidence of lymphoma was absent.

We were suspicious of a more distal site of obstruction and ordered an MR enterography (Figure 1) that revealed a transition point with focal thickening of the proximal jejunum. The decision was made to pursue endoscopic balloon dilation. On push enteroscopy, we encountered an ulcerated stricture with only 2-3 mm in luminal diameter (Figure 2).

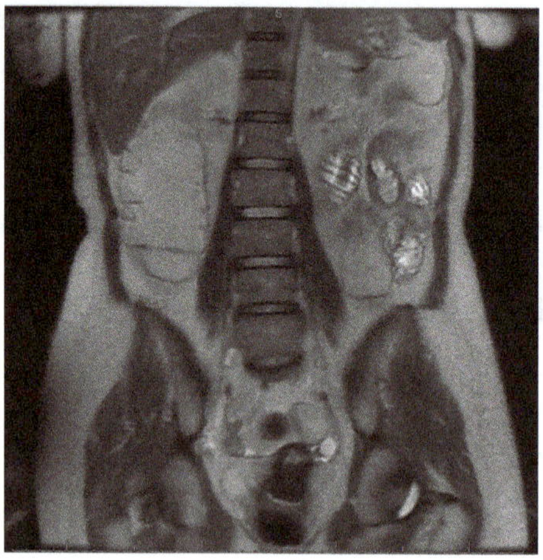

Figure 1: MR enterography showing small bowel obstruction with a transition point at focal thickening of the proximal jejunum (arrow).

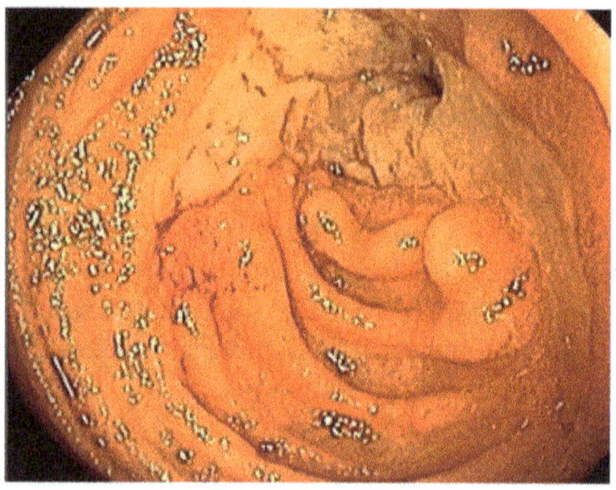

Figure 2: EGD showing a clean-based circumferential ulceration in the proximal jejunum with an ulcerated stricture estimated 2 mm in luminal diameter.

The site of stricture appeared to be the same segment of jejunal ulceration on initial enteroscopy that likely healed with scarring after chemotherapy. Decision was made to proceed with endoscopic dilation using a 6 mm biliary dilation balloon catheter, the smallest dilation catheter available via long pediatric colonoscope instrument channel. Roughly 4 mm diameter distention was reached before notable resistance was felt and evidence of trauma was seen. Patient tolerated a full liquid diet postprocedure and was discharged with a plan for a repeat dilation. To date, patient completed two additional endoscopic dilation procedures, followed by a small bowel resection, and remains alive after completion of total 6 rounds of R-CHOP without additional gastrointestinal complications.

3. Discussion and Conclusions

PTLD is a heterogeneous lymphoid proliferation that occurs after solid-organ or hematopoietic transplantation in the setting of prolonged immunosuppression [1–3]. The median time to diagnosis after transplantation is 2.5 years, and the incidence of PTLD in cardiac transplant patients ranges from 5 to 9% [4–6]. The clinical manifestations vary from nonspecific symptoms to sudden enlargement of nodal and extranodal lymphoid organs [7]. Lymphoid proliferations range from benign collections to malignant lymphomas involving T cells, B cells, and/or plasma cells [8]. PTLD is categorized based on the WHO classification of lymphoid neoplasm, and three main stages of evolution are recognized: early, polymorphic, and monomorphic lesions [9]. Polymorphic and monomorphic B-cell PTLD are the two most common histologic subsets, with increasing proportion of monomorphic cases noted in recent decades [8]. Of note, our patient had monomorphic-type PTLD with negative EBV stain, germinal center B-cell type with immunohistochemistry negative for NYC and positive for BCL2.

PTLD can also involve other organs such as central nervous system, bone marrow, spleen, lung, liver, and kidney [7]. PTLD involvement of small bowel in the form of GI bleed and viral infection has been reported previously [10–13]. However, a stricture in the small bowel from healed lymphomatous ulcer causing obstruction and needing endoscopic dilation has not been reported to our knowledge.

Our case highlights a rare diagnosis of small bowel stricture caused by healed lymphomatous ulcers in a patient with orthotopic heart transplantation and PTLD diagnosed 25 years after initial transplantation. We demonstrate successful endoscopic balloon dilations that improved the patient's obstructive symptoms. A multidisciplinary care involving oncology, pathology, gastroenterology, and colorectal surgery service was crucial to addressing gastrointestinal complications of PTLD. It is important to consider stricture from healed lymphomatous ulcers in posttransplant patients presenting with obstructive symptoms.

Abbreviations

PTLD: Posttransplant lymphoproliferative disorder
CHOP: Cyclophosphamide, doxorubicin, vincristine, and prednisone
GOO: Gastric outlet obstruction
MR: Magnetic resonance.

References

[1] D. Hayes, D. Tumin, R. E. Foraker, and J. D. Tobias, "Posttransplant lymphoproliferative disease and survival in adult heart transplant recipients," *Journal of Cardiology*, vol. 69, no. 1, pp. 144–148, 2017.

[2] C. C. Tai, J. L. Curtis, J. R. Szmuszkovicz et al., "Abdominal involvement in pediatric heart and lung transplant recipients with posttransplant lymphoproliferative disease increases the risk of mortality," *Journal of Pediatric Surgery*, vol. 43, no. 12, pp. 2174–2177, 2008.

[3] M. J. Aull, J. F. Buell, J. Trofe et al., "Experience with 274 cardiac transplant recipients with posttransplant lymphoproliferative disorder: a report from the Israel Penn international transplant tumor registry," *Transplantation*, vol. 78, no. 11, pp. 1676–1682, 2004.

[4] S. A. Webber, D. C. Naftel, F. J. Fricker et al., "Lymphoproliferative disorders after paediatric heart transplantation: a multi-institutional study," *The Lancet*, vol. 367, no. 9506, pp. 233–239, 2006.

[5] B. Z. Katz, E. Pahl, S. E. Crawford et al., "Case-control study of risk factors for the development of post-transplant lymphoproliferative disease in a pediatric heart transplant cohort," *Pediatric Transplantation*, vol. 11, no. 1, pp. 58–65, 2007.

[6] G. E. Wilde, D. J. Moore, and R. D. Bellah, "Post-transplantation lymphoproliferative disorder in pediatric recipients of solid organ transplants: timing and location of disease," *American Journal of Roentgenology*, vol. 185, no. 5, pp. 1335–1341, 2005.

[7] H. A. H. Ibrahim and K. N. Naresh, "Posttransplant lymphoproliferative disorders," *Advances in Hematology*, vol. 2012, Article ID 230173, 11 pages, 2012.

[8] D. E. Tsai, S. Bagley, R. Reshef et al., "The changing face of adult posttransplant lymphoproliferative disorder: changes in histology between 1999 and 2013," *American Journal of Hematology*, vol. 93, no. 7, pp. 874–881, 2018.

[9] S. H. Swerdlow, "Post-transplant lymphoproliferative disorders: a working classification," *Current Diagnostic Pathology*, vol. 4, no. 1, pp. 28–35, 1997.

[10] A. Siegel, J. Boike, I. Trivedi, and R. Yadlapati, "Posttransplant lymphoproliferative disorder of the small bowel as an unexpected cause of iron deficiency anemia decades after heart transplantation," *ACG Case Reports Journal*, vol. 4, p. e86, 2017.

[11] D. Nitta, K. Kinugawa, T. Imamura et al., "How should we treat early post-transplant lymphoproliferative disease after heart transplantation?" *International Heart Journal*, vol. 56, no. 6, pp. 676–678, 2015.

[12] P. Burra, A. Buda, U. Livi et al., "Occurrence of post-transplant lymphoproliferative disorders among over thousand adult recipients: any role for hepatitis C infection?" *European Journal of Gastroenterology & Hepatology*, vol. 18, no. 10, pp. 1065–1070, 2006.

[13] U. Allen and J. Preiksaitis, "Post-transplant lymphoproliferative disorders, epstein-barr virus infection, and disease in solid organ transplantation: guidelines from the American society of transplantation infectious diseases community of practice," *Clinical Transplantation*, vol. 33, no. 9, Article ID e13652, 2019.

18

Massive Hematochezia from a Large Bleeding Duodenal Diverticulum

Marcus Juan Esteban ,[1] Amit Sureen,[2] Daniel Herlihy,[1] Sherif Elhanafi,[1] and Marc J. Zuckerman[1]

[1]*Division of Gastroenterology, Texas Tech University Health Sciences Center, El Paso, TX, USA*
[2]*Department of Internal Medicine, Texas Tech University Health Sciences Center, El Paso, TX, USA*

Correspondence should be addressed to Marcus Juan Esteban; marcus.esteban@ttuhsc.edu

Academic Editor: Yoshifumi Nakayama

Background. Duodenal diverticula are a rare cause of gastrointestinal (GI) bleeding despite being a common finding in the GI tract. We present a case of a patient who had massive hematochezia due to a complex duodenal diverticulum. *Case Presentation.* A 74-year-old Hispanic female presented initially with generalized weakness. During admission, the patient had an episode of a large amount of hematochezia and had to be transferred to the intensive care unit (ICU). Upper endoscopy was done using a forward-viewing endoscope which revealed a bleeding complex duodenal diverticulum. Successful hemostasis was achieved through epinephrine injection followed by placement of hemostatic clips. *Conclusion.* Although rare, gastroenterologists need to be aware of duodenal diverticulum as a possible cause of gastrointestinal bleed. It could be life-threatening, and thus, prompt diagnosis and management is necessary.

1. Introduction

Diverticula are common findings in the adult GI tract and are mostly found in the colon [1]. The duodenum is the second most common location for GI tract diverticula [2]. Duodenal diverticula are often asymptomatic [1–3]. Possible complications include mechanical obstruction of the duodenum, biliary tract or pancreatic duct, inflammation causing perforation, abscess and fistula formation, and hemorrhage [1, 2]. We present a rare case of a patient who had massive hematochezia due to a complex duodenal diverticulum. Successful hemostasis was achieved with epinephrine injection followed by placement of hemostatic clips.

2. Case

A 74-year-old Hispanic female with a past medical history of type 2 diabetes mellitus and hypertension presented with generalized weakness. She initially denied any gastrointestinal bleeding. She had no history of aspirin or NSAID use and was not on any anticoagulants. On admission, vital signs were normal and she had pale conjunctiva. Her abdomen was mildly tender to palpation. Laboratory findings were significant for Hgb 6.7 g/dL and blood glucose of 494 mg/dL. INR was 1.0 on admission. She was admitted for transfusion and blood sugar management. After admission, she had an episode of a large amount of bright red blood per rectum. She became hypotensive and Hgb dropped to 3.7 g/dL. She was intubated, transferred to the intensive care unit, and started on continuous pantoprazole infusion. Gastric lavage gave a clear aspirate. Repeat Hgb was 10.5 g/dL after transfusion with 4 units of packed RBCs. Esophagogastroduodenoscopy (EGD) using a forward-viewing endoscope was done which showed a 30 mm diverticulum in the area of the major papilla with multiple smaller diverticula within the main diverticulum. There were several angiodysplasias within the diverticulum that were oozing blood (Figure 1). The lesions were injected with epinephrine (1 : 10,000 dilution) and four hemostatic clips were placed (Figure 2). There was no further bleeding after the

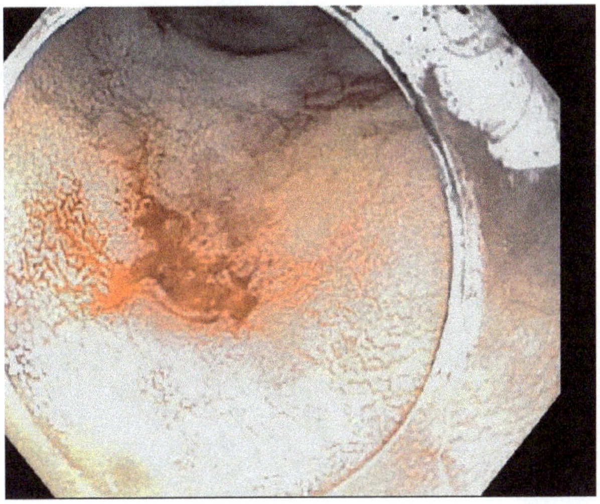

FIGURE 1: Actively oozing angiodysplasias within the diverticulum.

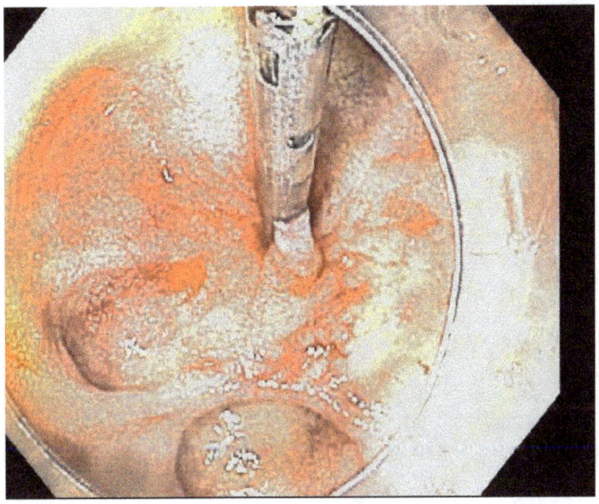

FIGURE 2: Angiodysplasias after injection and hemostatic clip placement. No bleeding was seen postintervention.

intervention. Hemoglobin remained stable throughout the rest of admission and she was eventually discharged home. The patient had no gastrointestinal issues at the 3-month follow-up.

3. Discussion

Diverticula are common findings in the adult GI tract and are found predominantly in the large colon [1]. The duodenum is the second most common location for GI tract diverticula after the colon [2]. In a retrospective review of patients over 23 years, 208 patients were identified with small bowel diverticula. Of these, 79% were in the duodenum, 18% were in the jejunum or ileum, and 3% were in the duodenum, jejunum, and ileum [4]. The precise incidence of duodenal diverticula is unknown, but based on autopsy data, it ranges from 3% to 22%. Radiologic findings on the upper gastrointestinal series estimate it at 2% to 5% [3, 5]. In a large series of 624 patients who underwent endoscopic retrograde cholangiopancreatography, the reported incidence was 23% [6]. There are two types of duodenal diverticula: endoluminal and extraluminal. The latter type is the most frequent. Endoluminal diverticula, as in our patient's case, are caused by congenital webs of the second duodenum. Extraluminal diverticula are known to be associated with bile duct disorders [3].

Duodenal diverticula are often asymptomatic [1–3]. Complications that have been reported include mechanical obstruction of the biliary tract causing obstructive jaundice and cholangitis, mechanical obstruction of the pancreatic duct causing pancreatitis, mechanical obstruction of the duodenum, inflammation causing perforation, abscess and fistula formation, and hemorrhage, which can be occult or profuse [1, 2]. The exact incidence of hemorrhage from duodenal diverticula is unknown [7, 8]. In the abovementioned retrospective study of 208 patients with small bowel diverticula, bleeding complications were reported in 14 patients [6] Diverticular bleeding can be due to an inflamed diverticulum, erosion of a diverticulum into a major vessel, arteriovenous malformations within the diverticulum, aortoenteric fistula formation, or angiodysplasia [6]. Less common causes of bleeding duodenal diverticula include Dieulafoy lesions in the diverticulum and bleeding secondary to intradiverticular polyps [9, 10]. Bleeding due to diverticular angiodysplasia, such as in our case, is exceptionally rare [5].

Given its rarity, a bleeding duodenal diverticulum may be unsuspected and can be difficult to diagnose. Diagnosis has been facilitated with the advent of endoscopy [11]. Upper endoscopy is the preferred modality of diagnosis for bleeding duodenal diverticulum as it also provides the opportunity to perform therapeutic interventions. Upper endoscopy may fail to reveal diverticula in the fourth portion of the duodenum, but it is recommended that the examination of the duodenum be extended as far as possible when the indication for endoscopy is gastrointestinal hemorrhage [3, 11]. In our case, we were fortunate to locate the bleeding source with a forward-viewing scope. In some cases, however, a side-viewing duodenoscope may be necessary [5, 11, 12]. Diverticulectomy previously was the primary treatment for the duodenal diverticulum [3, 13]. With the advances in endoscopy, various endoscopic therapeutic strategies such as injection with epinephrine, bipolar coagulation, argon plasma coagulation (APC), and hemostatic clips have been used for the treatment of bleeding duodenal diverticula [5, 9, 11, 12, 14]. In our case, successful hemostasis was achieved with epinephrine injection followed by placement of hemostatic clips. Surveillance endoscopy is not indicated for bleeding duodenal diverticulum.

4. Conclusion

Duodenal diverticula should be included in the consideration of rare causes of hematochezia. Prompt diagnosis and treatment is necessary to avoid life-threatening complications as was demonstrated in our case.

Authors' Contributions

ME, AS, and DH wrote the case report and the discussion part for the manuscript. They also did the literature review. SE and MZ helped in refining the case and providing expert opinions in the manuscript. All authors read and approved the final manuscript.

References

[1] C. Bierton and A. Gupta, "Giant duodenal diverticulum-an incidental finding," *Journal of Surgical Case Reports*, vol. 2019, p. 4, 2019.

[2] J. Balkissoon, B. Balkissoon, L. D. Leffall, and D. A. Posey, "Massive upper gastrointestinal bleeding in a patient with a duodenal diverticulum: a case report and review of the literature," *Journal of the National Medical Association*, vol. 84, no. 4, pp. 365–367, 1992.

[3] L. Rioux, S. Des Groseilliers, M. Fortin, and D. O. Mutch, "Massive upper gastrointestinal bleeding originating from a fourth-stage duodenal diverticulum: a case report and review of the literature," *Canadian journal of surgery. Journal canadien de chirurgie*, vol. 39, no. 6, pp. 510–512, 1996.

[4] R. Akhrass, M. B. Yaffe, C. Fischer, J. Ponsky, and J. M. Shuck, "Small-bowel diverticulosis: perceptions and reality," *Journal of the American College of Surgeons*, vol. 184, no. 4, pp. 383–388, 1997.

[5] A. T. Chatila, E. Gou, H. Abdulla, and S. Merwat, "Two cases of bleeding angiodysplasias within duodenal diverticulum," *ACG Case Reports Journal*, vol. 6, no. 3, Article ID e00027, 2019.

[6] M. Osnes, T. Løotveit, S. Larsen, and S. Aune, "Duodenal diverticula and their relationship to age, sex, and biliary calculi," *Scandinavian Journal of Gastroenterology*, vol. 16, no. 11, pp. 103–107, 1981.

[7] E. Perdikakis, E. G. Chryssou, and A. Karantanas, "Diagnosis of periampullary duodenal diverticula: the value of new imaging techniques," *Annals of Gastroenterology*, vol. 24, pp. 192–199, 2011.

[8] M. I. Yildirgan, M. Başoğlu, I Yilmaz et al., "Periampullary diverticula causing pancreaticobiliary disease," *Digestive Diseases and Sciences*, vol. 49, no. 11–12, p. 5, 2004.

[9] M. De Benito Sanz, M. Cimavilla Román, and R. Torres Yuste, "A Dieulafoy's lesion in a duodenal diverticulum. An infrequent cause of UGIB," *Revista Espanola De Enfermedades Digestivas*, vol. 110, no. 4, pp. 266-267, 2018.

[10] W. S. Lee, S. B. Cho, S. Y. Park et al., "Successful side-viewing endoscopic hemoclipping for dieulafoy-like lesion at the brim of a periampullary diverticulum," *BMC Gastroenterology*, vol. 10, no. 1, p. 24, 2010.

[11] A. A. Dalal, S. J. Rogers, and J. P. Cello, "Endoscopic management of hemorrhage from a duodenal diverticulum," *Gastrointestinal Endoscopy*, vol. 48, no. 4, pp. 418–420, 1998.

[12] N. Nishiyama, H. Mori, K. Rafiq et al., "Active bleeding from a periampullary duodenal diverticulum that was difficult to diagnose but successfully treated using hemostatic forceps: a case report," *Journal of Medical Case Reports*, vol. 6, no. 1, p. 367, 2012.

[13] N. G. Economides, R. P. McBurney, and F. H. Hamilton, "Intraluminal duodenal diverticulum in the adult," *Annals of Surgery*, vol. 185, no. 2, pp. 147–152, 1977.

[14] A. S. Soudagar, A. Abdinoor, O. Khan, and N. Gupta, "Use of side-viewing endoscope to treat a bleeding duodenal diverticulum," *Gastrointestinal Endoscopy*, vol. 81, no. 1, pp. 232-233, 2015.

19

Renal Cell Carcinoma in Fistulizing Crohn's Disease Patient Who Received Anti-TNF α Therapy

Abdullah Mohammed Albishi,[1] **Rafaat Chakik**,[1] **and Mohammed Bazeed**[2]

[1]*Gastroenterology and Endoscopy Department, Armed Forces Hospital Southern Region, Khamis Mushayt, Saudi Arabia*
[2]*Radiology Department, Armed Forces Hospital Southern Region, Khamis Mushayt, Saudi Arabia*

Correspondence should be addressed to Abdullah Mohammed Albishi; dr.abdullah6975@gmail.com

Academic Editor: Chia-Tung Shun

Inflammatory bowel diseases are chronic inflammatory diseases affecting the gastrointestinal tract with different clinical presentations. These chronic inflammatory diseases are associated with an increased risk for both intestinal and different types of extra-intestinal malignancies. In this case report, we describe the condition of a 29-year-old Saudi male diagnosed with fistulizing ileal Crohn's disease 7 years ago. The patient presented to the gastroenterology clinic with left flank pain for the last 2 months, which started gradually. The pain was dull, intermittent, and without a history of fever, dysuria, or hematuria. The patient was passing 3-4 times bowel motion, watery without blood or mucus. On examination, the patient looked well. Abdomen examination revealed a soft and lax abdomen with no tenderness or organomegaly. CT abdomen showed a well-defined hypodense focal lesion originally from the left kidney near the hilum region with a clue sign. Colonoscopy was performed and showed only terminal ileitis. The patient was referred to a urologist for further action. The patient was seen by the urologist, and they are planning for partial left nephrectomy. The renal surgical specimen histopathology was reported later as renal cell carcinoma.

1. Introduction

Renal cell carcinoma (RCC) originates in the lining of the proximal tubule in the kidneys. RCC is considered the commonest type of kidney malignancy in adults, and it is around 90–95% of all cases diagnosed as kidney cancers [1–3]. RCC is usually an asymptomatic disease, so the cases of RCC often have advanced course by the time of diagnosis [4]. Symptoms of RCC are different, but often include blood in the urine which is around 40% of the cases at the time they first seek medical attention, flank pain (40%), a mass in the abdomen or flank (25%), weight loss (33%), high blood pressure (20%), and fatigue [5]. The first step needed to diagnose RCC is a combination of patient symptoms, signs, and checking for any risk factors for RCC development. Based on the symptoms and signs presented, a range of laboratory tests (using blood and/or urine samples) may also be considered as an initial screening process to provide sufficient quantitative analysis of any abnormalities in electrolytes, renal and liver function, and blood clotting times. On physical examination, the abdomen palpation may reveal the presence of a mass or organ enlargement [6]. The main diagnostic tools for detecting RCC include ultrasound, computed tomography (CT), and magnetic resonance imaging (MRI) of the kidneys [7].

Chronic inflammation as well as drug-induced immunosuppression associated with inflammatory bowel disease especially Crohn's diseases particularly immunosuppressive medications such as thiopurines and methotrexate may play an important role in the development of different types of extra-intestinal malignancies by inducing DNA damage or impairing immunosurveillance of tumor cells [8, 9].

2. Case Presentation

A 29-year-old Saudi male was diagnosed with fistulizing ileal Crohn's disease 7 years ago and received adalimumab 40 mg subcutaneous every 2 weeks since being diagnosed. The patient was presented to the gastroenterology clinic for follow-up. He was complaining of left flank pain for the last 2 months, which started gradually. The pain was dull, intermittent, and without a history of fever, dysuria, or hematuria. The patient was passing 3-4 times bowel motion, watery without blood or mucus. He had no history of skin rash, joint pain, eye pain, redness, or jaundice and no history of NSAID use or recent intake of antibiotics.

Family history similar condition was negative. The patient gave a history of perianal complex fistulae which were managed surgically before diagnosed with Crohn's disease. The last colonoscopy showed terminal ileitis.

3. Clinical Examination

The patient looked well, with no pallor, no jaundice, or lymphadenopathy. The patient was vitally stable, afebrile. Cardiac and chest examinations were free. Abdomen examination revealed a soft and lax abdomen with no tenderness or organomegaly. Left and right renal angles were normal with no tenderness and no palpable masses. PR examination was normal with no obvious fistulae or hemorrhoids.

4. Investigation

WBC = 11, Hb = 15.2 g/dl, PLT = 320, and INR = 1.0.

Liver function tests and renal profile were normal. CRP = 14.5.

Urine analysis: normal, no nitrate, no WBC or RBC, and no cast.

4.1. Imaging. CT abdomen was performed and showed well-defined hypodense focal lesion originally from the left kidney near hilum region with clue sign. The renal lesion shows inhomogeneous enhancement in the arterial phase with partial wash out in delayed phase, it measured 2,6 cm × 2,6 cm, to rule out the possibility of renal cell carcinoma as shown in Figure 1.

Colonoscopy was performed and showed normal colonic mucosa up to terminal ileum. Terminal ileum biopsy showed acute on top of chronic ileitis.

The patient was referred to a urologist for further action. The patient was seen by the urologist, and they are planning for partial left nephrectomy. The surgical specimen histopathology was reported later as renal cell carcinoma.

4.2. Treatment. The patient has fistulizing ileal Crohn's disease and he needed treatment definitely, but a continuation on anti-TNF was not advised due to a history of malignancy. The patient started on anti-integrin medication (vedolizumab).

4.3. Outcome and Follow-Up. Follow-up after 6 months revealed that the patient was doing well with no abdominal pain. He was passing 2-3 times bowel motion. No extra-intestinal manifestation was observed. CBC, calprotectin, and CRP were normal. A follow-up CT of the abdomen was normal. The patient was advised to continue current medications with regular follow-up.

5. Discussion

Inflammatory bowel diseases (IBDs), including Crohn's disease (CD), ulcerative colitis (UC), and indeterminate colitis, are chronic inflammatory diseases affecting the gastrointestinal tract with different various clinical presentations. These kinds of chronic inflammatory diseases are associated with an increased risk for both intestinal and different extra-intestinal malignancies as well [10, 11]. The malignancy risk in IBD patients is mainly related to chronic inflammation and/or immunosuppression medications induced as shown in Figure 2 [12]. Especially immunosuppressive drugs may play an important role in the development of different types of extra-intestinal malignancies by inducing DNA damages or impairing immunosurveillance of tumor cells [13, 14]. The potential associated risk of malignancy is an important growing concern given the need for prolonged immunosuppressive therapy in IBD patients, especially given the aging IBD population.

The current case report was done to add more evidence for the association between Crohn's disease as one of the inflammatory bowel disorders (IBD) and renal malignancies. The association between renal cell carcinoma and IBD was reported in a cohort study including 180 patients [15]. However, the association with multilocular cystic renal neoplasm (MCRN) of low malignant potential has not been described previously. Soumaya et al. [16] reported that a patient with Crohn's disease and incidental multilocular cystic renal neoplasm (MCRN) of low malignant potential who presented with complicated Crohn's disease with the deep collection was treated with antibiotic including cefotaxime and metronidazole. After 2 weeks of treatment, the patient underwent a renal lumpectomy. The specimen gross examination revealed a well encapsulated, multiseptate tumor mass of 2.5 cm.

Wauters et al. [17] conducted a retrospective case-control and cohort study to detect the risk of renal cell carcinoma (RCC) with anti-tumor necrosis factor (anti-TNF) therapy in inflammatory bowel disease (IBD) and rheumatic diseases. The study revealed that RCC was confirmed in seven anti-TNF-exposed (TNF+) and 21 anti-TNF-naive (TNF-) IBD and one TNF+ and 26 TNF- RD patients.

The main differential diagnosis of a renal mass in a patient with Crohn's disease is pyelonephritis, renal malignancy, and inflammatory pseudotumor. Pyelonephritis can be caused by either bacterial or fungal infections due to the effect of immunosuppressive treatments. Imaging features such as enlargement of the kidney, perinephric stranding, and collection or abscess formation may be an indicator to have a biopsy [18]. The involvement of perinephric space, renal vein invasion, and metastases are gold patterns that may differentiate renal tumor which is confirmed by histology [19]. Renal inflammatory pseudotumor may be also considered as the main presentation for Wegener's granulomatosis in cases with Crohn's disease [20].

A considerable portion incidentally had asymptomatic and low-stage tumors in patients with inflammatory bowel

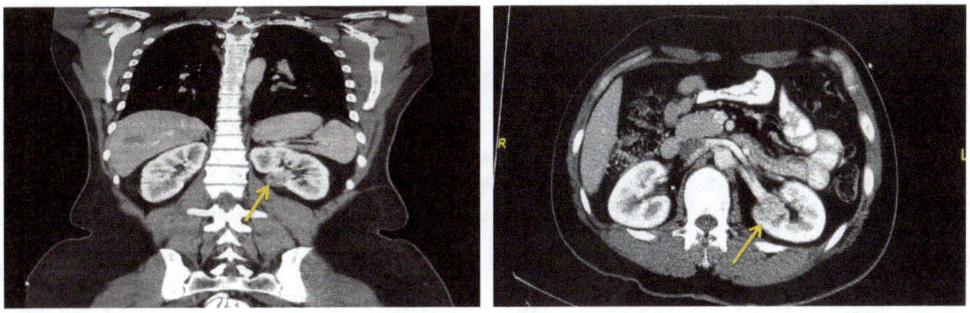

Figure 1: Axial and coronal view of abdominal CT scan showed a well-defined hypodense focal lesion originally from left kidney near hilum region with clue sign. The renal lesion showed inhomogeneous enhancement in the arterial phase with partial wash out in delayed phase, and it measured 2.6 cm × 2.6 cm.

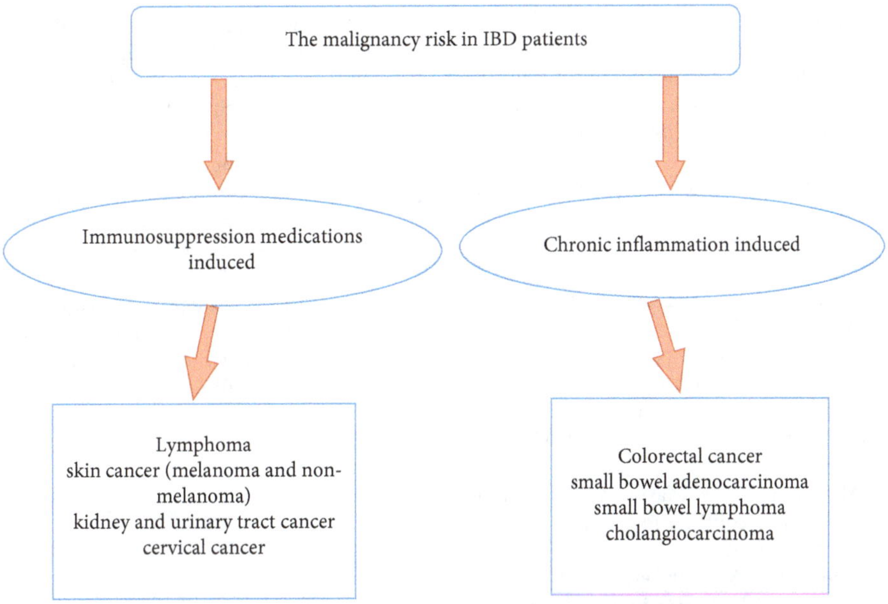

Figure 2: The risk of malignancies in IBD patients and related factors.

disease who require periodic abdominal imaging at a relatively young age especially patients on TNF treatment as well as rheumatic and general populations. However, potential treatment-related or disease-related risks cannot be excluded as patients with severe disease courses are more likely to receive concomitant immunosuppressive therapy.

Use of thiopurines carries a high rate of risk of kidney and bladder cancers in transplant recipients as well as the IBD patients; although the risk is almost restricted to older smoker males, no such increase was seen in patients who use anti-TNF [21].

Once the malignancy is diagnosed in IBD patients with biologics, the risk of IBD exacerbation if medication is stopped, versus the risk of progression of the malignancy if medication is continued, needs to be balanced. If a localized malignancy can be resected by the surgery, the immunosuppressive therapy could be maintained, but biologics should be stopped if chemotherapy will be started for the treatment of a solid tumor as chemotherapy which has an immunosuppressive effect and can induce and maintain IBD remission [22].

The treatment of IBD with biologics is not totally contraindicated in a patient with past history of malignancy, and decisions should be individualised. A delay of at least 2 years after successful malignancy eradication is appropriate, but for those malignancies with a high risk of late metastatic spread (including breast, malignant melanoma, and renal cell carcinoma) this should be extended to 5 years [23].

ECCO Guideline/Consensus Paper demonstrates that there is currently no evidence that the overall risk of malignancy is increased in patients being treated with anti-TNF agents alone [24].

6. Conclusion

Our case report focused on IBD as a risk factor to develop renal complications including renal cell carcinoma. IBD patients who are diagnosed with RCC are usually at a younger age as well as at an earlier stage of the disease. Immunosuppressive medications and anti-TNFα therapy may be the contributing agents and not adversely affect the survival. Patients if treated properly may show clinical improvement after treatment modifications. Periodic abdominal examination and imaging are required for IBD patients to help in the early diagnosis of any extra-intestinal complications with better survival.

References

[1] B. Curti, B. R. P. Jana, M. Javeed et al., *Renal Cell Carcinoma*, J. E. Harris, Ed., Medscape Reference, 2014, https://emedicine.medscape.com/article/281340-overview.

[2] B. I. Rini, W. K. Rathmell, and P. Godley, "Renal cell carcinoma," *Current Opinion in Oncology*, vol. 20, no. 3, pp. 300–306, 2008.

[3] NHS, *Kidney Cancer*, nhs.uk, Leeds, UK, 2017.

[4] V. A. Master, "Renal cell carcinoma," *Merck Manual Professional*, Merck Sharp & Dohme Corp, Kenilworth, NJ, USA, 2014.

[5] B. I. Rini, S. C. Campbell, and B. Escudier, "Renal cell carcinoma," *The Lancet*, vol. 373, no. 9669, pp. 1119–1132, 2009.

[6] L. S. Wood, "Renal cell carcinoma," *Clinical Journal of Oncology Nursing*, vol. 13, pp. 3–7, 2009.

[7] E. D. Agabegi and S. S. Agabegi, *Step-Up to Medicine (Step-Up Series)*, Lippincott Williams & Wilkins, Hagerstwon, MD, 2008.

[8] O. Bernheim, J.-F. Colombel, T. A. Ullman, D. Laharie, L. Beaugerie, and S. H. Itzkowitz, "The management of immunosuppression in patients with inflammatory bowel disease and cancer," *Gut*, vol. 62, no. 11, pp. 1523–1528, 2013.

[9] L. Beaugerie, F. Carrat, J. F. Colombel et al., "For the CSG Risk of new or recurrent cancer under immunosuppressive therapy in patients with IBD and previous cancer," *Gut*, vol. 63, no. 9, pp. 1416–1423, 2013.

[10] J. A. Eaden, K. R. Abrams, and J. F. Mayberry, "The risk of colorectal cancer in ulcerative colitis: a meta-analysis," *Gut*, vol. 48, no. 4, pp. 526–535, 2001.

[11] N. Pedersen, D. Duricova, M. Elkjaer, M. Gamborg, P. Munkholm, and T. Jess, "Risk of extra-intestinal cancer in inflammatory bowel disease: meta-analysis of population-based cohort studies," *American Journal of Gastroenterology*, vol. 105, no. 7, pp. 1480–1487, 2010.

[12] L. Biancone, S. Onali, C. Petruzziello, E. Calabrese, and F. Pallone, "Cancer and immunomodulators in inflammatory bowel diseases," *Inflammatory Bowel Diseases*, vol. 21, no. 3, pp. 674–698, 2015.

[13] L. Beaugerie, "Use of immunosuppressants and biologicals in patients with previous cancer," *Digestive Diseases*, vol. 31, no. 2, pp. 254–259, 2013.

[14] L. Beaugerie, N. Brousse, A. M. Bouvier et al., "Lymphoproliferative disorders in patients receiving thiopurines for inflammatory bowel disease: a prospective observational cohort study," *The Lancet*, vol. 374, no. 9701, pp. 1617–1625, 2009.

[15] A. A. P. Derikx Lauranne, H. C. Nissen Loes, P. H. Drenth Joost, M. van Herpen Carla, K. Wietske, and H. A. Verhoeven Rob, "Better survival of renal cell carcinoma in patients with inflammatory bowel disease," *Oncotarget*, vol. 6, no. 35, 2015.

[16] M. Soumaya, K. Mehdi, M. Nadia et al., "Crohn's disease and multilocular cystic renal neoplasm of low malignant potential: an unusual association," *Urology Case Reports*, vol. 16, pp. 79-80, 2018.

[17] L. Wauters, T. Billiet, K. Papamichael et al., "Incidence of renal cell carcinoma in inflammatory bowel disease patients with and without anti-TNF treatment," *European Journal of Gastroenterology & Hepatology*, vol. 29, no. 1, pp. 84–90, 2017.

[18] W. D. Craig, B. J. Wagner, and M. D. Travis, "Pyelonephritis: radiologic-pathologic review," *Radiographics*, vol. 28, no. 1, pp. 255–276, 2008.

[19] S. Sheth, J. C. Scatarige, K. M. Horton, F. M. Corl, and E. K. Fishman, "Current concepts in the diagnosis and management of renal cell carcinoma: role of multidetector ct and three-dimensional CT," *Radiographics*, vol. 21, no. suppl_1, pp. S237–S254, 2001.

[20] K. D. Fairbanks, D. B. Hellmann, E. K. Fishman, S. Z. Ali, and J. H. Stone, "Wegener's granulomatosis presenting as a renal mass," *American Journal of Roentgenology*, vol. 174, no. 6, pp. 1597-1598, 2000.

[21] T. Greuter, S. Vavricka, A. O. König, S. Beaugerie, and M. Scharl, "Malignancies in inflammatory bowel disease," *Digestion*, vol. 101, no. Suppl1, pp. 136–145.

[22] A. Jauregui-Amezaga, S. Vermeire, and H. Prenen, "Use of biologics and chemotherapy in patients with inflammatory bowel diseases and cancer," *Annals of Gastroenterology*, vol. 29, no. 2, pp. 127–136, 2016.

[23] C. A. Lamb, N. A. Kennedy, T. Raine et al., "British Society of Gastroenterology consensus guidelines on the management of inflammatory bowel disease in adults," *Gut*, vol. 68, no. Suppl 3, pp. s1–s106, 2019.

[24] V. Annese, L. Beaugerie, L. Egan et al., "European evidence-based consensus: inflammatory bowel disease and malignancies," *Journal of Crohn's and Colitis*, vol. 9, no. 11, pp. 945–965, 2015.

20

The Off-Label use of a Lumen-Apposing Metal Stent (LAMS) for a Benign Colon Anastomotic Stricture Causing Recurrent Bowel Obstruction in a Patient with Keloids

Michael Coles[1] **Pearl Uy,**[2] **Victoria Madray,**[3] **John Erikson Yap**[2] **and Subbaramiah Sridhar**[2]

[1]*Augusta University, Department of Internal Medicine, 1120 15th Street, Augusta, Georgia, USA*
[2]*Augusta University, Department of Gastroenterology and Hepatology, 1120 15th Street, Augusta, Georgia, USA*
[3]*Augusta University, Medical College of Georgia, 1120 15th Street, Augusta, Georgia, USA*

Correspondence should be addressed to Michael Coles; michaeljohncoles@gmail.com

Academic Editor: Hirotada Akiho

Anastomotic strictures are a known complication of colorectal surgery. Despite a wide range of medical devices that have been deployed for this complication, outcomes remain challenging. Lumen-apposing metal stents (LAMSs) have recently emerged as a potentially superior therapeutic option. We herein report a patient with a past medical history of pT3, N0 adenocarcinoma of the colon with anastomotic stricture recurrence who underwent successful placement of an LAMS. We suggest that patients with a predisposition for keloid formation or fibrosis-prone anastomotic wound healing should be considered for LAMS deployment early in the treatment course.

1. Introduction

Benign colon anastomotic strictures can lead to recurrent hospitalizations from bowel obstruction. Most benign gastrointestinal (GI) strictures are managed endoscopically with balloon dilation, intralesional steroid injection, incisional therapy, and/or self-expanding metal stents (SEMSs) [1]. However, strictures affecting the GI tract can be recalcitrant. We present the successful treatment of a benign recurrent sigmoid anastomotic stricture with a Lumen-Apposing Metal Stent (LAMS).

2. Case Report

We present a 67-year-old African-American male patient who underwent sigmoidectomy, diverting ostomy, and then, subsequent reversal under adjuvant chemotherapy for a pT3, N0 adenocarcinoma of the colon. His ostomy was complicated by recurrent keloid formation causing bowel obstruction prior to the ostomy reversal. He presented to the emergency department with abdominal pain, nausea, and constipation of two-week duration. He had tried multiple over-the-counter laxatives, which failed to abate his symptoms. He was not receiving opioid therapy.

Upon presentation, the patient's vital signs were normal. On physical examination, the patient had a significantly distended, nontender abdomen and hyperactive bowel sounds with tympany. His laboratory parameters were unremarkable. The abdominal X-ray demonstrated a dilated colon, and a follow-up CT scan demonstrated significant dilation of the colon measuring approximately 20 cm in diameter just proximal to the colonic anastomosis concerning for an obstructing anastomotic stricture (Figure 1). A flexible sigmoidoscopy revealed a 10 mm-long anastomotic stricture at 20 cm from the anal verge (Figure 2) with a luminal diameter of 8 mm. The stricture was subsequently dilated over multiple endoscopic sessions in a stepwise manner to attain a maximal stricture luminal diameter of 20 mm. However, over the following 6 months, the anastomotic stricture recurred, causing colonic obstruction requiring at least 4 more dilatation sessions.

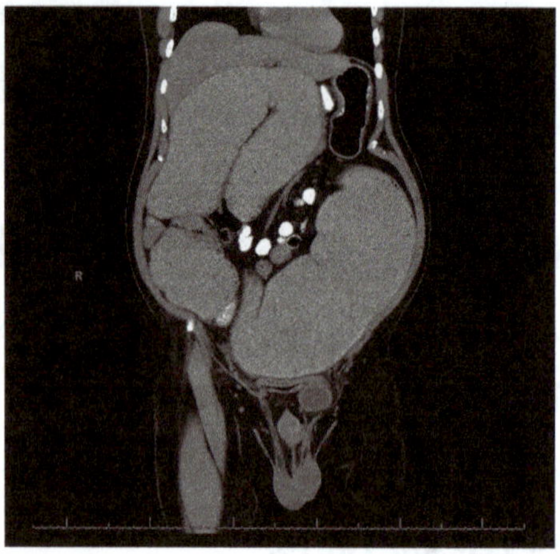

FIGURE 1: Coronal section of computed tomography without contrast of the abdomen and pelvis demonstrating significant dilation of the colon proximal to the colonic anastomosis from prior sigmoidectomy consistent with an obstructing anastomotic stricture.

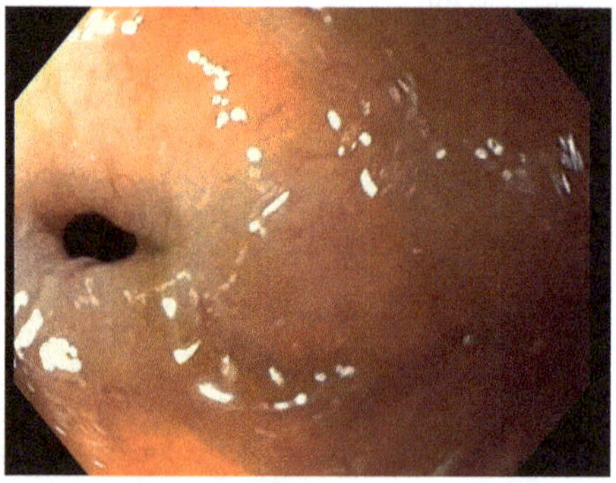

FIGURE 2: Flexible sigmoidoscopy 20 cm from the anal verge demonstrating a 10 mm-long anastomotic stricture with a luminal diameter of 8 mm.

Given the recalcitrant nature of the patient's anastomotic stricture, he was offered alternative therapies including placement of a Lumen-Apposing Metal Stent (LAMS) or surgical resection of the stricture. Due to the history of keloid formation, the patient elected to undergo LAMS placement. A flexible sigmoidoscopy was performed, and a 20 mm × 10 mm LAMS was successfully deployed at the anastomotic stricture site. The proximal aspect of the deployed LAMS was inspected with retroflexion with an ultrathin upper endoscope to ensure appropriate positioning of the stent (Figure 3).

The patient did well for 6 months following the stent placement. Subsequent flexible sigmoidoscopy showed the stent to be in good position with maintained patency (Figure 4). He had no abdominal pain, constipation, or rectal bleeding. He reported one normal bowel movement every 2-3 days while on a laxative. A flexible sigmoidoscopy with removal of the LAMS was performed with notable clean base ulcerations at the previous location of the stent. This was followed by injection of 40 mg of triamcinolone (10 mg into each of the four quadrants) into the previously strictured area. A follow-up flex sigmoidoscopy was performed after 13 months, which showed a patent anastomotic site, and repeat 4-quadrant triamcinolone injection was performed. The patient continues to remain asymptomatic without any hospitalizations for obstructive symptoms 5 months since his last flex sigmoidoscopy.

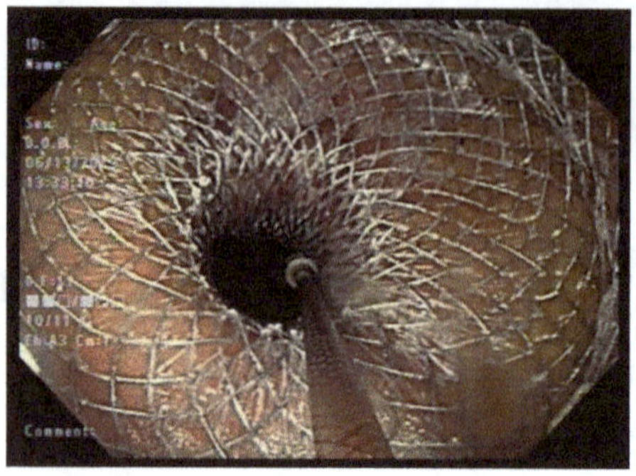

FIGURE 3: Retroflexion perspective demonstrating the proximal aspect of the deployed LAMS.

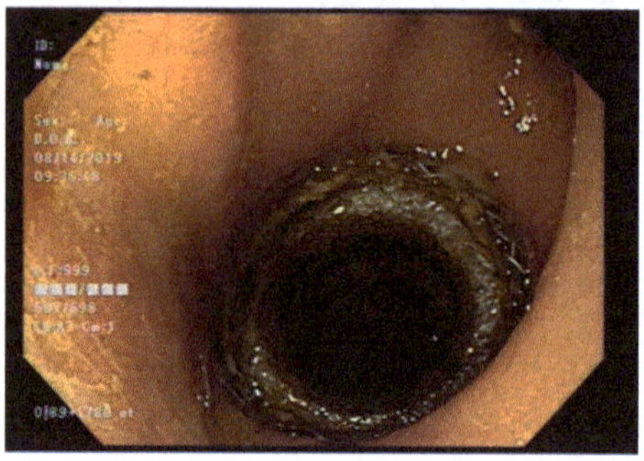

FIGURE 4: Flexible sigmoidoscopy illustrating a patent LAMS in place over an anastomotic stricture.

3. Discussion

Anastomotic strictures resulting from colorectal surgery are therapeutically challenging and often resistant to the established therapies including balloon dilations, incisional therapy, and deployment of biodegradable (BDS) or fully covered self-expanding metal stents (FC-SEMS) [1]. Lumen-apposing metal stents (LAMSs) were originally indicated to facilitate access and drainage of pancreatic fluid collections [1]. However, LAMS have recently emerged as a potentially superior clinical alternative to FC-SEMS. The therapeutic benefit of FC-SEMS may be undermined by their high migration rates and limited efficacy demonstrated in several trials [2]. The LAMS imparts lumen apposition via its wide flanges, which provides an anchoring mechanism, features lacking in FC-SEMS. FC-SEMS can be anchored by means of stent suturing but it is both expensive [3] and more technically challenging for the endoscopist, ultimately affecting the likelihood of procedural success [4]. In esophageal stenting studies with suturing of stent in-situ, migration rates still ranged as high as 33% [5] and 50% when not sutured [6]. Furthermore, stent suturing with FC-SEMS is also described to cause stricture overgrowth [3]. LAMS also are manufactured with larger lumen diameters of 10, 15, and 20 mm compared to the 8 and 10 mm of FC-SEMS, theoretically reducing the likelihood of obstruction when relatively larger stents are selected for use. In a 2019 systematic review and meta-analysis by Mohan et al., management using LAMS demonstrated statistically better outcomes, including lower rates of stent migration and postprocedure pain relative to FC-SEMS and BDS [7]. Although LAMSs are less likely to migrate, their comparatively shorter length may result in misalignment of the stent lumen relative to the stricture axis resulting in obstructive symptoms [3]. As such, careful characterization of stricture morphology must be taken into consideration prior to selection of stent type. Given the off-label use of an LAMS in benign gastrointestinal strictures, no definitive guidelines exist when selecting an optimal stent size. We opted for a conservative approach, with the smallest LAMS size of 10 mm to which our patient responded well. The decision to place an LAMS was motivated by the history of suboptimal therapeutic response to serial dilations. Its recalcitrant nature was speculated to partially be a sequelae of abnormal proliferation of keloidal tissue at the anastomotic site to which the LAMS tubular structure could facilitate a tract formation while maintaining lumen patency.

Postintervention information is limited mostly to case series with only short follow-up duration; however, the possibility of LAMS placement as a destination therapy may warrant consideration an individualized basis. Reintervention rates of 75% were noted at 300 days after LAMS removal in one study [8], and given such a high rate, LAMSs placed indefinitely is a therapeutic option. While placement could obviate the need for further intervention, patients may be at increased risk for bleeding, migration, stent burial or occlusion [9], and infection. Future prospective controlled trials are required to determine the long-term efficacy and risks associated with such a strategy.

In summary, this case highlights the use of an LAMS as an effective approach in the management of refractory colonic stricture. This device features ease of deployment and favorable safety profile, which yields effective palliation, recommending it as an excellent treatment option for recurrent bowel obstruction associated with a refractory benign colonic stricture. Less than 20 cases have been reported in the literature regarding the off-label use of an LAMS in the treatment of colonic strictures [10]. The accrual of larger patient experience will be important to evaluate the long-term efficacy of LAMSs in specific disease indications. Drug-elution capability allowing locoregional drug delivery addressing a wide range of benign and malignant lesions represents a potential future design modification that may enhance the utility of this minimally invasive treatment approach. Interestingly, there are multiple instances in the literature of gastrointestinal keloidal manifestations with subsequent motility complications [11–13]. Predisposition for keloid formation and altered anastomotic wound healing in patients with a benign stricture may indicate early implementation of LAMSs to achieve effective and facile restoration of colonic patency.

References

[1] D. Walter, U. Will, A. Sanchez-Yague et al., "A novel lumen-apposing metal stent for endoscopic ultrasound-guided drainage of pancreatic fluid collections: a prospective cohort study," *Endoscopy*, vol. 47, no. 1, pp. 63–67, 2015.

[2] T. Baron, I. Grimm, and S. Irani, "Lumen-apposing covered self-expandable metal stents for short-length gastrointestinal strictures: will they take hold?" *Endoscopy*, vol. 49, no. 4, pp. 315-316, 2017.

[3] J. Santos-Fernandez, C. Paiji, M. Shakhatreh et al., "Lumen-apposing metal stents for benign gastrointestinal tract strictures: an international multicenter experience," *World Journal of Gastrointestinal Endoscopy*, vol. 9, no. 12, pp. 571–578, 2017.

[4] S. N. Stavropoulos, R. Modayil, and D. Friedel, "Current applications of endoscopic suturing," *World Journal of Gastrointestinal Endoscopy*, vol. 7, no. 8, pp. 777–789, 2015.

[5] L. L. Fujii, E. A. Bonin, T. H. Baron, C. J. Gostout, L. M. Wong Kee Song, and L. M. Song, "Utility of an endoscopic suturing system for prevention of covered luminal stent migration in the upper GI tract," *Gastrointestinal Endoscopy*, vol. 78, no. 5, pp. 787–793, 2013.

[6] D. T. Dan, B. Gannavarapu, J. G. Lee, K. Chang, and V. R. Muthusamy, "Removable esophageal stents have poor efficacy for the treatment of refractory benign esophageal strictures (RBES)," *Diseases of the Esophagus*, vol. 27, no. 6, pp. 511-517, 2014.

[7] B. P. Mohan, S. Chandan, R. Garg et al., "Lumen-apposing metal stents, fully covered self-expanding metal stents, and biodegradable stents in the management of benign of GI strictures," *Journal of Clinical Gastroenterology*, vol. 53, no. 8, pp. 560–573, 2019.

[8] F. Bazerbachi, J. Heffley, B. Abu Dayyeh et al., "Safety and efficacy of coaxial lumen-apposing metal stents in the management of refractory gastrointestinal luminal strictures: a multicenter study," *Endoscopy International Open*, vol. 5, no. 9, pp. E861–E867, 2017.

[9] M. L. DeSimone, A. W. Asombang, and T. M. Berzin, "Lumen apposing metal stents for pancreatic fluid collections: recognition and management of complications," *World Journal of Gastrointestinal Endoscopy*, vol. 9, no. 9, pp. 456–463, 2017.

[10] B. Larson and D. G. Adler, "Lumen-apposing metal stents for gastrointestinal luminal strictures: current use and future directions," *Annals of Gastroenterology*, vol. 32, no. 2, pp. 141–146, 2019.

[11] M. H. Chew, A. Chiow, C. L. Tang, and F. Boffi, "Correspondence," *Techniques in Coloproctology*, vol. 12, no. 4, pp. 351–353, 2008.

[12] M. Hertl, S. Binder, M. Megahed, G. N. Goerz, and T. Krieg, "Gemeinsames Auftreten einer extraabdominellen Fibromatose und posttraumatischer Keloide," *Der Hautarzt*, vol. 45, no. 2, pp. 113–116, 1994.

[13] K. Yasutake, M. Tokisue, T. Masuda et al., "[Study on endoscopic features in responders to systemic chemotherapy in advanced gastric cancer]," *Nihon Gan Chiryo Gakkai Shi*, vol. 25, no. 10, pp. 2519–2525, 1990.

21

A Rare Case of Eosinophilic Gastroenteritis and Ampullitis Leading to Benign Papillary Stenosis

Akwe Nyabera,[1] **Keya Shah**,[2] **Nso Nso**,[1] **Saphwat Eskaros**,[1] **and Negar Niknam**[1]

[1]*Icahn School of Medicine at Mount Sinai (NYC Health+Hospitals/Queens) Program, New York City, NY, USA*
[2]*NYIT College of Osteopathic Medicine, Old Westbury, NY, USA*

Correspondence should be addressed to Akwe Nyabera; nyaberaa@nychhc.org

Academic Editor: Hirotada Akiho

Eosinophilic gastroenteritis is characterized by eosinophilic infiltration of the gastrointestinal wall. There have been limited studies of eosinophilic infiltration involving the ampulla. We present a 70-year-old woman with a history of asthma, eosinophilic esophagitis, and eosinophilic sinusitis, who underwent work up for postprandial abdominal pain and abnormal liver function tests. The patient had various imaging studies done, including computed tomography (CT) scan, magnetic resonance imaging (MRI), and magnetic resonance cholangiopancreatography (MRCP). Dilated extrahepatic bile duct with distal tapering towards the ampulla was noted on MRCP and afterwards on endoscopic ultrasound (EUS). Endoscopic retrograde cholangiopancreatography (ERCP) revealed an inflamed major ampulla with benign papillary stenosis. The patient was treated with sphincterotomy, sphincteroplasty/dilation of distal common bile duct, and placement of an 11.5 Fr × 7 cm plastic stent into the bile duct. Additionally, she was started on prednisone, which was gradually tapered down. The patient demonstrated significant improvement with systemic steroid therapy. Liver function tests (LFTs) completely normalized after ERCP. Ampullitis leading to papillary stenosis secondary to eosinophilic infiltration of the major papilla is a rare manifestation of eosinophilic gastrointestinal disorders (EGIDs). Early diagnosis would lead to appropriate medical and endoscopic management.

1. Introduction

Eosinophilic gastroenteritis is characterized by eosinophilic infiltration of the gastrointestinal wall [1, 2]. The stomach and small intestine are the most commonly affected organs [3, 4]. There have been limited studies of eosinophilic infiltration involving the ampulla. We present a patient with abnormal liver function tests and abdominal pain who was found to have benign papillary stenosis secondary to eosinophilic infiltration of the major papilla. The clinical presentation of eosinophilic gastroenteritis varies widely. It may present similarly to irritable bowel syndrome, dyspepsia, pancreatitis, or appendicitis [3, 5]. Eosinophils are inhabitants of the gastrointestinal mucosal lining delivering a natural defense in cases of parasitic infections [2]. High cytotoxic granular proteins will release after excessive eosinophils and accumulate in the mucosal tissue causing serious tissue destruction [5]. Biopsy is an important tool for establishing a diagnosis [2, 6]. Multiple biopsies may be required due to the variable nature of the disease [2]. Eosinophilic gastroenteritis is a substantially treatable disease with the elimination of empirical food diets. A single course of steroid therapy is first line therapy; in cases of relapsing or refractory conditions, steroid-sparing immunosuppressive agents are recommended in association with biological agents [3, 5]. Treatment is largely dependent on the severity of symptoms and extent of disease [7].

2. Case Presentation

A 70-year-old woman with a history of asthma, eosinophilic esophagitis, and eosinophilic sinusitis underwent work-up for postprandial abdominal pain, bloating, and dyspepsia. Her symptoms had been ongoing intermittently for 2 years. Laboratory results were significant for elevated eosinophils (19.4%) lipase (376 U/L), ALT (247 U/L), AST (332 U/L), and alkaline phosphatase (131 U/L). Initial EGD showed a hypertrophic major papilla, antral gastritis, and superficial gastric ulcers (Figures 1(a) and 1(b)).

She underwent MRI/MRCP which revealed CBD dilatation without choledocholithiasis but with tapering of the distal CBD (Figure 2).

The common hepatic duct was dilated to 10 mm, and the CBD was dilated to 8 mm with tapering towards the ampulla. ERCP revealed an inflamed major ampulla with benign papillary stenosis.

The patient was treated with sphincterotomy, and placement of an 11.5 Fr × 7 cm plastic stent into the bile duct was done. After sphincterotomy, the sphincter tissue was thick and fibrotic. Biopsies were significant for squamous esophageal mucosa with mild chronic esophagitis and gastric mucosa with increased eosinophils (reaching 26/high power field). Ampullary tissue showed chronic inflammation with focal increased eosinophils in the lamina propria; however, the exact eosinophilic count in the ampulla was not reported. Repeat ERCP was performed with stent removal, as well as sphincteroplasty/dilation of the papilla and distal CBD resulting in resolution of the stenosis. Repeat biopsies of the stomach and the ampulla showed benign glandular tissue with no eosinophils. Colonoscopy had been performed 5 years prior to presentation; findings were benign and did not show any eosinophilic infiltration of the colon.

Additionally, she was started on prednisone 40 mg daily, which was gradually tapered down by 10 mg a week. The patient demonstrated significant improvement with systemic steroid therapy. Liver function tests completely normalized, and eosinophil count trended down, but remained persistently elevated (13%). She was kept on 40 mg of pantoprazole twice a day and 2 mg of budesonide daily. Patient was monitored over six months, LFTs remained normal, and symptoms were controlled.

3. Discussion

We present a rare case of eosinophilic infiltration of the major ampulla which resulted in benign papillary stenosis. EGIDs represent a spectrum of inflammatory conditions classified by the infiltration of eosinophils in the gastrointestinal tract that manifests with variable clinical features [8]. Eosinophilic infiltration can involve any part of the gastrointestinal tract from the mouth to the anus and can infiltrate the gastrointestinal wall from the mucosa to the serosa [6]. Prevalence of EGIDs shows a primarily female predominance. Overall, EGIDs are rare, with less than 50,000 people affected in the US [9]. Manifestations are dependent on the location and extent of gastrointestinal involvement and more commonly present with abdominal pain, nausea, early satiety, vomiting, diarrhea, and weight loss [10]. Extraintestinal manifestations can be present in many patients such as seasonal allergies, atopy, and eczema [8].

Several imaging modalities and endoscopic procedures such as CT, MRI/MRCP, EGD, and EUS can be utilized to provide further insight into the condition when it involves the pancreatobiliary system [2]. In our patient, magnetic MRI/MRCP and EUS revealed CBD dilatation without choledocholithiasis but tapering of distal CBD towards the ampulla. EGD revealed antral gastritis, superficial gastric ulcers, and prominent major ampulla. ERCP revealed an inflamed major ampulla and benign papillary stenosis.

Biopsy is an important tool for establishing a diagnosis [2, 6]. Diagnosis of EGIDs often involves the presence of eosinophilic infiltration of the gastrointestinal tract on multiple biopsies as well as the absence of another disease process causing intestinal eosinophilia [2]. Similar to the patient's findings, gross endoscopic findings are generally nonspecific and may reveal mucosal edema, patchy erythematous changes, and superficial ulcerations, often mistaken for other gastrointestinal disorders [7]. The pathogenesis of EGIDs is not well understood and is thought to be related to the interaction between chemokines and eosinophils causing the release of cytokines such as interleukin-3, interleukin-5, and granulocyte colony-stimulating factor [11]. High cytotoxic granular proteins will release after excessive eosinophils accumulate in the mucosal tissue causing serious tissue destruction [5].

Treatment may vary depending on organ involvement, severity of symptoms, and extent of the disease [7]. In our patient, secondary to papillary stenosis, treatment was targeted to the biliary tree. The patient underwent endoscopic therapy with sphincterotomy, sphincteroplasty, and stent placement, as well as administration of systemic steroids. Systemic steroid therapy usually improves the symptoms of eosinophilic gastroenteritis, but in our patient, the ampulla was fibrotic appearing (likely secondary to sequalae of chronic inflammation), and the benign papillary stenosis was unlikely to resolve with steroid therapy alone. It required additional sphincterotomy, stent placement, and sphincteroplasty (balloon dilation of the papillae and the distal CBD). The same mechanism is also observed in esophageal stenosis in patients with eosinophilic esophagitis. A fibrotic stenosis of esophagus in the setting of eosinophilic esophagitis would require dilation as well as medical treatment with steroids and proton pump inhibitor [12].

Other treatment options include modified diets due to food sensitivities, glucocorticoids, and azathioprine to inhibit inflammatory eosinophilic growth factors, leukotriene receptor antagonists to diminish eosinophil chemoattraction, and biologic agents against targeted inflammatory mediators [7]. Lirentelimab, a newer agent, is an anti-Siglec-8 antibody that depletes eosinophils and inhibits mast cells. It has been used in phase 2 clinical trials with favorable outcomes. However, further studies are needed to validate these results [13].

Ampullitis leading to papillary stenosis secondary to eosinophilic infiltration in the major papilla is a rare manifestation of EGIDs. Early diagnosis would lead to appropriate medical and endoscopic management and perhaps prevention of sever strictures.

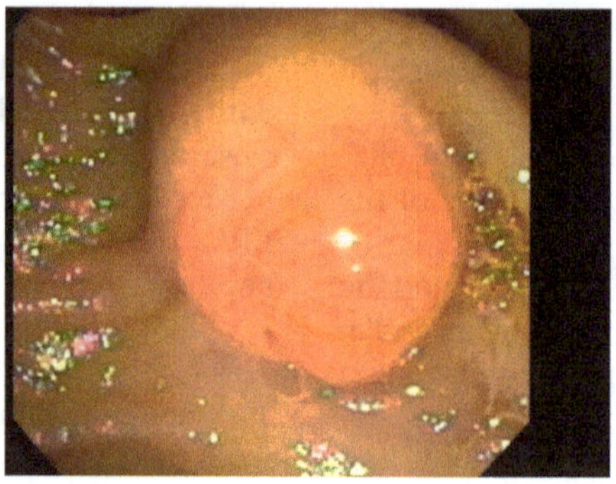

(a)

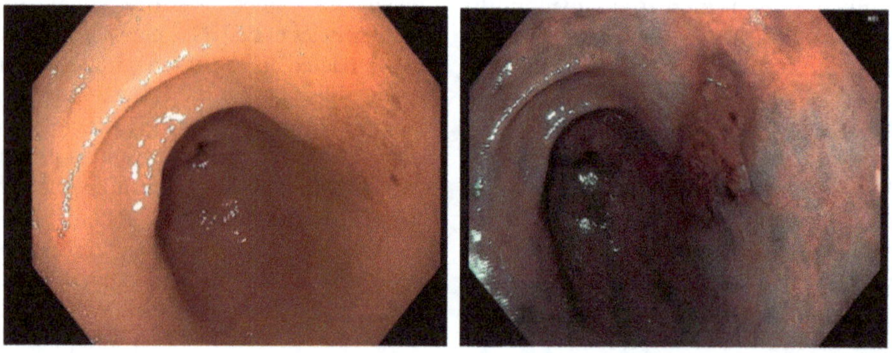

(b)

FIGURE 1: (a) Prominent and bulging major ampulla and (b) antral gastritis (superficial gastric ulcers).

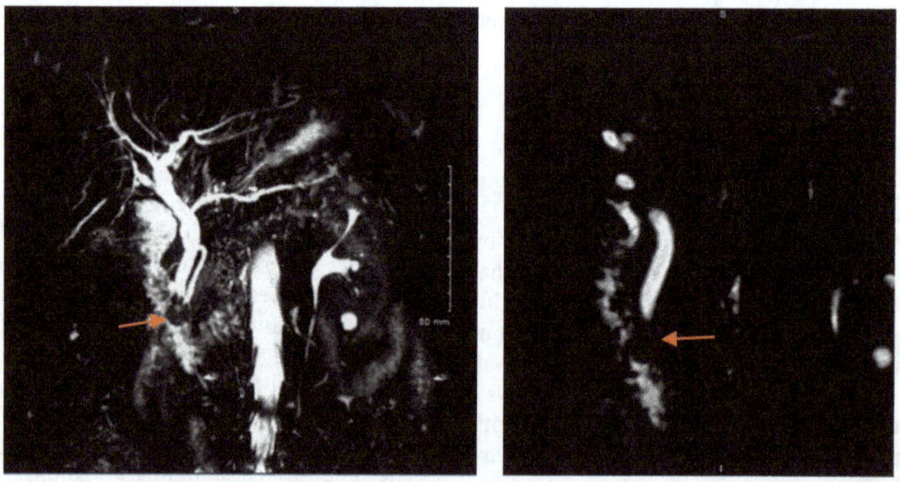

(a) (b)

FIGURE 2: MRI/MRCP showing CBD dilatation without choledocholithiasis as well as papillary stenosis.

Authors' Contributions

Dr. Akwe Nyabera, Dr. Nso Nso, and Keya Shah wrote the first draft of the manuscript. Dr. Akwe Nyabera and Dr. Nso Nso were involved in the concept and design. Dr. Akwe Nyabera, Dr. Nso Nso, Keya Shah, Dr. Saphwat Eskaros, and Dr. Negar Niknam performed the critical revision.

References

[1] N. Méndez-Sánchez, N. C. Chávez-Tapia, G. Vazquez-Elizondo, and M. Uribe, "Eosinophilic gastroenteritis: a review," *Digestive Diseases and Sciences*, vol. 52, no. 11, pp. 2904–2911, 2007.

[2] R. A. Sheikh, T. P. Prindiville, R. E. Pecha, and B. H. Ruebner, "Unusual presentations of eosinophilic gastroenteritis: case series and review of literature," *World Journal of Gastroenterology*, vol. 15, no. 17, pp. 2156–2161, 2009.

[3] M. M. Walker, M. Potter, and N. J. Talley, "Eosinophilic gastroenteritis and other eosinophilic gut diseases distal to the oesophagus," *The Lancet Gastroenterology & Hepatology*, vol. 3, no. 4, pp. 271–280, 2018.

[4] M. Y. Yun, Y. U. Cho, I. S. Park et al., "Eosinophilic gastroenteritis presenting as small bowel obstruction: a case report and review of the literature," *World Journal of Gastroenterology*, vol. 13, no. 11, pp. 1758–1760, 2007.

[5] R. Daneshjoo and N. J. Talley, "Eosinophilic gastroenteritis," *Current Gastroenterology Reports*, vol. 4, no. 5, pp. 366–372, 2002.

[6] V. Uppal, P. Kreiger, and E. Kutsch, "Eosinophilic gastroenteritis and colitis: a comprehensive review," *Clinical Reviews in Allergy & Immunology*, vol. 50, no. 2, pp. 175–188, 2016.

[7] A. A. Alfadda, M. A. Storr, and E. A. Shaffer, "Eosinophilic colitis: epidemiology, clinical features, and current management," *Therapeutic Advances in Gastroenterology*, vol. 4, no. 5, pp. 301–309, 2011.

[8] H. E. Oh and R. Chetty, "Eosinophilic gastroenteritis: a review," *Journal of Gastroenterology*, vol. 43, no. 10, pp. 741–750, 2008.

[9] E. T. Jensen, C. F. Martin, M. D. Kappelman, and E. S. Dellon, "Prevalence of eosinophilic gastritis, gastroenteritis, and colitis," *Journal of Pediatric Gastroenterology & Nutrition*, vol. 62, no. 1, pp. 36–42, 2016.

[10] K. J. Kelly, "Eosinophilic gastroenteritis," *Journal of Pediatric Gastroenterology and Nutrition*, vol. 30, no. 1, pp. 28–35, 2000.

[11] S. P. Hogan, A. Mishra, E. B. Brandt, P. S. Foster, and M. E. Rothenberg, "A critical role for eotaxin in experimental oral antigen-induced eosinophilic gastrointestinal allergy," *Proceedings of the National Academy of Sciences*, vol. 97, no. 12, pp. 6681–6686, 2000.

[12] W. J. Ravich, "Endoscopic management of benign esophageal strictures," *Current Gastroenterology Reports*, vol. 19, no. 10, p. 50, 2017.

[13] E. S. Dellon, K. A. Peterson, J. A. Murray et al., "Anti-Siglec-8 antibody for eosinophilic gastritis and duodenitis," *New England Journal of Medicine*, vol. 383, no. 17, pp. 1624–1634, 2020.

22

Systemic Lupus Erythematosus Presenting with Ischemic Proctitis and Abdominal Compartment Syndrome

Yousaf Bashir Hadi,[1] John Lindsay IV,[2] Syeda Fatima Zehra Naqvi,[1] and Hatim Al-Jaroushi[3]

[1]*Department of Medicine, West Virginia University, Morgantown, WV, USA*
[2]*West Virginia University School of Medicine, Morgantown, WV, USA*
[3]*Department of Medicine, Section of Pulmonary and Critical Care Medicine, West Virginia University, Morgantown, WV, USA*

Correspondence should be addressed to Yousaf Bashir Hadi; yousaf.hadi@hsc.wvu.edu

Academic Editor: Olga I. Giouleme

Ischemic colitis and proctitis is a rare manifestation of systemic lupus erythematosus (SLE) and results from mesenteric vasculitis. Owing to diverse blood supply and presence of multiple collaterals, rectum is the least effected site in SLE enteritis. Ischemic proctocolitis as the presenting feature of SLE is exceedingly rare, with only three cases reported in the published scientific literature. We present the first case of SLE presenting as ischemic proctitis, leading to intraperitoneal hemorrhage and abdominal compartment syndrome. A young lady presented with ischemic proctitis and a hematoma masquerading as a pelvic mass, with subsequent development of massive intraperitoneal hemorrhage, shock, and rectal perforation. The patient required urgent surgery and was initiated on high-dose steroids.

1. Introduction

Ischemic colitis and proctitis is a rare manifestation of systemic lupus erythematosus (SLE). It results from small-vessel vasculitis and is accompanied by high SLE disease activity, and can affect the small or large intestine. Diagnosis is confirmed with sigmoidoscopy and histopathology. Ischemic proctocolitis as the presenting feature of SLE is exceedingly rare, with only three cases reported in the published scientific literature [1–3]. No prior reports of hemorrhagic shock and perforations in this setting exist in the current literature. We present the first reported case of ischemic proctocolitis leading to massive intraperitoneal hemorrhage and hemorrhagic shock, with subsequent perforation as the initial presentation of SLE.

2. Case Presentation

A 39-year-old female presented to West Virginia University Hospitals' Intensive care unit as a transfer from an outside facility. She had initially presented to the outside facility with abdominal pain of 2 weeks' duration. The patient experienced worsening abdominal pain and weakness on the day of presentation, which prompted her to report to the outside facility. She was found to have a skin rash, involving her arms and face, which was biopsied, revealing a leukocytoclastic vasculitis. She was also found to have severe anemia and ascites. A computed tomography (CT) scan without contrast was concerning for an irregularity in the rectal lumen with a perirectal pelvic mass or hematoma. Over the course of her stay there, she developed hypotension and shock; she was intubated and transferred to our facility for further evaluation and management.

On presentation to West Virginia University, she was found to be in shock. She endorsed a past history of thrombocytopenia; the patient had been told that she had idiopathic thrombocytopenic purpura and splenectomy. She reported lower abdominal pain. Her initial blood pressure was 82/50, and she was pale on examination with large, tense ascites. Her hemoglobin on arrival was 4.4 gram/dl, white

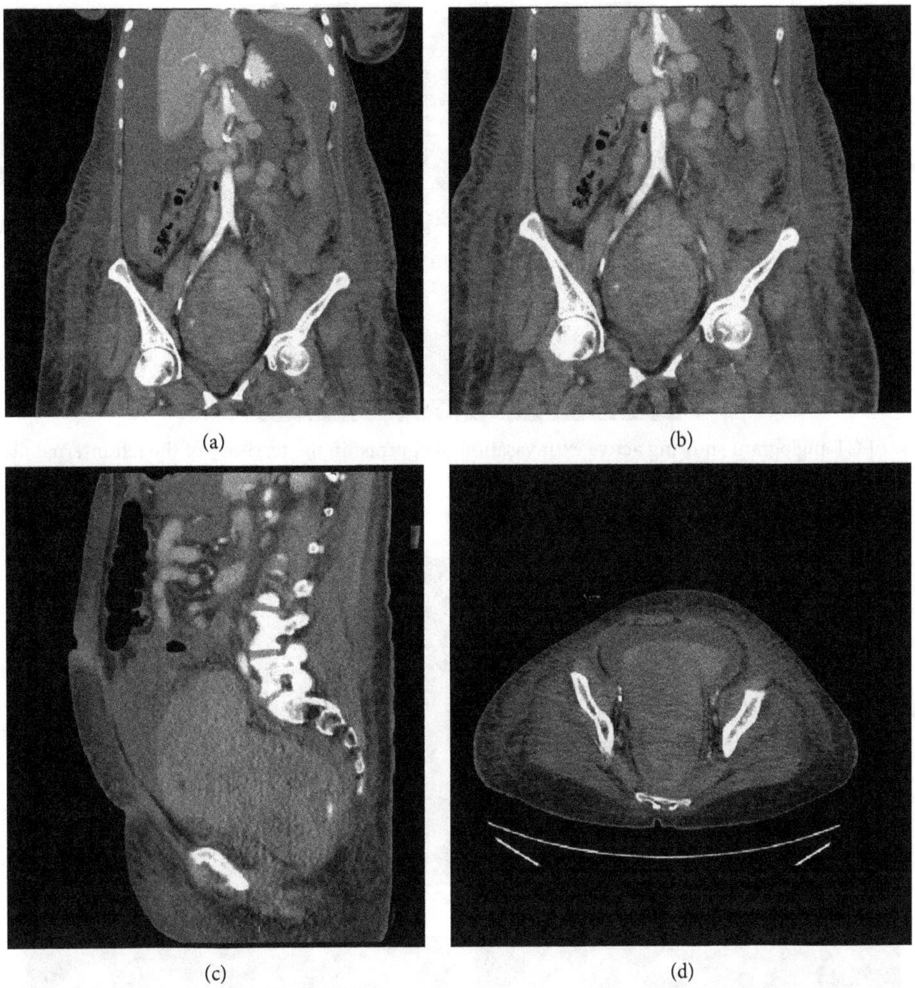

Figure 1: a, b) Coronal views of CT abdomen and pelvis with contrast show a heterogeneous, mass-like appearance of an organized rectal hematoma. (c) Sagittal view shows prominent rectal dilatation with high intensity signal showing probable active contrast extravasation. (d) Axial view of the hematoma.

blood cell count was 8500, and she had a fever of 101 degrees Fahrenheit. She was volume resuscitated with crystalloids and blood products, broad spectrum antibiotics were administered, and due to a concern for intra-abdominal bleeding, she was rushed to CT scanning. A CT scan of the abdomen and pelvis with contrast was obtained that revealed prominent distention of the rectum with heterogeneous density material within. It could represent a hematoma or a mass originating from a pelvic organ or the rectum itself. Large volume ascites was also noted, which likely represented hemorrhagic ascites. These findings can be seen on Figures 1(a)–1(d).

After returning from the scanner, the patient's hemodynamic state worsened; norepinephrine, vasopressin, and then phenylephrine were serially added subsequently. Her hemoglobin count was monitored closely, and she continued to require blood transfusions.

After 10 hours of presentation, the patient had received 7 blood transfusions, and she remained in hemorrhagic shock. Her abdominal pressures continued to worsen, and the patient was developing abdominal compartment syndrome; she had developed anuria and renal failure with no urine output since presentation, and her respiratory status was worsening, requiring higher positive end expiratory pressures. General surgery service did not find her a candidate for exploratory laparotomy due to hesitation from the patient and her family and the unclear diagnosis at that time. A paracentesis was performed at the bedside, with removal of 4 liters of bloody fluid. The patient had considerable improvement in her hemodynamic and respiratory status after her paracentesis and was weaned off vasopressors. However, her bleeding failed to resolve, and she continued to require blood transfusions with redevelopment of hemorrhagic shock. A detailed discussion was held with the family, and the surgical service and surgery was deferred. The patient was sent for a CT angiogram after a second paracentesis and removal of 4 liters of blood from her peritoneal cavity. The CT angiogram revealed active contrast extravasation, and

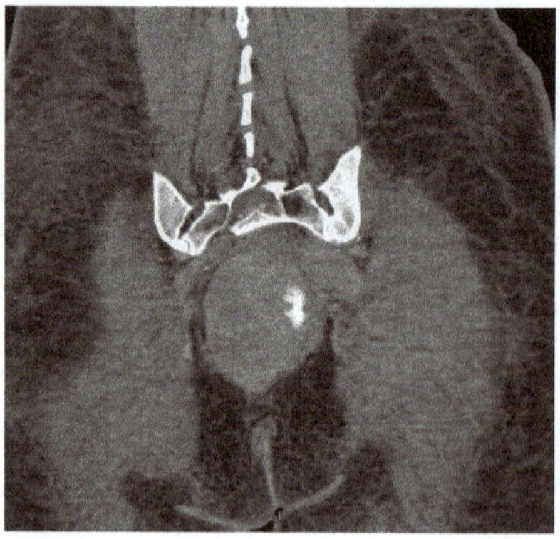

Figure 2: Sagittal view of CT angiogram showing active extravasation of contrast in the territory of the left internal iliac artery and inferior rectal artery.

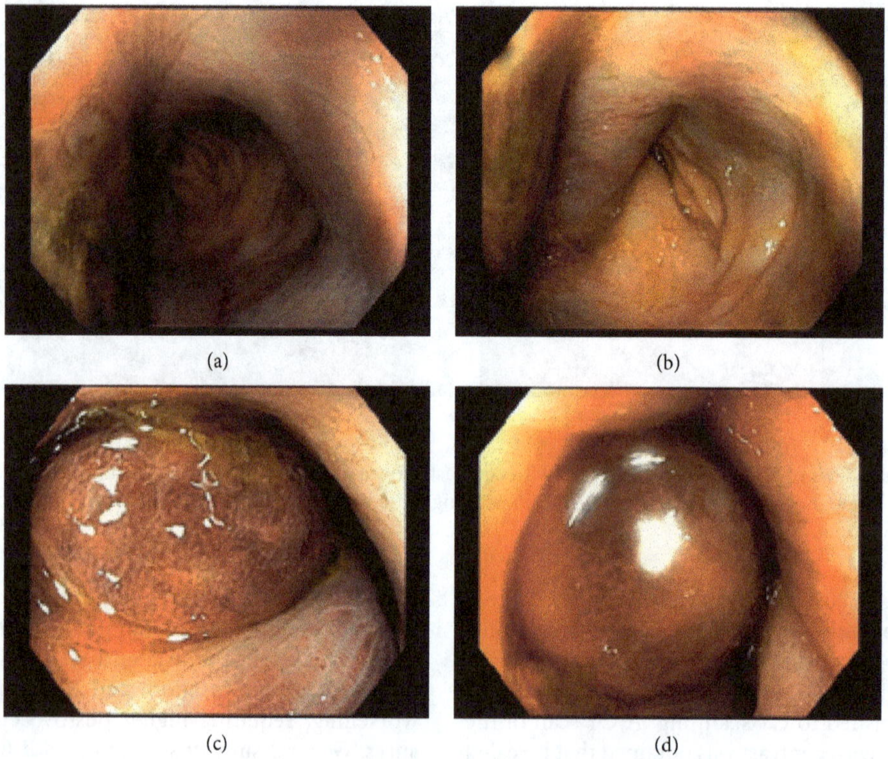

Figure 3: (a–d) Sigmoidoscopy images; an ischemic rectum with a bulging, tense hematoma in the rectal wall can be seen.

selective embolization of branches of her left inferior rectal and internal iliac vessel was performed. Figure 2 shows the CT angiogram with active extravasation.

The patient received an urgent sigmoidoscopy on returning to her room from her angiogram that revealed an ischemic rectum with a bulging, tense hematoma in the rectal wall, and no associated mass was identified (Figure 3). Findings appeared consistent with ischemic proctitis. The patient's hemoglobin stabilized and her abdomen remained soft and nontender, with marked improvement in her respiratory and hemodynamic state after the embolization.

A serum vasculitis panel, antinuclear antibodies (ANA), Anti-double stranded DNA antibodies (Anti-DS DNA), anti-phospholipid antibodies, and complement levels were checked. However, the next day, the patient developed sudden abdominal pain and guarding, with abdominal exam consistent with peritonitis, and her hemodynamic state acutely worsened. A CT scan was obtained without contrast that revealed pneumoperitoneum out of proportion to the history of recent paracenteses, and she was emergently taken to the operating room for exploratory laparotomy and underwent proctectomy and colostomy with abdominal washout. A large amount of intraperitoneal clots were removed. The next day, the patient's ANA and DsDNA antibodies came back as positive at levels of 1 : 320 and 734 IU/dl (normal: <150 IU/

dl), respectively. Low complement levels were found; C4 was 2 mg/dl (normal: 12–39 mg/dl), and C3 was 14 mg/dl (normal: 81–157 mg/dl). Anti-myeloperoxidase antibodies and phospholipid antibodies were negative, and anti-SS-A and SS-B antibodies also returned negative. A transthoracic echocardiogram revealed a mild-to-moderate pericardial effusion. The patient's biopsy showed two gross transmural perforations, ischemic proctocolitis, with acute serositis, and fat necrosis. Lymphocytic infiltration was noted. The patient was definitively diagnosed with ishemic proctocolitis secondary to active systemic lupus erythematosus, leading to intraperitoneal hemorrhage.

Over the course of the next three weeks, the patient was initiated on pulse dose methylprednisolone. The patient's renal function recovered. Rheumatology service was consulted, and the patient was initiated on hydroxychloroquine and was discharged after 3 weeks of surgery. At a follow-up of 6 months, the patient is doing well and continues her treatment for SLE. She has now been diagnosed with lupus nephritis with a renal biopsy.

3. Discussion

Gastrointestinal tract manifestations of SLE include intestinal pseudo-obstruction, lupus mesenteric vasculitis (LMV), protein losing enteropathy, or thrombosis of vasculature [4, 5]. Small bowel, usually the jejunum or ileum, seems to be most commonly affected [6]. Rarely, gastric and rectal involvement has also been described in the literature. Owing to diverse blood supply and presence of multiple collaterals, rectum is the least effected site in SLE enteritis. Previously, there are a total of three reports of proctitis as the presenting manifestation of SLE [1–3].

Lupus mesenteric vasculitis is the likely underlying mechanism of gut involvement in most of these cases. Unfortunately, no established histopathological hallmark of SLE enteritis currently exists [7]. Macroscopically and endoscopically, the appearance usually reflects edema, ulceration, gangrene, and rarely, perforation. GI involvement in SLE is usually diagnosed clinically, with imaging evidence as an adjunct, after exclusion of other gastrointestinal insults. Although SLE enteritis, with its reported prevalence of 0.2 to 9.7%, [8] is highly suspected in patients with established SLE, diagnosing SLE enteritis is a big challenge in patients with no previous SLE diagnosis.

Ischemic colitis is rare in SLE, with a reported incidence of 0.2%. However, it can prove life-threatening in cases where there is a delay in diagnosis and management [9, 10]. Our case resulted in a perforation and required emergent surgery, with significant associated morbidity. A high index of suspicion for SLE in patients presenting with fever and rash in an absence of infectious milieu can help expedite diagnosis and earlier initiation of immunosuppression. Our patient had initially presented with abdominal pain without ascites to the outside facility and developed shock and hemorrhage after a few days of presentation.

Treatment of SLE with vasculitis usually includes cyclophosphamide or some other immunosuppressant agent in addition to steroids. Our patient was initiated on methylprednisolone and hydroxychloroquine only. As the patient already showed a remarkable recovery, the addition of another agent was deferred. This level of response to steroids only is unusual.

Our patient was appropriately diagnosed with SLE based on serologic evidence; lack of probable alternate diagnoses, and fulfillment of the both the American College of Rheumatology (ACR) criteria and the Systemic Lupus International Collaborating Clinic (SLICC) criteria [11]. Initiation of steroids led to rapid recovery. Our patient had photosensitivity, rash, vasculitis, fever, and pericardial effusion, as well as positive serology. Although she self-reported being diagnosed with ITP in the past, serology from that time were not available.

In conclusion, we present an exceedingly rare presentation of SLE hitherto unreported in the published literature. Our patient presented with ischemic proctitis and a hematoma masquerading as a pelvic mass, with subsequent development of massive intraperitoneal hemorrhage, shock, and rectal perforation, as the presenting manifestation of SLE.

References

[1] P. Reissman, E. G. Weiss, T. A. Teoh, F. V. Lucas, and S. D. Wexner, "Gangrenous ischemic colitis of the rectum: a rare complication of systemic lupus erythematosus," *The American Journal of Gastroenterology*, vol. 89, no. 12, pp. 2234–2236, 1994.

[2] J. Teramoto, Y. Takahashi, S. Katsuki et al., "Systemic lupus erythematosus with a giant rectal ulcer and perforation," *Internal Medicine*, vol. 38, no. 8, pp. 643–649, 1999.

[3] P. Chattopadhyay, C. A. Philips, D. Dhua, and S. Saha, "Systemic lupus erythematosus presenting as ischaemic proctitis," *Lupus*, vol. 20, no. 6, pp. 653–655, 2011.

[4] X.-P. Tian and X. Zhang, "Gastrointestinal involvement in systemic lupus erythematosus: insight into pathogenesis, diagnosis and treatment," *World Journal of Gastroenterology*, vol. 16, no. 24, p. 2971, 2010.

[5] H. Chng, B. Tan, C. Teh, and T. Lian, "Major gastrointestinal manifestations in lupus patients in Asia: lupus enteritis, intestinal pseudo-obstruction, and protein-losing gastroenteropathy," *Lupus*, vol. 19, no. 12, pp. 1404–1413, 2010.

[6] C.-K. Lee, M. Ahn, E. Lee et al., "Acute abdominal pain in systemic lupus erythematosus: focus on lupus enteritis (gastrointestinal vasculitis)," *Annals of the Rheumatic Diseases*, vol. 61, no. 6, pp. 547–550, 2002.

[7] M. S. Cappell, "Intestinal (mesenteric) vasculopathy ii," *Gastroenterology Clinics of North America*, vol. 27, no. 4, pp. 827–860, 1998.

[8] J. H. Ju, J.-K. Min, C.-K. Jung et al., "Lupus mesenteric vasculitis can cause acute abdominal pain in patients with SLE," *Nature Reviews Rheumatology*, vol. 5, no. 5, pp. 273–281, 2009.

[9] S. Miyahara, S. Ito, A. Soeda et al., "Two cases of systemic lupus erythematosus complicated with colonic ulcers," *Internal Medicine*, vol. 44, no. 12, pp. 1298–1306, 2005.

[10] T.-C. Tan, G.-L. Wansaicheong, and B.-H. Thong, "Acute onset of systemic lupus erythematosus with extensive gas-

trointestinal and genitourinary involvement," *Lupus*, vol. 21, no. 11, pp. 1240–1243, 2012.

[11] J. Tiao, R. Feng, K. Carr, J. Okawa, and V. P. Werth, "Using the American College of Rheumatology (ACR) and Systemic Lupus International Collaborating Clinics (SLICC) criteria to determine the diagnosis of systemic lupus erythematosus (SLE) in patients with subacute cutaneous lupus erythematosus (SCLE)," *Journal of the American Academy of Dermatology*, vol. 74, no. 5, pp. 862–869, 2016.

23

Leukocytoclastic Vasculitis as a Rare Dermatologic Extraintestinal Manifestation of Ulcerative Colitis in an Elderly Patient with Positive PR3-ANCA

Jacky Ng,[1] David Zezoff,[2] and Hanadi Abou Dargham[2]

[1]*Touro University California, 1310 Club Dr, Vallejo, CA 94592, USA*
[2]*Graduate Medical Education, St. Joseph's Medical Center, 1800 N California St, Stockton, CA 95204, USA*

Correspondence should be addressed to Jacky Ng; jacky.ng2@tu.edu

Academic Editor: Hirotada Akiho

Ulcerative colitis is an inflammatory bowel disease that in rare cases may develop extraintestinal manifestations. This case report aims to add to the limited clinical data on leukocytoclastic vasculitis and possible ANCA-associated vasculitis as rare cutaneous and rheumatologic extraintestinal manifestations of IBD, particularly in elderly patients. Our case involves a 79-year-old male with a history of mild-moderate ulcerative colitis on oral mesalamine 2.4 g daily and pyoderma gangrenosum who presented with recurrent bilateral polyarthralgia, joint swelling, diffuse lower extremity purpura, acute kidney injury, and scrotal rash. Autoimmune titers were significant for positive ANA and PR3-ANCA. Biopsy of purpuric lesions demonstrated findings suggestive of leukocytoclastic vasculitis. The patient was promptly treated with pulse-dose methylprednisolone for 3 days with rapid improvement of symptoms.

1. Introduction

Ulcerative colitis (UC) is an inflammatory bowel disease (IBD) characterized by autoimmune damage to the colonic mucosa. It most commonly involves the rectum and may extend proximally to other portions of the colon. UC is known to have unique extraintestinal manifestations that frequently affect the joints, skin, or eyes. [1] However, it is rare for the coexistence of small-vessel vasculitis and these enteropathic symptoms without active bowel disease. [2] In our case, we present a 79-year-old male with a significant history of mild-moderate UC and pyoderma gangrenosum who presented with diffuse polyarthralgia with swelling, extensive bilateral lower extremity purpura, scrotal ulcerations, and acute kidney injury. Serological testing was significant for PR3-ANCA antibodies, and dermatological evaluation of the purpura was consistent with leukocytoclastic vasculitis. The patient was treated with pulse-dose methylprednisolone for 3 days with rapid improvements in arthralgias, bilateral leg rash, and renal function. The patient was eventually discharged to a skilled nursing facility for rehabilitation of deconditioning and advanced medical needs.

2. Case Description

A 79-year-old male with a significant history of mild-moderate ulcerative colitis on oral mesalamine 2.4 g daily and pyoderma gangrenosum, hypertension, coronary artery disease, and benign prostatic hypertrophy presented to the emergency department for evaluation of bilateral polyarthralgia with associated weakness and swelling (including the metacarpal joints and ankles; see Figure 1), diffuse lower extremity purpura, violaceous rash (see Figure 2), and scrotal ulcerations. He had similar pains 3 months prior to presentation, but symptoms resolved without medical intervention. Notably, he reported the rash on his lower extremities started one week prior to presentation and was initially pruritic. However, this too gradually abated.

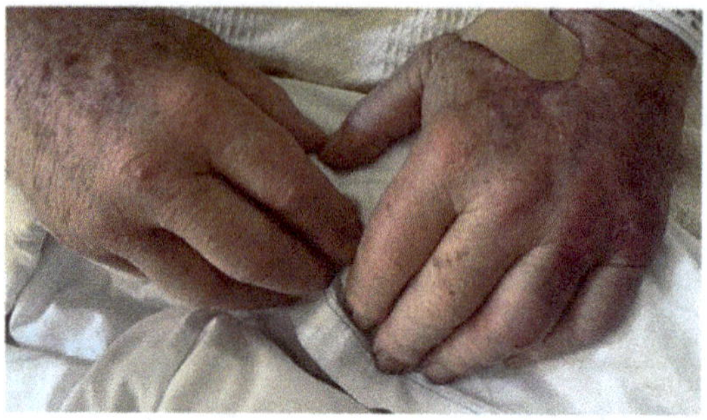

FIGURE 1: The patient had been prescribed oral mesalamine 2.4 g twice a day in the past as a treatment for his ulcerative colitis, but the patient admitted to noncompliance due to inability to care for himself.

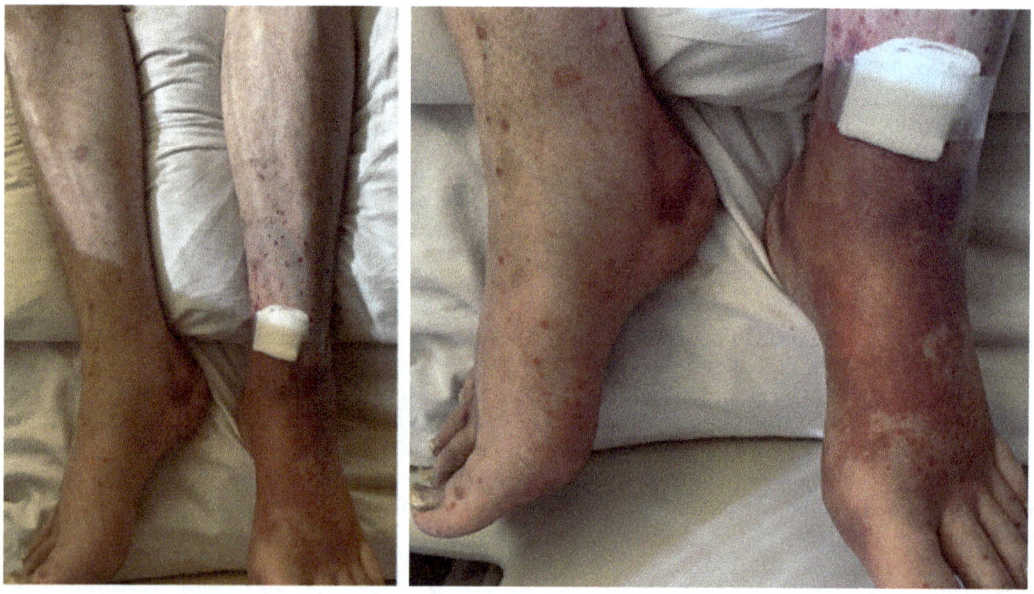

FIGURE 2: Status post skin biopsy, initiation of pulse-dose Solu-Medrol.

Initial lab work demonstrated acute kidney injury with a creatinine of 3.6 mg/dL (normal range: 0.7–1.3 mg/dL). Urinalysis was positive for gross hematuria and proteinuria. Coagulation studies showed elevated fibrinogen levels at 882 mg/dL (normal range: 200–393 md/dL), elevated PT/INR at 16.2 and 1.4, respectively, and elevated PTT at 41.4. Inflammatory markers such as ESR and CRP were also elevated at 84 mm/hr (NR < 20 mm/hr) and 32.53 mg/dL (NR: 0.01–0.82 mg/dL), respectively. CT abdomen and pelvis without IV contrast demonstrated no evidence of diverticulitis, colitis, or ischemic bowel disease, no mechanical bowel obstruction, perforation, or free air, + air-fluid levels within the rectum without wall thickening, marked distention of the urinary bladder, and prostatomegaly. CT chest w/o contrast and CXR were unremarkable.

Given these diagnostic findings and the patient's subacute onset purpura with confluence below the waist and worsening bilateral MCP, shoulder, knee, and dorsal foot joint swelling and pain, rheumatology was consulted. Autoimmune/vasculitis-related titers were sent, which were grossly unremarkable except for positive antinuclear antibodies (ANA), anti-chromatin/nucleosome antibodies, and proteinase-3 antineutrophil cytoplasmic antibodies (PR3-ANCA/c-ANCA). Nephrology was onboard due to concerns for pauci-immune glomerulonephritis, but the patient did not exhibit symptoms specific to granulomatosis polyangiitis (GPA), such as nasal or respiratory complications. Additionally, no casts were present in urinalysis. Because of the patient's age and elevated PSA, he was not a candidate for cyclophosphamide or any other immunosuppressive therapy. Rheumatology postulated the cause to be extraintestinal manifestations of poorly controlled ulcerative colitis, but due to the unclear diagnosis, skin biopsy was taken by general surgery and sent to pathology. The patient was treated empirically with high-dose Solu-Medrol for 3 days. Patient's joint pain, skin rash (see Figure 3), and kidney function continued to improve day to day under the high-dose Solu-Medrol regimen. Final pathology of left leg skin biopsy, along with clinical correlates, demonstrated findings compatible with leukocytoclastic vasculitis. The patient was discharged to SNF for rehabilitation, and it was recommended that he follows with his primary care, gastroenterologist, cardiologist, and rheumatologist. Unfortunately, the patient shortly thereafter was infected with the deadly

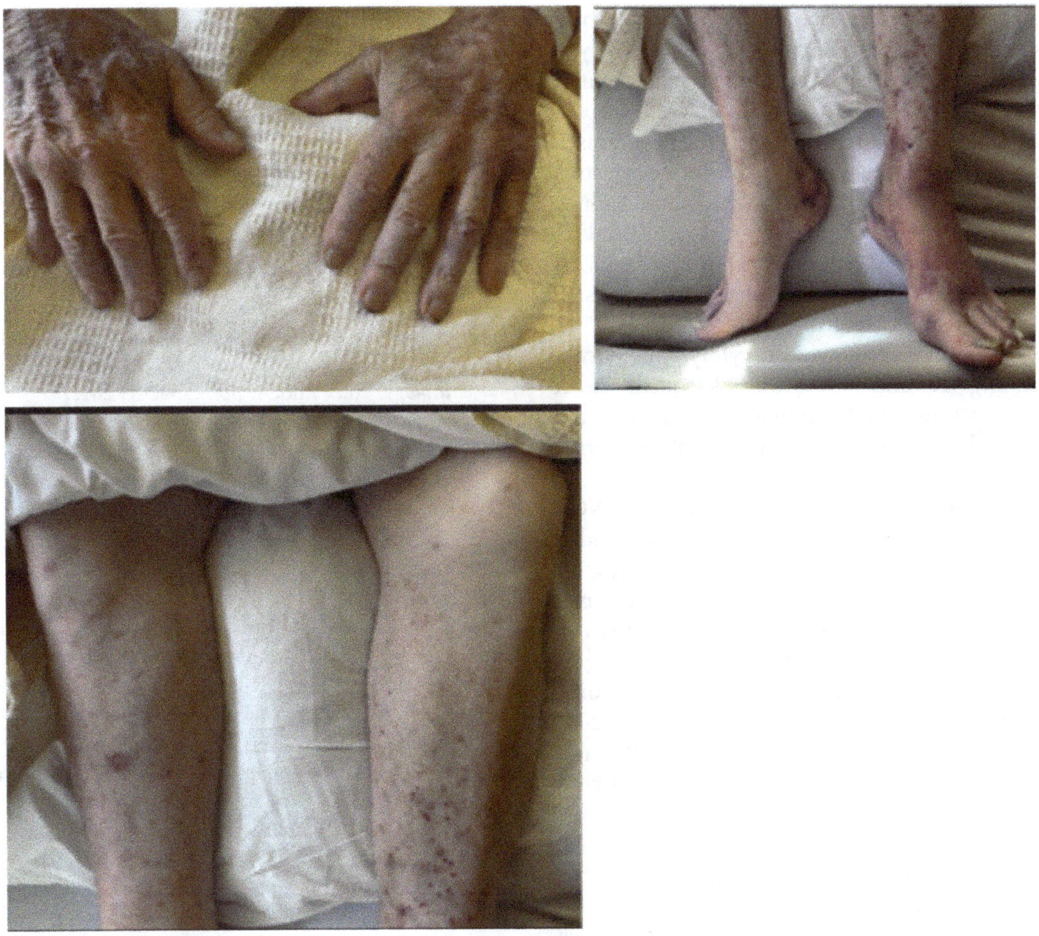

FIGURE 3: 3 days post-Solu-Medrol treatment with improvement in purpura and arthralgias.

virus SARS-CoV-2 and was placed on hospice after he developed complications of COVID-19.

3. Discussion

Ulcerative colitis (UC) is an inflammatory bowel disease (IBD) that commonly causes continuous colonic inflammation and lesions, but is also known to be associated with extraintestinal manifestations (EIM) including rash, such as pyoderma gangrenosum or erythema nodosum, arthritis, primary sclerosis cholangitis, ulcerations, and more. [3] The pathogenesis of EIM in IBD is still unclear, but is believed to be involved with an upregulated immune response at the extraintestinal site due to shared epitopes [1]. In the literature, multiple EIM may occur simultaneously and the presence of one EIM can confer a higher likelihood to develop further additional EIM [1]. It is reported that skin manifestations occur in about 15% of patients with IBD and is most commonly associated with pyoderma gangrenosum and erythema nodosum [4, 5]. Joint symptoms affecting peripheral large and small joints occur in up to 40% of patients with IBD and typically demonstrate minimal to no erosions [6–8]. They are classified into 2 types: type 1 (pauciarticular) arthralgia, which is typically asymmetric/migratory involvement affecting less than 5 large joints, or type 2 (polyarticular) arthralgia, which is frequently symmetrical involving 5 or more small joints. Type 1 is associated with active intestinal disease activity and high frequency of other EIM, whereas type 2 may be independent of active intestinal symptoms and is associated only with uveitis [6, 8]. Additionally, type 1 is usually self-resolving or improves with anti-inflammatory treatment whereas type 2 symptoms may be refractory to anti-inflammatory treatment and can persist for months to years. In our case, based on the above evidence and the patient's previous history of pyoderma gangrenosum, it is found that our patient presented with type 1 pauciarticular arthralgia.

A unique manifestation of our patient's ulcerative colitis flare-up was the vasculitis involvement with leukocytoclastic vasculitis (LCV). Leukocytoclastic vasculitis manifests as an exceedingly rare palpable, purpuric skin lesion, typically of the lower extremities, which was representative in our case [9, 10]. As of 2014, less than 20 cases of LCV have been reported in relation to UC in the English literature [11]. Upon the review of these cases in the literature, it was noticed that LCV involved juvenile to young adult patients; on the other hand, LCV manifested in an elderly patient in our case [11–14]. It appears that there is no apparent pattern in whether LCV precedes or succeeds intestinal symptoms [15]. Blanco et al. reported LCV as an immune complex-mediated disease in which the deposition of immune complexes within the subendothelial space in the wall of small dermal vessels leads to a cascade of events, triggering the activation of complement, leukostasis, release of lysosomal enzymes, and consequent rupture and extravasation of erythrocytes and tissue necrosis [16]. Ulcerative colitis shares a similar pathogenesis in which immune mechanisms and deposition of immune complexes occur in the intestinal mucosa instead of the vascular wall [17]. This would support the theory of how treating the underlying UC results in LCV remittance. However, the exact relationship between LCV and UC is still in debate [1, 13]. Miossec et al. proposed such a relational mechanism, stating that unregulated Th17 responses from interleukin-21 enhanced cytolytic activity as the culprit linking UC and LCV [18]. Subsequent downstream effects contribute to inflammation, ischemia, and impaired mucosal healing, resulting in intestinal and dermal damage [19].

Ulcerative colitis is typically associated with pANCA, which are antibodies directed against myeloperoxidase (MPO-ANCA), and is specific for microscopic polyangiitis. However, in this case, cANCA, or antibodies against proteinase-3 (PR3-ANCA), was demonstrated. cANCA is commonly associated with granulomatosis with polyangiitis (formerly Wegener's granulomatosis), for which this diagnosis was plausible [20]. Recent literature has used cANCA as a biomarker differentiating UC from CD [21, 22], and it has been associated with various systemic diseases such as lupus erythematosus (SLE), rheumatoid arthritis, IBDs, endocarditis, and other infections and malignancies [23]. To our knowledge, the current literature detailing the specific role of cANCA in relation to positive ANA and anticentromere antibodies is limited. However, cANCA positivity in this case likely represents UC with extensive disease as supported by Mahler et al [24]. This would be in concordance with the patient's lack of medical adherence with mesalamine coupled with his multiple EIMs. The argument supporting the differential of a pauci-immune glomerulonephritis, such as granulomatosis with polyangiitis, is less likely. The classical presentation of GPA typically involves nasal, pulmonary, or confirmed renal involvement, which were absent in this case [25]. The patient's acute kidney injury rapidly improved with resolution of his urinary retention after Foley catheter insertion, ruling out a glomerular cause of injury. A kidney biopsy was not performed during his hospital stay given the rapid improvement in his kidney function post steroid therapy.

4. Conclusion

Our case report adds to the limited clinical data on leukocytoclastic vasculitis and possible ANCA-associated vasculitis as rare cutaneous and rheumatologic extraintestinal manifestations of IBD, particularly in elderly patients. Patients with a history of ulcerative colitis presenting with a clinical picture of purpuric skin lesions, polyarthralgias, and acute kidney injury should be promptly evaluated for rare extraintestinal manifestations of inflammatory bowel disease. Definitive treatment of patient's underlying UC with high-dose systemic corticosteroids led to marked improvement of LCV, arthralgias, and kidney function.

References

[1] S. R. Vavricka, A. Schoepfer, M. Scharl, P. L. Lakatos, A. Navarini, and G. Rogler, "Extraintestinal manifestations of inflammatory bowel disease," *Inflammatory Bowel Diseases*, vol. 21, no. 8, pp. 1982–1992, 2015.

[2] S. Humbert, P. Guilpain, X. Puéchal et al., "Inflammatory bowel diseases in anti-neutrophil cytoplasmic antibody-associated vasculitides: 11 retrospective cases from the French Vasculitis Study Group," *Rheumatology*, vol. 54, no. 11, pp. 1970–1975, 2015.

[3] J. S. Levine and R. Burakoff, "Extraintestinal manifestations of inflammatory bowel disease," *Gastroenterology and Hepatology*, vol. 7, no. 4, pp. 235–241, 2011.

[4] A. J. Greenstein, H. D. Janowitz, and D. B. Sachar, "The extraintestinal complications of Crohn's disease and ulcerative colitis: a study of 700 patients," *Medicine (Baltimore)*, vol. 55, no. 5, pp. 401–412, 1976.

[5] R. S. W. Basler and H. V. Dubin, "Ulcerative colitis and the skin," *Archives of Dermatology*, vol. 112, no. 4, pp. 531–534, 1976.

[6] S. R. Vavricka, L. Brun, P. Ballabeni et al., "Frequency and risk factors for extraintestinal manifestations in the Swiss inflammatory bowel disease cohort," *American Journal of Gastroenterology*, vol. 106, no. 1, pp. 110–119, 2010.

[7] S. Smale, R. S. Natt, T. R. Orchard, A. S. Russell, and I. Bjarnason, "Inflammatory bowel disease and spondylarthropathy," *Arthritis & Rheumatism*, vol. 44, no. 12, pp. 2728–2736, 2001.

[8] T. R. Orchard, B. P. Wordsworth, and D. P. Jewell, "Peripheral arthropathies in inflammatory bowel disease: their articular distribution and natural history," *Gut*, vol. 42, no. 3, pp. 387–391, 1998.

[9] W. M. Sams, E. G. Thorne, P. Small, M. F. Mass, R. M. McIntosh, and R. E. Stanford, "Leukocytoclastic vasculitis," *Archives of Dermatology*, vol. 112, pp. 219–226, 1976.

[10] T. M. Lotti, C. Comacchi, and I. Ghersetich, "Cutaneous necrotizing vasculitis," *Rheumaderm*, vol. 455, pp. 115–125, 1999.

[11] G. T. Butts, P. R. Bishop, J. P. Wyatt, and M. J. Nowicki, "Leukocytoclastic vasculitis in an adolescent with ULCERATIVE colitis: report of a case and review of the literature," *SAGE Open Medical Case Reports*, vol. 2, Article ID 2050313X1454760, 2014.

[12] F. Iannone, C. Scioscia, and A. Musio, "Leucocytoclastic vasculitis as onset symptom of ulcerative colitis," *Annals of the Rheumatic Diseases*, vol. 62, no. 8, pp. 785-786, 2003.

[13] D. Martin, T. Handler, and J. McDermott, "Leucocytoclastic vasculitis in SEVERE ulcerative colitis," *Military Medicine*, vol. 176, no. 5, pp. 581–583, 2011.

[14] S. Akbulut, E. Ozaslan, F. Topal, L. Albayrak, B. Kayhan, and C. Efe, "Ulcerative colitis presenting as leukocytoclastic vasculitis of skin," *World Journal of Gastroenterology*, vol. 14, no. 15, p. 2448, 2008.

[15] F. Tripodi Cutrì, R. Salerno, A. Lo Schiavo, A. G. Gravina, M. Romano, and E. Ruocco, "Ulcerative colitis associated with leukocytoclastic vasculitis of the skin," *Digestive and Liver Disease*, vol. 41, no. 7, pp. e42–e44, 2009.

[16] R. Blanco, V. M. Martinez-Taboada, V. Rodriguez-Valverde, and M. Garcia-Fuentes, "Cutaneous vasculitis in children and adults," *Medicine (Baltimore)*, vol. 77, no. 6, pp. 403–418, 1998.

[17] B. R. Smoller, N. S. McNutt, and F. Contreras, "The natural history of vasculitis," *Archives of Dermatology*, vol. 126, no. 1, pp. 84–89, 1990.
[18] P. Miossec, T. Korn, and V. K. Kuchroo, "Interleukin-17 and type 17 helper T cells," *New England Journal of Medicine*, vol. 361, no. 9, pp. 888–898, 2009.
[19] A. Robinson, S. Keely, J. Karhausen, M. E. Gerich, G. T. Furuta, and S. P. Colgan, "Mucosal protection by hypoxia-inducible factor prolyl hydroxylase inhibition," *Gastroenterology*, vol. 134, no. 1, pp. 145–155, 2008.
[20] A. Wiik, "What you should know about PR3-ANCA. An introduction," *Arthritis Research*, vol. 2, no. 4, pp. 252–4, 2000.
[21] M. T. Arias-Loste, G. Bonilla, I. Moraleja et al., "Presence of anti-proteinase 3 antineutrophil cytoplasmic antibodies (ANTI-PR3 ANCA) as serologic markers in inflammatory bowel disease," *Clinical Reviews in Allergy and Immunology*, vol. 45, no. 1, pp. 109–116, 2013.
[22] M. P. Horn, A. M. Peter, F. Righini Grunder et al., "PR3-ANCA and panel diagnostics in pediatric inflammatory bowel disease to distinguish ulcerative colitis from Crohn's disease," *PLoS One*, vol. 13, no. 12, Article ID e0208974, 2018.
[23] M. Weiner and M. Segelmark, "The clinical presentation and therapy of diseases related to Anti-Neutrophil Cytoplasmic antibodies (ANCA)," *Autoimmunity Reviews*, vol. 15, no. 10, pp. 978–982, 2016.
[24] M. Mahler, D. P. Bogdanos, P. Pavlidis et al., "Pr3-anca: a promising biomarker for ulcerative colitis with extensive disease," *Clinica Chimica Acta*, vol. 424, pp. 267–273, 2013.
[25] J. C. Jennette, R. J. Falk, and A. H. Gasim, "Pathogenesis of antineutrophil cytoplasmic autoantibody vasculitis," *Current Opinion in Nephrology and Hypertension*, vol. 20, no. 3, pp. 263–270, 2011.

24

Crohn's Disease Diagnosed in a Man with Sarcoidosis: Coincidence or Correspondence?

Krystal Mills, Shaheen Fatima, and Norberto Fas

Internal Medicine Program, Morehouse School of Medicine, 720 Westview Drive SW, Atlanta, GA 30310, USA

Correspondence should be addressed to Krystal Mills; kmills@msm.edu

Academic Editor: Yoshiro Kawahara

Crohn's disease and sarcoidosis are characterized by noncaseating granulomas, but rarely do they present in the same patient. Their coexistence presents a diagnostic challenge as they are often classified as clinically separate, despite their similarities. We present a case of a 59-year-old man previously diagnosed with pulmonary sarcoidosis who presented to the emergency room with abdominal pain and diarrhea. Colonoscopy revealed multiple ulcers in the colon, with histology in keeping with newly diagnosed Crohn's colitis. The patient had a good clinical response to initiation of steroid therapy and a tumor necrosis factor (TNF) inhibitor.

1. Background

Crohn's disease (CD) and sarcoidosis (SA) are both granulomatous disorders, but it is estimated that the concurrence of these diseases in the same patient may be as rare as one person in 10,000,000 [1, 2]. CD is characterized by gastrointestinal involvement [3], whereas SA is characterized by respiratory involvement [4]. However, there are overlapping clinicopathological features which support a possible correlation between these granulomatous disorders.

2. Case Report

A 59-year-old African American man with a medical history of pulmonary sarcoidosis presented to the emergency room with a one-month history of abdominal pain and diarrhea. He had been discharged four days prior to this index presentation, after presenting with similar symptoms that was treated as infectious colitis. The abdominal pain was greatest in the periumbilical region and cramping in character. Since the initial onset, the pain changed from intermittent to constant in duration and increased in severity from 4 out of 10 to 10 out of 10. He endorsed associated nausea, unintentional weight loss, bloating, loud bowel sounds, seven to ten loose stools per day, hematochezia, and tenesmus. He also reported a painful genital ulcer and endorsed pain in the distal interphalangeal joints of the fourth digits of his hands that was worse in the morning. He denied other skin changes, fever, chills, vomiting, exposure to ill contacts, new foods, or recent travel. He was a former smoker with a 39-year pack history, drank beer daily, but denied illicit drug use. He denied any personal or family history of inflammatory bowel disease or colon cancer. His colonoscopy three years prior was significant for diverticula and a benign polyp which was removed.

On examination, he was in painful distress and tachycardic with other vitals within normal limits. Abdominal examination revealed hyperactive bowel sounds and diffuse abdominal tenderness with voluntary and involuntary guarding. He had a right inguinal genital ulcer and scattered pustules on his back. Laboratory results revealed hemoglobin, 9.2 g/dL; hematocrit, 31.1%; MCV, 76.4 fL; platelet count, 503 K/cmm; ferritin, 13 L; total iron, 13 L; iron saturation, 4; PT, 16.5 sec; INR, 1.35; vitamin K, <50 mcg; albumin, 3.3 g/dL; C-reactive protein, 81.2 mg/L; ESR, >100 mm/hr; and negative tuberculosis skin test. CT abdomen showed asymmetric wall thickening with subtle adjacent pericolic fat stranding and mesenteric vessel engorgement involving the transverse and proximal sigmoid colon (Figures 1 and 2).

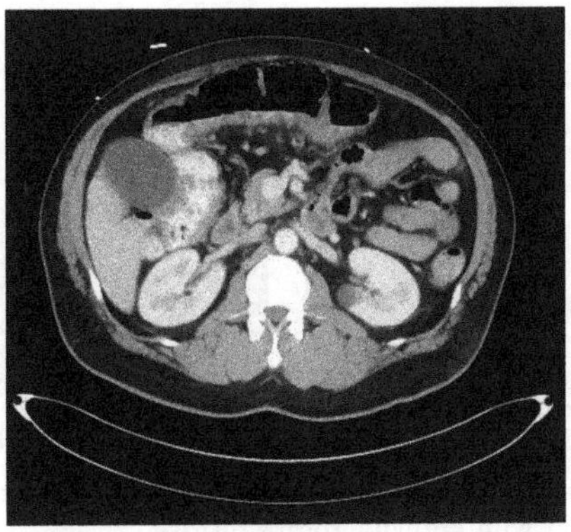

FIGURE 1: CT abdomen image showing asymmetric wall thickening with subtle adjacent pericolonic fat stranding and mesenteric vessel engorgement involving the transverse and proximal sigmoid colon.

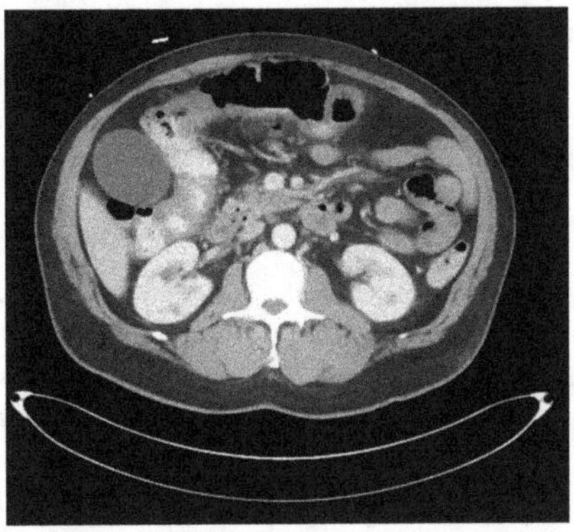

FIGURE 2: CT abdomen image showing multiple shotty mesenteric lymph nodes, which are nonspecific, possibly reactive related to the colonic process.

Stool studies were negative for infection. Punch biopsy of the genital ulcer done for H&E and infectious studies revealed fibrosis and inflammatory infiltrate, and tissue culture revealed no yeast or fungi. Colonoscopy revealed a large deep ulcer in the midtransverse colon and a few ulcers in the distal descending and sigmoid colon. Colon biopsies resulted as focal active colitis in the right colon, moderate active colitis with crypt abscess formation and ulceration in the transverse colon, and fragments of regenerative/hyperplastic colonic mucosa with ulceration in the descending colon. He was started on solumedrol 30 mg IV twice daily and then transitioned to oral steroids and anti-TNF-alpha therapy. The patient reported improvement in symptoms at one-month follow-up. He had a repeat colonoscopy eight months later that showed persistent active colitis that was improving, and he was continued on anti-TNF-alpha therapy (Figure 3).

3. Discussion

Although CD and SA are both granulomatous disorders, their coexistence in the same patient is exceptionally rare [3] and scarcely reported in the literature [5–8]. Noncaseating granulomas are considered the pathologic hallmark of CD and SA [9, 10], but the primary location of granulomas differs. The diseases sometimes mimic each other as respiratory involvement has been reported in up to 40–50% of inflammatory bowel disease (IBD) [4], and gastrointestinal involvement may occur in 10% of sarcoidosis [5].

SA of the digestive tract primarily involves the stomach, unlike the ileocolic involvement seen in CD. Respiratory involvement in IBD varies from airway disease to diseases of the lung parenchymal vessels or pleura and adverse drug reactions [2–4]. Extra-intestinal manifestations of CD parallel the systemic manifestations of SA. In this index case, the patient's groin ulcer was in keeping with pyoderma gangrenosum (PG), which is associated with CD and SA. PG occurs in only 0.5–5% of patients with IBD [11] and exhibits a female preponderance. It is even rarer in patients with SA and typically occurs after trauma. It is unclear whether PG is related to the disease activity of CD or SA, but the use of immunosuppressive agents, which this patient received, resolves the condition.

CD and SA are more common in women and exhibit a peak in the second to third decade of life [12, 13]. The patient in our case was male and older than 40 years, further underscoring his exceptionally unique presentation. The patient was African American, and this race is disproportionately affected by SA [13]. This differs from CD, which is

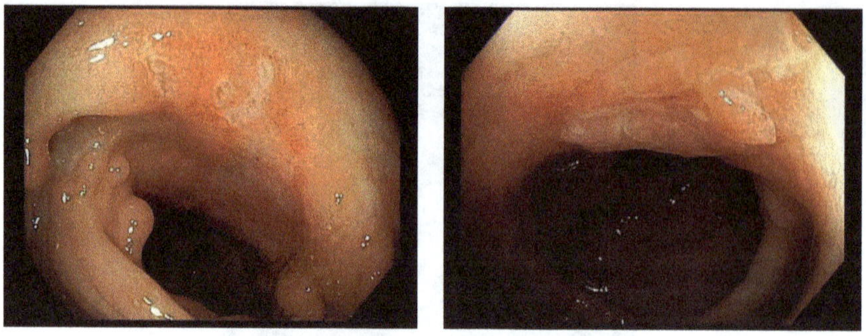

FIGURE 3: Elective colonoscopy repeated as outpatient was significant for multiple scattered pseudopolyps and discrete ulcerations seen from the transverse colon to sigmoid colon consistent with known Crohn's disease.

most common in non-Hispanic whites. His history of smoking was his most likely environmental risk factor for CD. His age at diagnosis of CD conferred a good prognosis as persons diagnosed after 60 years of age are less likely to develop complicated CD [12]. There were no granulomas seen on pathology, but they are found in only 30% of patients with CD, more commonly in women and often with more severe disease [14].

At the genetic level, the nucleotide-binding oligomerization domain-containing protein 2 (NOD2) polymorphisms present in CD have been found in a juvenile form of SA known as Blau syndrome [15, 16]. A genome-wide association study performed on CD and SA patients revealed that the most significant association was with the single-nucleotide polymorphism (SNP) rs1398024 on chromosome 10p12.2 and unidentified variants in the C10ORF67 gene region that may be underlying risk factors [17]. Other genetic associations between SA and CD include butyrophilin-like 2 (BTNL2), interleukin-23 receptor, and HERC2 [18].

Theories for coexistence include SA arising as a direct or indirect side effect of the medication used to treat CD. However, in our case, SA preceded CD. In patients with this temporal relation, there are theories that the conditions may be phenotypical manifestations of the same disease spectrum or arise from separate stimuli in which the inciting agent is inhaled in SA and ingested in CD [19]. This case serves to highlight similarities between CD and SA that are not well understood, underscoring the need for further research to identify whether they should remain clinically separate. Although their coexistence is exceptionally rare, new onset CD should be considered in patients with SA who develop gastrointestinal symptoms. Additionally, new onset SA should be considered in patients with CD who develop respiratory symptoms.

References

[1] G. C. Nguyen, C. A. Chong, and R. Y. Chong, "National estimates of the burden of inflammatory bowel disease among racial and ethnic groups in the United States," *Journal of Crohn's and Colitis*, vol. 8, no. 4, pp. 288–295, 2014.

[2] P. Ungprasert, C. S. Crowson, and E. L. Matteson, "Influence of gender on epidemiology and clinical manifestations of sarcoidosis: a population-based retrospective cohort study 1976–2013," *Lung*, vol. 195, no. 1, pp. 87–91, 2017.

[3] P. A. McCormick, D. P. O'Donoghue, and M. X. Fitzgerald, "Crohn's colitis and sarcoidosis," *Postgraduate Medical Journal*, vol. 62, no. 732, pp. 951–953, 1986.

[4] X. Q. Ji, L. X. Wang, and D. G. Lu, "Pulmonary manifestations of inflammatory bowel disease," *World Journal of Gastroenterology*, vol. 20, no. 37, Article ID 13501, 2014.

[5] M. Friedman, M. A. Ali, and M. L. Borum, "Gastric sarcoidosis: a case report and review of the literature," *Southern Medical Journal*, vol. 100, no. 3, pp. 301–303, 2007.

[6] A. J. Padilla and M. Sparberg, "Regional enteritis and sarcoidosis in one patient," *Gastroenterology*, vol. 63, no. 1, pp. 153–160, 1972.

[7] K. Izumikawa, N. Motoi, H. Takaya et al., "A case of concurrent sarcoidosis, aortitis syndrome and crohn's disease," *Internal Medicine*, vol. 50, no. 23, pp. 2915–2917, 2011.

[8] W. Fries, S. A. Grassi, L. Leone et al., "Association between inflammatory bowel disease and sarcoidosis: report of two cases and review of the literature," *Scandinavian Journal of Gastroenterology*, vol. 30, no. 12, pp. 1221–1223, 1995.

[9] V. Kumar, A. K. Abbas, and J. C. Aster, *Robbins Basic Pathology E-Book*, Elsevier Health Sciences, Amsterdam, Netherlands, 2017.

[10] D. G. James, "A clinicopathological classification of granulomatous disorders," *Postgraduate Medical Journal*, vol. 76, no. 898, pp. 457–465, 2000.

[11] A. V. Weizman, B. Huang, S. Targan et al., "Pyoderma gangrenosum among patients with inflammatory bowel disease: a descriptive cohort study," *Journal of Cutaneous Medicine and Surgery*, vol. 18, no. 5, p. 361, 2014.

[12] S. M. Quezada, E. K. Steinberger, and R. K. Cross, "Association of age at diagnosis and crohn's disease phenotype," *Age and Ageing*, vol. 42, no. 1, pp. 102–106, 2013.

[13] B. P. Little, "Sarcoidosis: overview of pulmonary manifestations and imaging," *Seminars in Roentgenology*, vol. 50, no. 1, pp. 52–64, 2015.

[14] T. Molnár, L. Tiszlavicz, C. Gyulai, F. Nagy, and J. Lonovics, "Clinical significance of granuloma in crohn's disease," *World Journal of Gastroenterology*, vol. 11, no. 20, p. 3118, 2005.

[15] C. D. Rosé, S. Pans, I. Casteels et al., "Blau syndrome: cross-sectional data from a multicentre study of clinical, radiological and functional outcomes," *Rheumatology*, vol. 54, no. 6, pp. 1008–1016, 2015.

[16] N. Kanazawa, I. Okafuji, N. Kambe et al., "Early-onset sarcoidosis and CARD15 mutations with constitutive nuclear factor-κB activation: common genetic etiology with blau syndrome," *Blood*, vol. 105, no. 3, pp. 1195–1197, 2004.

[17] A. Franke, A. Fischer, M. Nothnagel et al., "Genome-wide association analysis in sarcoidosis and crohn's disease unravels a common susceptibility locus on 10p12. 2," *Gastroenterology*, vol. 135, no. 4, pp. 1207–1215, 2008.

[18] E. Ghrenassia, A. Mekinian, C. Chapelon-Albric et al., "Digestive-tract sarcoidosis," *Medicine*, vol. 95, no. 29, Article ID e4279, 2016.

[19] J. M. T. Willoughby, "Crohn's disease and sarcoidosis in siblings: follow-up of a published report with a new case and brief review of the literature," *Frontline Gastroenterology*, vol. 8, no. 1, pp. 74–77, 2017.

25

A Rare Case of Pseudomembranous Colitis Presenting with Pleural Effusion and Ascites with Literature Review

Hossain Salehi[1] and **Amir Mohammad Salehi**[2]

[1]*Gastroenterology Ward, Baharlo Hospital, Tehran University of Medical Sciences, Tehran, Iran*
[2]*Medical Student, School of Medicine, Hamadan University of Medical Sciences, Hamadan, Iran*

Correspondence should be addressed to Amir Mohammad Salehi; amirchsalehi19171917@gmail.com

Academic Editor: Yoshihiro Moriwaki

Clostridium difficile infection usually results from long-term and irregular antibiotic intake. The high-risk individuals for this infection include the patients undergoing chemotherapy due to malignancy, immunocompromised patients, and hospitalized patients receiving broad-spectrum antibiotics. The most common clinical manifestation of *Clostridium difficile* infection is diarrhea. However, pleural effusion and ascites have rarely been observed. As mentioned, these manifestations can be developed in a patient being treated with broad-spectrum antibiotics. Therefore, the present study reports a rare case of *Clostridium difficile* infection manifesting with these rare manifestations who was a 78-year-old female patient with a history of COVID-19, orthopedic surgery, and antibiotic treatment with cefixime and gentamicin.

1. Introduction

Clostridium difficile infection (CDI) is a major public health issue. Despite the remarkable changes in its diagnosis and treatment in recent years, the incidence of this infection has increased in hospitalized patients, as well as the community [1]. *Clostridium difficile* is a Gram-positive bacillus and obligate anaerobe whose spores abundantly occurred in nature. These spores can easily be swallowed by humans and proliferate in the distal parts of the intestine. This organism can initiate the destruction of the epithelial cell barrier and create a pseudomembrane by secreting toxins A and B [2]. The main risk factor for *Clostridium difficile* infection is a recent antibiotic exposure [3], and the infection is often neglected due to the lack of sensitive diagnostic tests and most importantly the lack of clinical suspicion. Although diarrhea is the most common clinical manifestation of CDI, the related manifestations varied and include hypovolemia, electrolyte imbalance, hypoproteinemia, toxic megacolon, gastrointestinal perforation, diffuse intravascular coagulation (DIC), and sepsis [4]. However, hydrothorax and ascites are very rare manifestations of CDI.

2. Case Report

A 78-year-old woman presented to the Emergency Department of the Baharloo Hospital with hematemesis since two days before presentation. The patient reported a history of COVID-19 contraction about one month ago with decreased oxygen saturation, followed by an orthopedic surgery due to a femoral neck fracture caused by falling. Moreover, she reported postoperative treatment with cefixime and gentamicin for one week and had received favipiravir, corticosteroids, and aspirin for 20 days due to her COVID-19 infection. Also, she did not report any history of underlying diseases or smoking. In physical examination, the patient had normal respiratory rate, heart rate, and body temperature. She had no abdominal tenderness; however, she looked ill.

Afterward, the patient underwent an endoscopy and was diagnosed with mucosal tearing in the gastroesophageal junction (Mallory Weiss syndrome). Therefore, local injection of epinephrine (1 : 10,000), followed by argon plasma coagulation (APC), was performed for the patient to maintain the hemostasis. The patient was then transferred to the gastroenterology and hepatology ward. The day following the endoscopy, she complained of abdominal pain, diarrhea, and dyspnea. In physical examination, she had a temperature of 37.8°C, a heart rate of 85 per minute, and a respiratory rate of 22 per minute. There was no erythema in the pharyngeal examination, and there was no cervical lymphadenopathy. In addition, heart sounds were normal, while there were decreased pulmonary sounds at the base of the lungs. Also, the patient's abdomen was distended and tender and had shifting dullness in percussion.

Laboratory tests performed on the admission day showed leukocytosis (10400 per mm^3), elevated CRP levels (220 mg/L), hypoalbuminemia (2.39 gr/dl), and elevated lactate dehydrogenase levels (511 U/L). First, an abdominal ultrasound was requested for the patient, which reported ascites. Then, the patient underwent a pulmonary CT scan, which confirmed pleural effusion (Figure 1). The patient underwent thoracocentesis and paracentesis, and the sample analysis showed an exudative pleural effusion and low-SAAG ascites. In addition, cytological examination and culturing of the ascites sample did not show any malignancies or bacterial, mycobacterial, and fungal infection (Table 1). Also, the patient underwent bronchoscopy and bronchoalveolar lavage (BAL) after consultation with a pulmonology specialist, showing unremarkable results. Therefore, the underlying cause of ascites and pleural effusion was not still diagnosed. Finally, the patient underwent abdominal CT scan for her abdominal pain, tenderness, and distension. The CT scan report suggested the possibility of colorectal cancer. Therefore, the patient underwent colonoscopy. She had yellow plaques throughout the colon, which underwent a biopsy. Finally, histological examinations suggested CDI (Figures 2(a) and 2(b)). Thus, the patient was treated with metronidazole (500 mg TDS) and vancomycin (125 mg every 6 h) for 14 days, leading to gradual improvement of her symptoms and resolution of ascites and pleural effusion.

3. Discussion

Clostridium difficile infection is the leading cause of hospital-acquired diarrhea in developed countries. However, it is usually underdiagnosed, most importantly due to lack of clinical suspicion [5].

The main risk factor for this infection is antibiotic exposure, especially with clindamycin, ampicillin, and cephalosporins. The second and third-generation cephalosporins, especially cefotaxime, ceftriaxone, cefuroxime, and ceftazidime, are commonly associated with this infection [2]. Furthermore, prolonged treatment with proton pump inhibitors (PPIs) can lead to intestinal infections, including CDI. Therefore, the patients undergoing long-term PPI treatment should be evaluated for CDI if they develop diarrhea [6]. In addition to antibiotic exposure, other risk factors for CDI include old age (older than 55), recent hospitalization, the history of CDI, malignancy, CRF, use of immunosuppressive drugs, and ICU admission [7].

The CDI diagnosis is based on a combination of clinical (passing watery stool 3 times a day for more than 2 days without other explanations) and paraclinical (detection of toxins A or B, toxicogenic *Clostridium difficile* detection using PCR, or pseudomembrane observation using colonoscopy) findings [2].

Most cases of CDI infections primarily presented with hydrothorax or ascites have been reported in immunocompromised adults (8 out of 14 cases reported), and there are rare reports in children (2 out of 14 cases reported) or immunocompetent adults (4 out of 14 cases reported) [4]. Up to now, 14 cases of CDI with ascites or hydrothorax as clinical manifestations have been reported, as given in Table 2. From these 14 patients, only 6 patients developed ascites and pleural effusion simultaneously. The mechanism of pleura effusion and ascites due to CDI remains unclear; however, hypoalbuminemia, colonic inflammation with microperforation and infectious peritonitis, and toxin-mediated cytokines enhancing vascular permeability could be involved [4, 8].

Since there is no effective vaccination against *Clostridium difficile*, several strategies have been emphasized to prevent the spread of the infection, such as antibiotic use limitations, contamination prevention of sanitary equipment and facilities, and use of probiotics [9]. Minimizing the use of antibiotics in hospitalized patients can effectively reduce the incidence of *Clostridium difficile* infection. For example, restrictions on ceftriaxone and ciprofloxacin administration combined with related instructions could reduce the infection rate by 77% in a hospital with 952 beds in Scotland [9]. Also, probiotic bacteria can replace the natural flora of the gastrointestinal tract, thus preventing diarrhea induced by *Clostridium difficile*. However, the evidence on the effectiveness of probiotics in CDI prevention is weak, despite the numerous clinical studies performed on this topic [10]. A large study investigating the effects of high-dose probiotic administration did not find clear evidence of the effectiveness of these drugs in CDI prevention. Therefore, the effective role of these agents has not yet been confirmed [10]. However, a systematic review including 38 randomized controlled trials on a total of more than 8000 patients showed that the use of the yeasts in the genus *Brassica* could regulate the intestinal flora and exert antitoxic effects. In addition, it has higher therapeutic effects on the CDI compared to other probiotics [11].

Since 1970, metronidazole and vancomycin have been introduced as the medications of choice for CDI treatment. Moreover, no clinically significant resistance to any of these drugs has been observed despite their administration for millions of patients [9]. Vancomycin is preferred in severe infections; however, these two are not significantly different in treating mild to moderate infections [9]. In 2011, fidaxomicin was approved by the Food and Drug Administration (FDA) of the United States for CDI treatment. The clinical studies performed showed the almost equal effectiveness of fidaxomicin and vancomycin in acute CDI treatment. Moreover, the recurrence risk was reportedly

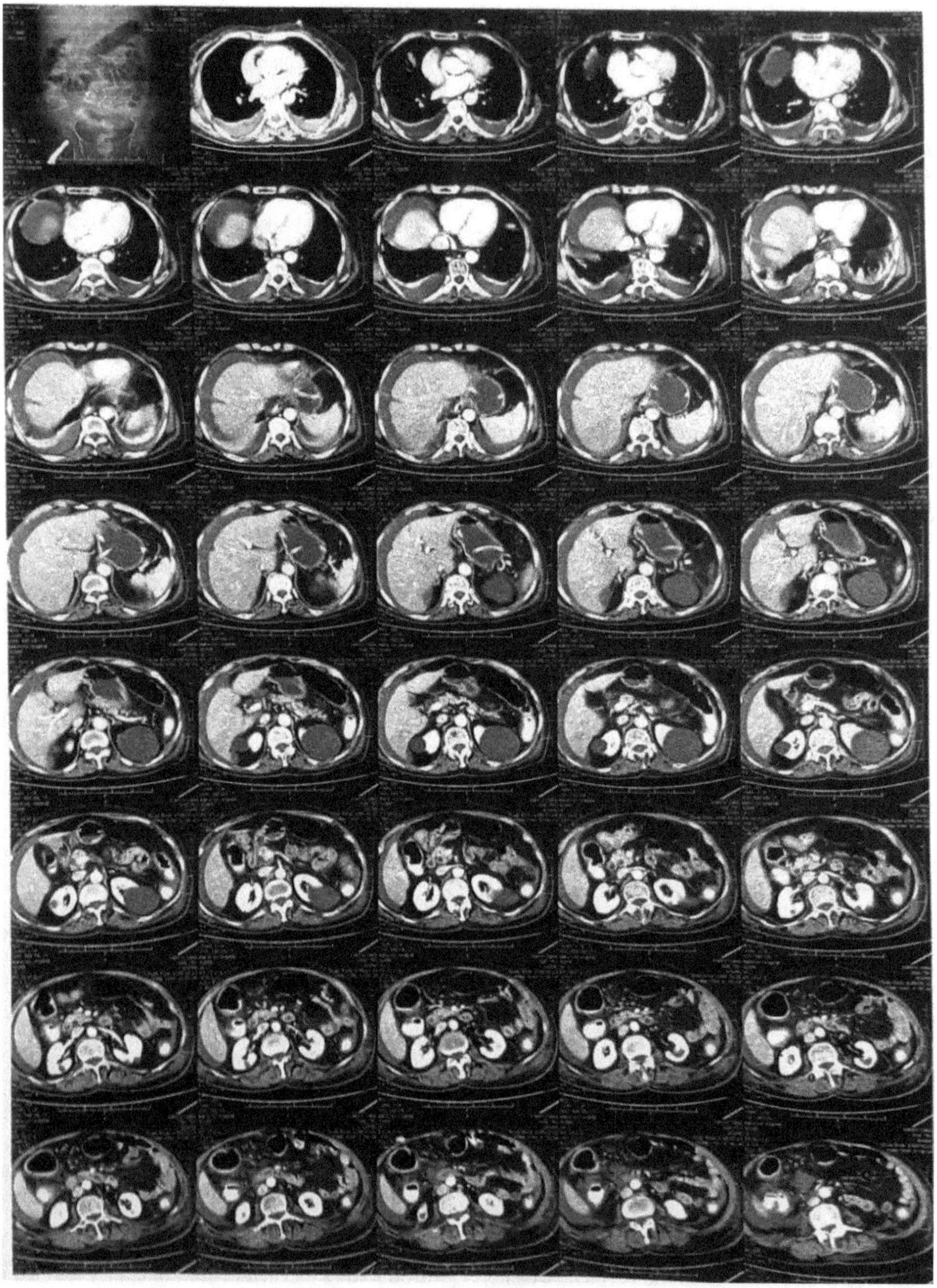

FIGURE 1: Computed tomography (CT) showing the presence of ascites and pleural effusion.

lower in patients treated with fidaxomicin [9]. Recently, fecal microbial transplant (FMT) has been introduced as the most recent therapeutic strategy for CDI, which is performed more than 3 times a day in the form of enema for patients with recurrent CDI. However, to treat the hydrothorax and ascites induced by CDI, the underlying disease should be treated, and the fluid should be drained if necessary [4].

TABLE 1: The analysis of pleural and peritoneal fluid samples.

Factor	Ascites	Pleural effusion
Color	Yellow	Yellow
Appearance	Turbid	Semiclear
Leukocyte count (per mm^3)	1312	400
Neutrophil (%)	80%	70%
Lymphocyte (%)	20%	30%
Glucose	125 mg/dl	81 mg/dl
Protein	3140 mg/dl	2100 mg/dl
RBC	610 mm^3	250 mm^3
Albumin	1900 mg/dl	1300 mg/dl
LDH	771 IU/L	344 IU/L
Ratio	SAAG: 0/49 (low SAAG)	Pleural LDH/serum LDH: 0.67 (exudative)

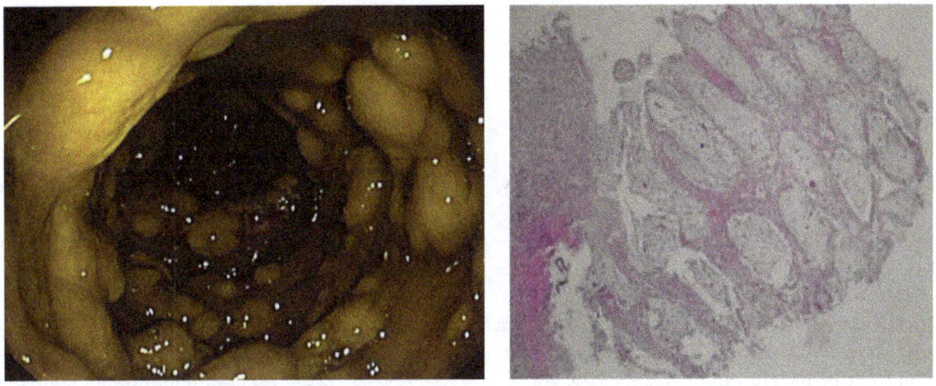

(a) (b)

FIGURE 2: Patient colonoscopic findings (a). The presence of mucopurulent exudates (pseudomembrane) in pathological examinations indicates CDI (b).

TABLE 2: Summary of case reports on CDI presenting with hydrothorax and ascites as the main symptoms.

Study by	Year	Age (y)	Primary disease	Antibiotics treatment before CDI/duration	Pleural effusion	Ascites	Antibiotic/duration	Outcome
Shen et al. [12]	2009	61	Ulcerative colitis/10 d after intestinal operation	Ampicillin IV/NG	–	+	Vancomycin PO/NG metronidazole IV/NG	Died
Dong in nam et al. [13]	2015	80	Hypertension	Ceftriaxone 2.0 g/ day	+	+		Cured
Tsourous et al. [14]	2007	60	Type 2 diabetes/PAOD/ soft tissue infection combined with osteomyelitis	Amoxicillin, clindamycin PO/ 40 d	–	+	Vancomycin PO/NG	Cured
Boaz et al. [15]	2000	25	Oral cavity infection	Clindamycin PO/ 10 d	+	+	Vancomycin PO/NG	Cured
Pang et al. [4] (according to the narration)	2015	71	Gastrointestinal bleeding due to cirrhosis	Ceftriaxone IV/ 14 d	–	+	Ornidazole PO/14 d	Cured
Zukerman et al. [16]	1997	54	AIDS/pneumocystosis	SMX, RMP PO/7 m	–	+	–	Died
		48	Heroin IV usage/URI	Erythromycin NG/ 7d	–	+	Metronidazole NG/NG	Cured
		30	AIDS/*P. aeruginosa* pneumonia	Ceftazidime, gentamicin IV/NG	–	+	Vancomycin PO/14 d	Cured
		33	AIDS	SMX, fluconazole NG/NG	–	+	Metronidazole/PO/14 d	Cured
		58	CAP	Erythromycin NG/ 6 d	–	+	Metronidazole PO/21 d	Cured

TABLE 2: Continued.

Study by	Year	Age (y)	Primary disease	Antibiotics treatment before CDI/duration	Pleural effusion	Ascites	Antibiotic/duration	Outcome
Zwiener et al. [17]	1982	2.5	Otitis media	Amoxicillin NG/ 10 d	+	+	Vancomycin PO/14 d	Relapsed
Yujian Liang et al. [4]	2020	6	Diffuse large B cell lymphoma	Vancomycin, imipenem IV/3 d	+	+	Vancomycin PO/12 d	Cured
Alsultan MH et al. [18]	2021	25	End-stage renal disease (ESRD)	Levofloxacin, ceftazidime, metronidazole	+	+	vancomycin (250 mg/4 times daily) metronidazole (500 mg/3 times daily)	Cured
Our case	2021	72	COVID-19	Cefixime, gentamicin	+	+	Vancomycin PO/14 d metronidazole/PO/14d	Cured

References

[1] F. Marra and K. Ng, "Controversies around epidemiology, diagnosis and treatment of *Clostridium difficile* infection," *Drugs*, vol. 75, no. 10, pp. 1095–1118, 2015.

[2] S. H. Cohen, D. N. Gerding, S. Johnson et al., "Clinical practice guidelines for *Clostridium difficile* infection in adults: 2010 update by the society for healthcare epidemiology of America (SHEA) and the infectious diseases society of America (IDSA)," *Infection Control and Hospital Epidemiology*, vol. 31, no. 5, pp. 431–455, 2010.

[3] K. Brown, K. Valenta, D. Fisman, A. Simor, and N. Daneman, "Hospital ward antibiotic prescribing and the risks of clostridium difficile infection," *JAMA Internal Medicine*, vol. 175, no. 4, pp. 626–633, 2015.

[4] Y. Liang, X. He, T. Wang et al., "Massive hydrothorax and ascites as the primary manifestation of infection with *Clostridium difficile*: a case report and literature review," *Frontiers in Pediatrics*, vol. 8, Article ID 254, 2020.

[5] L. Alcalá, E. Reigadas, M. Marín, A. Martín, P. Catalán, and E. Bouza, "Impact of clinical awareness and diagnostic tests on the underdiagnosis of *Clostridium difficile* infection," *European Journal of Clinical Microbiology & Infectious Diseases: Official Publication of the European Society of Clinical Microbiology*, vol. 34, no. 8, pp. 1515–1525, 2015.

[6] N. Parikh and C. W. Howden, "The safety of drugs used in acid-related disorders and functional gastrointestinal disorders," *Gastroenterology Clinics of North America*, vol. 39, no. 3, pp. 529–542, 2010.

[7] C. Van Werkhoven, J. Van Der Tempel, R. Jajou, S. Thijsen, R. Diepersloot, and M. Bonten, "Identification of patients at high risk for *Clostridium difficile* infection: development and validation of a risk prediction model in hospitalized patients treated with antibiotics," *Clinical Microbiology and Infection*, vol. 21, no. 8, pp. e1–e8, Article ID 786, 2015.

[8] S. Di Bella, P. Ascenzi, S. Siarakas, N. Petrosillo, and A. Di Masi, "*Clostridium difficile* toxins A and B: insights into pathogenic properties and extra intestinal effects," *Toxins*, vol. 8, no. 5, Article ID 134, 2016.

[9] E. Bass, E. Steinberg, and R. Luthra, "*Clostridium difficile* infection," *Hospital Medicine*, vol. 22, pp. 162–215, 2015.

[10] S. J. Allen, "The potential of probiotics to prevent *Clostridium difficile* infection," *Infectious Disease Clinics of North America*, vol. 29, no. 1, pp. 135–144, 2015.

[11] S. E. Madoff, M. Urquiaga, C. D. Alonso, and C. P. Kelly, "Prevention of recurrent clostridioides difficile infection: a systematic review of randomized controlled trials," *Anaerobe*, vol. 61, Article ID 102098, 2020.

[12] B. Shen, F. H. Remzi, and V. W. Fazio, "Fulminant clostridium difficile-associated pouchitis with a fatal outcome," *Nature Reviews Gastroenterology & Hepatology*, vol. 6, no. 8, pp. 492–495, 2009.

[13] D. I. Nam, C. Kang, I. H. Jung, H. G. Moon, B. R. Youn, and N. H. Lee, "Pseudomembranous colitis: a complicated case with transient increase of carcinoembryonic antigen," *The Ewha Medical Journal*, vol. 38, no. 1, pp. 54–58, 2015.

[14] G. I. Tsourous, L. G. Raftopoulos, E. E. Kafe, E. K. Manoleris, K. P. Makaritsis, and S. G. Pinis, "A case of pseudomembranous colitis presenting with massive ascites," *European Journal of Internal Medicine*, vol. 18, no. 4, pp. 328–330, 2007.

[15] A. Boaz, M. Dan, I. Charuzi, O. Landau, Y. Aloni, and S. Kyzer, "Pseudomembranous colitis," *Diseases of the Colon & Rectum*, vol. 43, no. 2, pp. 264–266, 2000.

[16] E. Zuckerman, G. Kanel, C. Ha, J. Kahn, B. Gottesman, and J. Korula, "Low albumin gradient ascites complicating severe pseudomembranous colitis," *Gastroenterology*, vol. 112, no. 3, pp. 991–994, 1997.

[17] R. J. Zwiener, W. M. Belknap, and R. Quan, "Severe pseudomembranous enterocolitis in a child," *The Pediatric Infectious Disease Journal*, vol. 8, no. 12, pp. 876–882, 1989.

[18] M. Alsultan and Q. Hassan, "A rare culture-negative ascites induced by clostridium difficile in a patient with end-stage renal disease: a case report and literature review," *Austin Journal of Nephrology and Hypertension*, vol. 8, no. 2, Article ID 1097, 2021.

An Alarming Mimicry of Intra-Abdominal Infections: Acute Appendiceal Diverticulitis

Youseung Kim,[1] Varun Kesar,[2] Douglas Grider,[1,3,4] and Maithili V. Chitnavis[2]

[1] *Virginia Tech Carilion School of Medicine, Department of Internal Medicine, Roanoke, VA, USA*
[2] *Virginia Tech Carilion School of Medicine, Department of Internal Medicine, Division of Gastroenterology and Hepatology, Roanoke, VA, USA*
[3] *Virginia Tech Carilion School of Medicine, Department of Basic Science Education, Roanoke, VA, USA*
[4] *Dominion Pathology Associates, Roanoke, VA, USA*

Correspondence should be addressed to Youseung Kim; ykim1@carilionclinic.org

Academic Editor: Olga I. Giouleme

A 65-year-old woman presented with three days of colicky abdominal pain. Abdominal imaging illustrated small bowel enteritis, ascites in both paracolic gutters, and incidental hepatic steatosis. Although ascites fluid demonstrated high neutrophil count consistent with peritonitis and the patient received adequate antibiotics, she clinically deteriorated. Subsequent exploratory laparotomy revealed necrotic appendix and multiple intra-abdominal abscesses. Histopathology showed acute suppurative appendicitis with multiple other intact small diverticula, indicating likely perforation of inflamed appendiceal diverticula with subsequent abscess formation and abdominal peritonitis. This case highlights the importance of ascites fluid analysis and continued clinical correlation, especially in cases of rare entities with atypical presentations.

1. Introduction

Diverticula are small protrusions formed from the walls of the tubular gastrointestinal tract and can be associated with several complications such as hemorrhage, inflammation, and perforation. Anatomically, there are two types of diverticula—true and false. True diverticula involve all three layers of the intestinal wall, which consists of the mucosa, submucosa, and muscularis propria, and are most recognized in congenital diverticula such as Meckel's diverticula. False diverticula consist of only mucosa and submucosa without the involvement of the muscularis propria and are associated with acquired diverticulosis. Not surprisingly, many colonic diverticula are false diverticula and originate from weak points in the intestinal wall [1]. Acute appendiceal diverticulitis is a rare pathology of the appendix with the incidence of 0.004–2.1% [2] and is described in the literature by isolated case reports [3, 4]. We present a case of acute appendiceal diverticulitis with delayed diagnosis complicated by perforation of the diverticulum, abscess formation, and peritonitis.

2. Case Presentation

A 65-year-old woman with a history of essential hypertension presented with three days of intermittent, left lower quadrant colicky abdominal pain and nonbilious vomiting, a few hours after an outdoor barbecue, along with subjective fever, chills, and dizziness. Abdominal and pelvic computed tomography (CT) with contrast showed signs of small bowel enteritis (Figure 1). Incidental findings included diffuse hepatic steatosis and small amounts of ascites in both paracolic gutters.

At admission, the emergency general surgery service was consulted and recommended intravenous hydration and treatment for infectious enteritis under the general medicine service. A diagnostic paracentesis on the second day of hospitalization revealed an ascitic fluid white blood cell (WBC) count of 18,800 cells/mm^3 with 75% neutrophils, 12% lymphocytes, 13% mononuclear cell, glucose of 94 mg/dL, protein of 3.9 g/dL, and LDH of 459 IU/L. The patient was continued on cefepime for possible spontaneous bacterial peritonitis (SBP). However, by the third day of

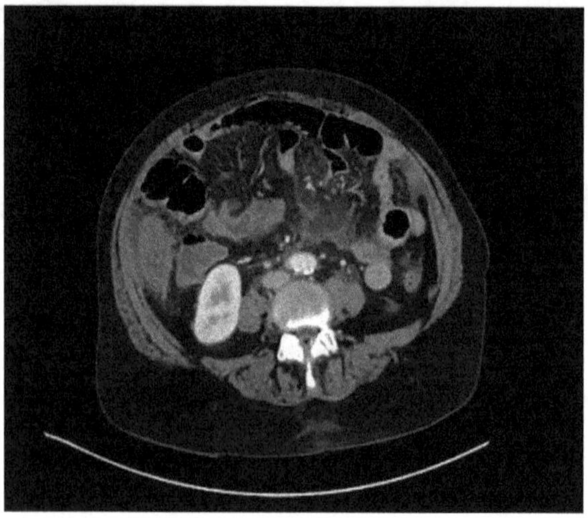

Figure 1: Initial computed tomography (CT) of the abdomen and pelvis with small bowel enteritis and fluid collections in paracolic gutters.

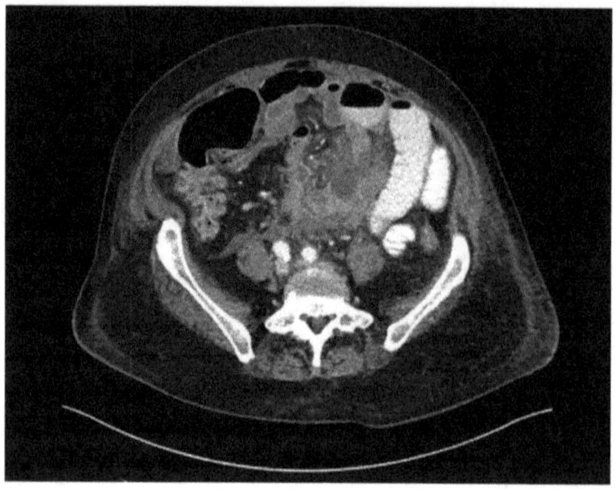

Figure 2: Repeat computed tomography (CT) of the abdomen and pelvis with new peritoneal enhancement suggestive of peritonitis.

admission, the patient's abdominal pain had intensified. The gastroenterology team was consulted for the management of ascites. On examination, the patient had a distended, rigid abdomen with voluntary abdominal guarding and diffuse significant tenderness to palpation suggestive of peritonitis. Given that diagnostic paracentesis was also suspicious for secondary bacterial peritonitis by Runyon's criteria [5], a repeat CT of the abdomen and pelvis with contrast and surgical reconsultation were recommended. CT illustrated worsening moderate ascites without free air, but with new peritoneal enhancement, suggestive of peritonitis (Figure 2), along with the concern for small bowel obstruction (SBO) in the left lower abdominal quadrant.

The patient was initially treated conservatively for a possible SBO, but due to continued worsening abdominal pain, she subsequently underwent diagnostic laparoscopy. This revealed multiple pockets of pus and purulent peritonitis. Consequently, the laparoscopy was converted to open laparotomy with drainage of intraloop, right lower quadrant, and pelvic abscesses. Appendectomy for a necrotic-appearing appendix was also performed. Histopathology showed acute suppurative appendicitis and periappendicitis with multiple small diverticula along the length of the remaining viable appendix, supporting the likely perforation of one or more diverticula secondary to acute inflammation with subsequent abscess formation and abdominal peritonitis (Figure 3). The patient completed a total of ten days of antibiotics and was discharged with clinical improvement.

3. Discussion

There are two classifications of diverticula: congenital or acquired. Congenital diverticulum, or true diverticulum, is a rare entity, with minimal incidence of perforation because it includes all the layers of mucosa, submucosa, and muscularis propria. By comparison, an acquired diverticulum is a false diverticulum that does not involve the muscularis propria and therefore has higher tendency for perforation [6, 7].

In retrospect, this patient presented with nonspecific symptoms of appendiceal diverticulitis of false diverticula. The patient's nonspecific gastrointestinal symptoms including abdominal pain and ascites along with initial imaging concerning for parenchymal liver disease led to a suspicion for SBP. Despite antibiotic therapy, the patient continued to worsen with peritoneal signs on abdominal exam and persistent leukocytosis. Moreover, elevated ascitic total protein and LDH were highly concerning for secondary peritonitis by fulfilling two of three Runyon's criteria, which has a sensitivity and specificity of 67 and 96%, respectively [5]. This prompted repeat imaging and subsequent laparotomy revealing purulent peritonitis, the likely source being perforated suppurative appendiceal diverticulitis.

Delay in the diagnosis and treatment of appendiceal diverticulitis is not uncommon. Appendiceal diverticulitis is often difficult to distinguish from other intra-abdominal infections of the right-sided colon such as infectious ileocecitis caused by *Yersinia*, *Campylobacter*, and *Salmonella* and pseudomembranous colitis caused by *Clostridium difficile* and especially from acute appendicitis, both clinically and radiologically [8]. Clinically, patients with either acute appendicitis or appendiceal diverticulitis will typically present with nonspecific gastrointestinal symptoms, including abdominal pain, nausea, vomiting, and diarrhea. Radiographically, both disease processes illustrate inflammation of the appendix on contrast-enhanced CT studies, though the rate of incidence may differ between them [9]. A retrospective cohort study conducted by Ito et al. reported only 24% visualization of appendiceal diverticulum and 16% of fluid collection in the appendiceal lumen in patients with a pathologically proven diagnosis of appendiceal diverticulitis compared to 100% visualization of the appendix with 88% of fluid collection in the appendiceal lumen in patients with acute appendicitis [9]. Furthermore, the appendix could not be visualized in the CT findings of 48% of the patients in the appendiceal diverticulitis group [9]. Nonspecific clinical and radiological findings can lead to delay in diagnosis as well as treatment of appendiceal diverticulitis, thus increasing the rate of severe complications such as perforation compared to acute appendicitis (65.8% vs. 10.2%) [10].

Recent studies suggest that there may be subtle characteristics in patient presentation that help differentiate

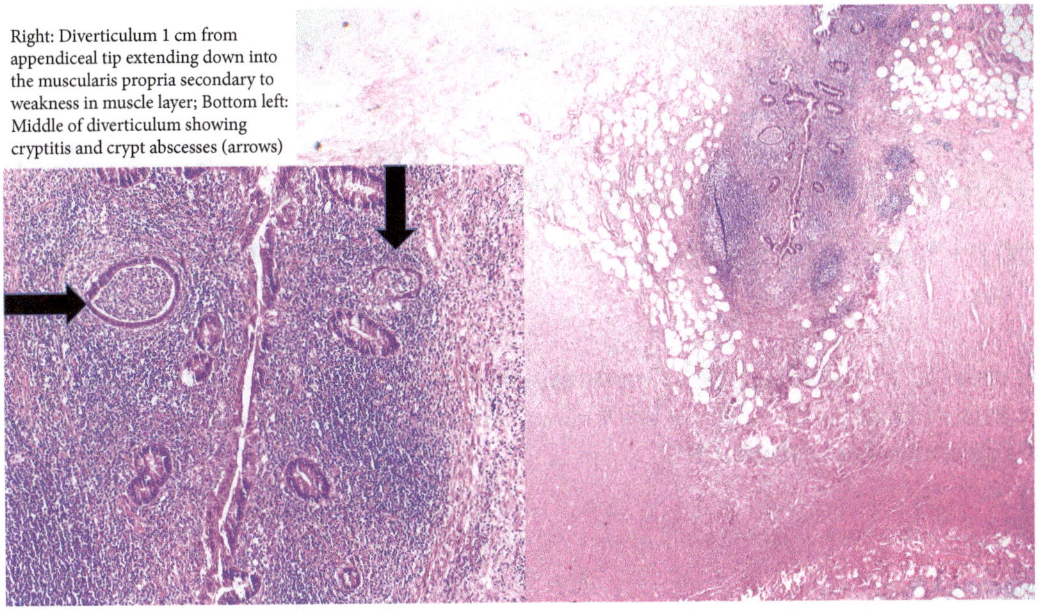

FIGURE 3: Histopathology of appendiceal diverticulitis in the portion of the remaining viable appendix.

between appendiceal diverticulitis and acute appendicitis. For example, appendiceal diverticulitis more commonly presents in older patients compared to acute appendicitis, with an average of 43 versus 29 years, respectively [4]. Also, patients with appendiceal diverticulitis have a longer average duration of time before emergency department presentation compared to that of acute appendicitis, 71 versus 37 hours [11]. These factors lead to an increased rate of severe complications associated with appendiceal diverticulitis, such as perforation, compared to acute appendicitis [10]. Although appendiceal diverticulitis is a rarer entity as compared to acute appendicitis, further characterization and consideration of this entity may benefit to decrease complications and mortality associated with this condition.

Authors' Contributions

Youseung Kim and Varun Kesar composed the first draft of the manuscript which was then critically reviewed by the remaining authors.

References

[1] J. A. Maykel and F. G. Opelka, "Colonic diverticulosis and diverticular hemorrhage," *Clinics in Colon and Rectal Surgery*, vol. 17, no. 3, pp. 195–204, 2004.

[2] B. Abdullgaffar, "Diverticulosis and diverticulitis of the appendix," *International Journal of Surgical Pathology*, vol. 17, pp. 231–237, 2019.

[3] D. Seker, G. Seker, S. Kahramanca, M. Gurler, A. Turker, and H. Kulacoglu, "A rare but distinctive cause of acute abdomen: appendiceal diverticulitis," *Journal of Emergency Medicine*, vol. 44, pp. 61-62, 2013.

[4] I. Yamana, S. Kawamoto, K. Inada, S. Nagao, T. Yoshida, and Y. Yamashita, "Clinical characteristics of 12 cases of appendiceal diverticulitis: a comparison with 378 cases of acute appendicitis," *Surgery Today*, vol. 42, no. 4, pp. 363–367, 2012.

[5] M. L. R. Lu, A. Agarwal, J. Sloan, and A. Kosmin, "Infected ascites: distinguishing secondary peritonitis from spontaneous bacterial peritonitis in a cirrhotic patient with classic symptoms," *ID Cases*, vol. 8, pp. 29–31, 2017.

[6] D. C. Collins, "A study of 50,000 specimens of the human vermiform appendix," *Surgery Gynecology & Obstetrics*, vol. 101, no. 4, pp. 437–445, 1955.

[7] K. C. Chong, "Diverticula of the vermiform appendix: a report of nine cases," *Postgraduate Medical Journal*, vol. 52, no. 610, pp. 504–510, 1976.

[8] S. J. Tang and R. Wu, "Ilececum: a comprehensive review," *Canadian journal of gastroenterology & hepatology*, vol. 2019, Article ID 1451835, 21 pages, 2019.

[9] D. Ito, K. Miki, S. Seiichiro et al., "Clinical and computed tomography findings of appendiceal diverticulitisvsacute appendicitis," *World Journal of Gastroenterology*, vol. 21, no. 13, pp. 3921–3927, 2015.

[10] T. J. Sohn, Y. S. Chang, J. H. Kang et al., "Clinical characteristics of acute appendiceal diverticulitis," *Journal of the Korean Surgical Society*, vol. 84, no. 1, pp. 33–37, 2013.

[11] I. Lobo-Machin, L. Delgado-Plasencia, I. Hernandez-Gonzalez et al., "Appendiceal diverticulitis and acute appendicitis: differences and similaries," *Revista Española de Enfermedades Digestivas*, vol. 106, no. 7, pp. 452–458, 2014.

Ulcerative Colitis in Hematological Malignancies: Paraneoplastic Manifestation or Coincidental Bystander?

Gregorios Christodoulidis,[1] Konstantinos Perivoliotis,[1] Anastasios Manolakis,[2] Alexandros Diamantis,[1] Apostolos Koffas,[2] Dimitrios Magouliotis,[1] Vasiliki Pappi,[3] and Dimitrios Zacharoulis[1]

[1]*Department of Surgery, University Hospital of Larissa, Mezourlo 41110, Larissa, Greece*
[2]*Department of Gastroenterology, University Hospital of Larissa, Mezourlo 41110, Larissa, Greece*
[3]*Department of Hematology, General Hospital of Volos, Volos, Greece*

Correspondence should be addressed to Konstantinos Perivoliotis; kperi19@gmail.com

Academic Editor: Gregory Kouraklis

Evidence of coexistence of diverse hematological malignancies—lymphoma, leukemia, multiple myeloma, and myelodysplastic syndromes—and either ulcerative colitis or Crohn's disease can be found in the literature. However, a more "systemic" effort to reach further and examine the potential of either one as paraneoplastic manifestation has not been performed. Based on these, three cases of ulcerative colitis manifesting before, simultaneously, and after the onset of different hematological malignancies are presented and critically evaluated.

1. Introduction

The term "paraneoplastic" has been coined to describe a series of manifestations resulting from biologically active substances or immune responses, induced by solid tumors or hematological malignancies. Evidence of coexistence of diverse hematological malignancies—lymphoma, leukemia, multiple myeloma, and myelodysplastic syndromes—and either ulcerative colitis (UC) or Crohn's disease (CD) can be found in the literature [1–3]. However, a more "systemic" effort to reach further and examine the potential of either one as potential paraneoplastic manifestation has not been performed. Based on these, three cases of UC manifesting before, simultaneously, and after the onset of different hematological malignancies are presented and critically evaluated.

2. Case Presentation

2.1. Case 1. A 71-year-old male Caucasian with a history of multiple myeloma (MM) treated with lenalidomide and dexamethasone was referred to our department with episodes of hematochezia. Lenalidomide was ceased one month ago, due to mild diarrhea. The patient was on a 100 mg/day acetylsalicylic acid thromboprophylaxis regimen. Endoscopic and histopathologic findings indicative of ulcerative pancolitis as well as laboratory parameters are presented in Table 1. A partial response of MM was recorded, and bone marrow biopsy revealed a 15% monoclonal plasmocyte infiltration. The patient was treated with antibiotics, prednisone, and 5-aminosalicylates (5-ASA), reaching clinical remission. Two months later, upper extremity lytic lesions consistent with MM recurrence were detected. When lenalidomide and dexamethasone were reintroduced later, no UC flare-ups were recorded, despite the lack of a more UC-specific therapy, as the patient, on his own initiative, discontinued 5-ASA. During the next four years, both UC and MM remained in remission.

2.2. Case 2. A 57-year-old male Caucasian was admitted for fatigue, low-grade fever, and bloody diarrhea. Endoscopic

Table. 1: Laboratory parameters recorded in each patient

	Case 1	Case 2	Case 3
WBC	9500/μL	Pre-t 2580/μL Post-t 3500/μL	12000/μL
Hct	35%	Pre-t 22.9% Post-t 26.7%	36.6%
Plt	WNR	Pre-t 138000/μL Post-t 226000/μL	452000/μL
Reticulocyte count	WNR	Pre-t 0.02×10^6 Post-t 0.028×10^6	WNR
ESR (mm)	40	78	38
CRP (mg/dL)	9	13	1.3
IgG (mg/dL)	WNR	WNR	1890
IgA (mg/dL)	WNR	385	363
ASCA (U/mL)	— 20.9 U/mL (IgA)	62.2 (IgG) 38.1 (IgA)	— —
ANCA	—	1 : 40 (a-ANCA)	1 : 320 (c-ANCA)
Anti-EBV	+ (IgG)	+ (IgG)	+ (IgG)
Anti-CMV	+ (IgG)	+ (IgG)	+ (IgG)
Anti-VZV	+ (IgG)	+ (IgG)	+ (IgG)
Anti-HSV-1	+ (IgG)	+ (IgG)	+ (IgG)
HLA typing	B35, B55	B51, B55	B07, B35
Cultures (blood/fecal)	Negative	Negative	Negative
Additional	High avidity	Coombs (−) Anti-platelet antibodies (−)	High avidity
Endoscopy	Continuous pattern involvement of all colonic segments' friability, petechial bleeding, edema, and granularity	Continuous pattern involvement of all colonic segments' mucous friability, petechial bleeding, oedema, and granularity	Similar to case 2
Histopathology	Crypt atrophy, crypt abscesses, and LP mononuclear cell infiltration	Similar to case 1	Similar to cases 1, 2

WBC: white blood cell; Hct: hematocrit; Plt: platelet; t: treatment; ESR: erythrocyte sedimentation rate; CRP: C-reactive protein; Ig: immunoglobulin; ASCA: anti-*Saccharomyces cerevisiae* antibodies; ANCA: anti-neutrophil cytoplasm antibodies; EBV: Epstein-Barr; CMV: cytomegalovirus; HSV-1: herpes simplex virus-1; VZV: varicella-zoster virus; HLA: human leukocyte antigen; WNR: within normal range; LP: lamina propria.

findings and histopathology, consistent with UC pancolitis and laboratory parameters, are included in Table 1. Due to concomitant pancytopenia, a bone marrow biopsy was performed, which established the diagnosis of myelodysplastic syndrome (MDS). More specifically, an intermediate risk I MDS was diagnosed, with a 10% bone marrow infiltration by blast cells with normal karyotype. Following treatment with antibiotics, prednisone and 5-ASA, remission was established also accompanied by an improvement in blood count analyses (Table 1). The patient did not receive any transfusion and was conservatively supported with erythropoiesis-stimulating agents.

2.3. Case 3. A 44-year-old male Caucasian was admitted to our department, with low-grade fever, mild diffuse abdominal pain, and bloody diarrhea. Three years ago, due to episodes of mild diarrhea, and after positive bone marrow biopsies, the diagnosis of systemic mastocytosis (SM) was confirmed. In addition to this, UC was diagnosed 2 months prior to current hospitalization. He was under 5-ASA and tapering doses of prednisone. Laboratory, endoscopic, and histopathologic findings are presented in Table 1. The patient exhibited a UC pancolitis for which he received treatment with prednisone, 5-ASA, budesonide enemas, and azathioprine (AZA). After clinical remission, the patient was closely followed being asymptomatic under AZA and 5-ASA. After 12 months, endoscopy for therapeutic evaluation and biopsies were carried out. All findings were once more suggestive of UC, and the possibility of an SM-diseased colon was histopathologicaly ruled out.

3. Discussion

A rather serious turmoil has been created with respect to hematological malignancies complicating inflammatory bowel disease (IBD), and although data from large studies indicate an increased risk for UC patients to develop myeloid leukemia, it is not yet clear whether the disease itself or the different therapeutic agents used are to be held accountable [1, 4]. In contrast, little is known about the prevalence of IBD in patients with hematopoietic malignancies [1–3] while the notion that UC may represent a paraneoplastic manifestation in such cases is "terra incognita." Motivated by the admission in our tertiary center, during a 2½-year period, of three patients with three different hematological malignancies accompanied by UC at an almost identical extent and severity, it seemed fit to further examine this association.

The close link between inflammation and cancer is well studied, with autoimmune disorders predisposing to malignancies and autoimmune phenomena manifesting more frequently on the setting of cancer. This idea has been recently enriched through the recognition of chronic antigenic stimulation as a major player for the onset of diverse malignancies, including hematological as well as autoimmune disorders such as IBD either occurring independently or in conjunction. Immune-stimulating conditions involving activation of immune cells may lead eventually to pro-oncogenic mutations in actively dividing cells while immune dysregulation taking place in the setting of hematopoietic cancer may lead to cross-linking reactions and recognition of endogenous molecules thus triggering several autoimmune phenomena [5–7]. Moreover, the biological pathways involved in hematological malignancies and UC are interlinked, with several mediators of inflammation and cellular populations with an altered response profile being shared among these entities [8]. Indeed, tumor necrosis factor-alpha (TNF-α), nuclear factor kappa-light-chain-enhancer of activated B cells (NF-kB), interleukins (IL-1, -5, -6, and -8), angiogenesis factors (i.e., vascular endothelial growth factor (VEGF)), irregular plasmatoid cells inducing pronounced TNF-α and reduced interferon-gamma production, and eosinophils are key-components of the pathogenesis of MM, MDS, SM, and UC [3, 7–12]. Further details pertaining to each case are also presented below.

In the first case, UC was associated with MM while its manifestation preceded by almost 2 months the diagnosis of recurrent MM. In addition, adequate "control" of MM was accompanied by a lack of UC relapse. Acting together, the molecular and cellular components described earlier may have favored the onset of UC, before ultimate diagnosis of MM recurrence. At this point, it is important to underline that all cases of IBD accompanying MM pertain to CD alone. In these cases, the treatment regimens did not, however, include lenalidomide, a thalidomide analogue with a×2000 greater potency for TNFα inhibition [9]. Thalidomide has been used in some studies for the induction or maintenance of CD remission, whereas no benefits whatsoever were recorded with respect to UC. Based on these, we cannot exclude the possibility that the thalidomide analog may have conditioned the IBD-genic potential of MM, discouraging the onset of CD while leaving intact those biological pathways ultimately leading to the UC phenotype. Likewise, it seemed quite reasonable to include pharmaceutic colitis in differential diagnosis. Against these notions are the observations that during a 4-year follow-up the diagnosis of UC has not changed and, in addition, when lenalidomide was readministered, no adverse events implicating the colon were recorded.

The link of MDS with several autoimmune phenomena is well established. This close association is such that pharmacologically induced suppression of these manifestations is accompanied by partial MDS improvement, as in our case [10]. Another finding replicated in our study is the association of MDS with an extensive UC (pancolitis) [3]. In terms of pathogenesis, impaired mitogenic response, diminished CD4-positive cell numbers, and functional abnormalities in B cell subset accompanied by hyper- or hypogammaglobulinemia or impaired antibody-dependent killing have been recorded in MDS. Similarly, impairment in mitogenic, CD4-positive, and B cell response has been reported in UC patients. Moreover, certain potent inhibitors of hematopoiesis inducing accelerated cell death, such as TNF-α, may also be markedly upregulated in both MDS and UC [3, 10]. Hence, it is not surprising that treatment targeting UC and its biological pathways may exert a favorable effect in hematological status of MDS.

As for the cosegregation of SM with ulcerative colitis is not surprising as both disorders may share a common Th2 pathogenetic background. Moreover, the colon may be implicated in mastocytosis, posing a serious challenge in terms of differential diagnosis, as it is mimicking IBD [11]. According to the published literature, the presence of mast cells may modulate IBD through participation in normal immunity, increase in intestinal permeability and sensitivity, eosinophil chemoattraction, release of vasoactive mediators, and superoxide dismutase colonic injury. In this case, the SM-related increased presence of mast cells and their products could have exerted these phenomena, thus disrupting mucosal epithelial barrier, initiating and sustaining an inappropriate inflammatory process subsequently leading to UC [13].

In view of all three cases, patients were male Caucasians with no family history of IBD. A male predominance in MDS, MM, and lately IBD has already been recorded and is probably reflected in our series, too [8, 10, 14]. Likewise, the common ethnic background of all patients most likely results from the Caucasian predominance in our district, although the presence of certain ethnic/race-related genes conferring susceptibility cannot be excluded. An altered immunogenic profile has been documented, as increased levels of immunoglobulins (IgG and IgA) were recorded. Moreover, the notorious autoimmune disorders, including IBD, cross-reactive c-ANCA, a-ANCA, and ASCA were found, suggesting an altered pattern recognition status, targeting both endogenous as well as microbial components [14–16]. What might be of importance is that c-ANCA and ASCA, are not commonly encountered in UC, and their presence has been associated in some cases with distinct UC phenotype—usually pancolitis [15, 16]. Moreover, positivity for these markers has been shown to be a genetic trait, cosegregating in families irrespective of the presence of IBD in individual relatives [14]. Apart from the evident immune dysregulation, the three cases described above seem to share a common immunogenetic background through major histocompatibility complex class I (MHC-I), HLA B* alleles (B07, B35, B51, and B55), known for their involvement in the presentation of intracellular and viral components as well as the attempt of cancer cells to evade the anticancer immune response of T cells, through intensified expression of HLA products, also recorded in patients with hematologic malignancies [17]. The B07, a rather frequent allele, already linked to hematological malignancies [18], is also frequently encountered among Greek UC patients and associated with greater disease extent [19]. The presence of B35 has been documented in cases of cosegregated autoimmune disorders, such as UC and Takayasu arteritis, as well as UC and postinfectious Guillain-Barré syndrome (GBS) [20–23]. B51 shows a strong link with Adamantiades-Behcet [24] while B55 is involved in hepatitis C virus patient progress [25]. Interestingly, all alleles presented above are also classified under the same HLA B7 "supertype" based on their shared peptide binding motifs [26]. What might be of some importance is that all three patients were tested positive for IgG antibodies against EBV, CMV, HSV-1, and VZV. EBV has been associated with hematological malignancies, mainly lymphoma while EBV and CMV were also related to MM [27]. None of the patients, however, had signs of acute infection or viral reactivation and at this point it is impossible to extend this finding as these seropositivities are very common.

When co-evaluating all the data presented above, it is vital to proceed cautiously in order to avoid any misinterpretations. In clinical practice, a paraneoplastic manifestation often serves as an alarm signal for additional work-up aiming at revealing the presence of an underlying malignancy [28]. Based on the available literature, routine investigation for malignant disorders in patients diagnosed with UC, to date, is not justifiable. The association recorded in our cases although thought-provoking is not adequate on its own to change this notion, and it does, however, seem to raise some issues and encourage further hypotheses. For instance, this "paraneoplastic" UC emerged while being tightly linked to diverse malignancies, yet all of a hematologic "origin." Interestingly, UC manifested in an identical extent and severity in patients bearing HLA B7 supertype components, an identical viral serology profile, while exhibiting an uncommon, for UC, autoimmune serologic pattern (ASCA and c-ANCA in two cases). In addition, this link was further strengthened as a therapeutic benefit was recorded on the malignancy during effective control of UC and inversely on the maintenance of UC remission with successful treatment of the malignancy. Based on the experience drawn from these cases, a clinician should stay alert during differential diagnosis of common conditions in those disorders. Thus, anemia a common manifestation in UC should not be easily attributed solely to the chronicity of the disorder, blood or ferrum loss, malabsorption, and drug-induced or autoimmune hemolysis, especially if accompanied by additional cytopenias. Vice versa, diarrhea in a patient with known hematological malignancy should not be merely attributed to infection or drug toxicity. For the authors, two additional, important, and quite provocative hypotheses remain to be thoroughly examined. Could the association of UC with hematological malignancies be due to a genetic predisposition, implicating the components of the MHC-I, HLA B7 supertype, as in these cases? Similarly, could this "paraneoplastic" extensive UC represent a distinct entity, a unique or specific UC phenotype similar to the one described for GBS associated with *Campylobacter jejuni* infection [20]?

Taking into account the abovementioned evidence, we can safely conclude that the coexistence of inflammatory bowel disease in hematological malignancies patients that present with gastrointestinal tract symptoms should be acknowledged and investigated. Furthermore, in order to enhance the treatment efficacy outcomes and facilitate medical and pathogenetic research, a multidisciplinary and multicenter approach should be applied.

References

[1] L. C. Huang and A. Merchea, "Dysplasia and cancer in inflammatory bowel disease," *Surgical Clinics of North America*, vol. 97, no. 3, pp. 627–639, 2017.

[2] J. Cosnes, "What should be done in inflammatory bowel disease patients with prior malignancy?" *Digestive Diseases*, vol. 35, no. 1-2, pp. 50–55, 2017.

[3] Z. Wang, Y. Zhou, and Y. Liu, "Concurrent inflammatory bowel disease and myelodysplastic syndrome: report of nine new cases and a review of the literature," *Digestive Diseases and Sciences*, vol. 53, no. 7, pp. 1929–1932, 2008.

[4] J. Xie and S. H. Itzkowitz, "Cancer in inflammatory bowel disease," *World Journal of Gastroenterology*, vol. 14, no. 3, p. 378, 2008.

[5] J. J. Jin, J. H. Butterfield, and C. R. Weiler, "Hematologic malignancies identified in patients with hypereosinophilia and hypereosinophilic syndromes," *The Journal of Allergy and Clinical Immunology: In Practice*, vol. 3, no. 6, pp. 920–925, 2015.

[6] K. C. Söderberg, L. Hagmar, J. Schwartzbaum, and M. Feychting, "Allergic conditions and risk of hematological malignancies in adults: a cohort study," *BMC Public Health*, vol. 4, no. 1, p. 51, 2004.

[7] B. B. Aggarwal, S. Shishodia, S. K. Sandur, M. K. Pandey, and G. Sethi, "Inflammation and cancer: how hot is the link?" *Biochemical Pharmacology*, vol. 72, no. 11, pp. 1605–1621, 2006.

[8] G. J. Reynolds, K. A. Annis, and W. J. S. de Villiers, "Review article: multiple myeloma and inflammatory bowel disease," *Digestive Diseases and Sciences*, vol. 52, no. 9, pp. 2022–2028, 2007.

[9] G. W. Muller, R. Chen, S.-Y. Huang et al., "Amino-substituted thalidomide analogs: potent inhibitors of TNF-α production," *Bioorganic & Medicinal Chemistry Letters*, vol. 9, no. 11, pp. 1625–1630, 1999.

[10] S. Giannouli, M. Voulgarelis, E. Zintzaras, A. G. Tzioufas, and H. M. Moutsopoulos, "Autoimmune phenomena in myelodysplastic syndromes: a 4-yr prospective study," *Rheumatology*, vol. 43, no. 5, pp. 626–632, 2004.

[11] A. Bedeir, D. M. Jukic, L. Wang, D. K. Mullady, M. Regueiro, and A. M. Krasinskas, "Systemic mastocytosis mimicking inflammatory bowel disease: a case report and discussion of gastrointestinal pathology in systemic mastocytosis," *The American Journal of Surgical Pathology*, vol. 30, no. 11, pp. 1478–1482, 2006.

[12] S.-H. He, "Key role of mast cells and their major secretory products in inflammatory bowel disease," *World Journal of Gastroenterology*, vol. 10, no. 3, pp. 309–318, 2004.

[13] G. Boeckxstaens, "Mast cells and inflammatory bowel disease," *Current Opinion in Pharmacology*, vol. 25, pp. 45–49, 2015.

[14] V. Neudecker, S. P. Colgan, and H. K. Eltzschig, "Novel therapeutic concepts for inflammatory bowel disease—from bench to bedside," *Journal of Molecular Medicine*, vol. 95, no. 9, pp. 899–903, 2017.

[15] F. Zhou, B. Xia, F. Wang et al., "The prevalence and diagnostic value of perinuclear antineutrophil cytoplasmic antibodies and anti-*Saccharomyces cerevisiae* antibodies in patients with inflammatory bowel disease in mainland China," *Clinica Chimica Acta*, vol. 411, no. 19-20, pp. 1461–1465, 2010.
[16] J. Xu, C.-H. Yang, X.-Y. Chen, X.-H. Li, M. Dai, and S.-D. Xiao, "A subset of ulcerative colitis with positive proteinase-3 antineutrophil cytoplasmic antibody," *World Journal of Gastroenterology*, vol. 14, no. 45, p. 7012, 2008.
[17] M. Bassani-Sternberg, E. Barnea, I. Beer, I. Avivi, T. Katz, and A. Admon, "Soluble plasma HLA peptidome as a potential source for cancer biomarkers," *Proceedings of the National Academy of Sciences*, vol. 107, no. 44, pp. 18769–18776, 2010.
[18] J. Bae, T. Hideshima, G. L. Zhang et al., "Identification and characterization of HLA-A24-specific XBP1, CD138 (Syndecan-1) and CS1 (SLAMF7) peptides inducing antigens-specific memory cytotoxic T lymphocytes targeting multiple myeloma," *Leukemia*, vol. 32, no. 3, pp. 752–764, 2018.
[19] C. Papasteriades, C. Spiliadis, A. Emmanouilidis, C. Papadimitriou, J. Economidou, and O. Manousos, "Histocompatibility antigens (HLA-A, B) and ulcerative colitis in a Greek population," *Digestion*, vol. 33, no. 4, pp. 229–232, 1986.
[20] V. K. Wachira, H. M. Peixoto, and M. R. F. de Oliveira, "Systematic review of factors associated with the development of Guillain-Barré syndrome 2007–2017: what has changed?" *Tropical Medicine & International Health*, vol. 24, no. 2, pp. 132–142, 2019.
[21] B. Mishu and M. J. Blaser, "Role of infection due to *Campylobacter jejuni* in the initiation of guillain-barre syndrome," *Clinical Infectious Diseases*, vol. 17, no. 1, pp. 104–108, 1993.
[22] K. Tominaga, A. Tsuchiya, H. Sato et al., "Co-existent ulcerative colitis and Guillain-Barré syndrome: a case report and literature review," *Clinical Journal of Gastroenterology*, vol. 12, no. 3, pp. 243–246, 2019.
[23] A. Hokama, F. Kinjo, T. Arakaki et al., "Pulseless hematochezia: takayasu's arteritis associated with ulcerative colitis," *Internal Medicine*, vol. 42, no. 9, pp. 897-898, 2003.
[24] J. Karasneh, A. Gül, W. E. Ollier, A. J. Silman, and J. Worthington, "Whole-genome screening for susceptibility genes in multicase families with Behçet's disease," *Arthritis & Rheumatism*, vol. 52, no. 6, pp. 1836–1842, 2005.
[25] S. Nishiguchi, S. Kaneshiro, M. Tanaka et al., "Association of HLA alleles with response (especially biochemical response) to interferon therapy in Japanese patients with chronic hepatitis C," *Journal of Interferon & Cytokine Research*, vol. 23, no. 3, pp. 135–141, 2003.
[26] A. Sette and J. Sidney, "Nine major HLA class I supertypes account for the vast preponderance of HLA-A and -B polymorphism," *Immunogenetics*, vol. 50, no. 3-4, pp. 201–212, 1999.
[27] M. Csire, G. Mikala, M. Pető et al., "Detection of four lymphotropic herpesviruses in Hungarian patients with multiple myeloma and lymphoma," *FEMS Immunology & Medical Microbiology*, vol. 49, no. 1, pp. 62–67, 2007.
[28] L. C. Pelosof and D. E. Gerber, "Paraneoplastic syndromes: an approach to diagnosis and treatment," *Mayo Clinic Proceedings*, vol. 85, no. 9, pp. 838–854, 2010.

28

Pseudomonas aeruginosa: An Uncommon Cause of Antibiotic-Associated Diarrhea in an Immunocompetent Ambulatory Adult

Ryan T. Hoff, Ami Patel, and Alan Shapiro

Department of Medicine, Division of Gastroenterology, Advocate Lutheran General Hospital, Park Ridge, USA

Correspondence should be addressed to Ryan T. Hoff; ryan.hoff@aah.org

Academic Editor: Hideto Kawaratani

Pseudomonas aeruginosa is an opportunistic Gram-negative pathogen known to cause enterocolitis in children, amongst other types of infections. *Pseudomonas aeruginosa* has been widely reported as a cause of antibiotic-associated diarrhea in adult immunocompromised hosts. We present an 81-year-old previously healthy female as the first reported case of *Pseudomonas aeruginosa* antibiotic-associated diarrhea in an immunocompetent host in the United States.

1. Introduction

Pseudomonas aeruginosa is an opportunistic Gram-negative pathogen known to cause enterocolitis in children and nosocomial infections, including hospital-acquired pneumonia and catheter-associated urinary tract infections (UTIs). Rarely, *Pseudomonas aeruginosa* causes antibiotic-associated diarrhea in immunocompromised hosts, but this has not been reported in immunocompetent ambulatory adults.

2. Case Presentation

An 81-year-old previously healthy woman presented to the emergency department (ED) with diarrhea for 2 days. A week prior to symptom onset, she completed a 17-day course of ciprofloxacin for a UTI, with resolution of dysuria. She described frequent, watery, nonbloody bowel movements with nausea and emesis. Her last colonoscopy 5 years prior showed only diverticulosis. She was treated with intravenous saline and ondansetron and discharged. The next day, she developed bloody bowel movements associated with weakness and mild lower abdominal pain. With ongoing diarrhea, she returned to the ED. Physical exam showed very mild left lower quadrant abdominal tenderness, without rebound or guarding. Laboratory studies showed white blood cell count 11,800 cells/mcL, potassium 3.3 meq/dL, lactate 1.0 mmol/L, and lipase 67 units/L. Electrolytes and liver enzymes were otherwise normal. *Clostridioides difficile* (*C. difficile*) stool toxin PCR was negative. CT abdomen and pelvis without contrast showed diverticulosis and mild inflammation surrounding the sigmoid colon (Figures 1 and 2). Empiric ciprofloxacin and metronidazole were started, and the patient was admitted to the medical floor. Over the next 3 days, she gradually improved. Stool culture grew *Pseudomonas aeruginosa*, with absence of normal fecal flora. Sensitivities showed resistance to ciprofloxacin and levofloxacin and sensitivity to all other antibiotics tested. Given her clinical improvement, antibiotics were discontinued after 7 days.

3. Discussion

We report a case of *Pseudomonas aeruginosa* as a cause of bacterial colitis. Our patient's recent long course of antibiotic therapy likely increased her susceptibility to this infection via loss of normal fecal microbiota, leading to a loss of competitive exclusion and diminished colonic barrier protection. While the episode of bleeding and abdominal discomfort could be manifestations of

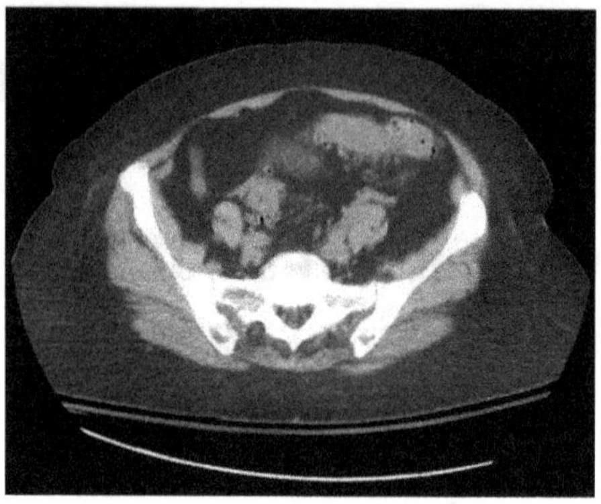

FIGURE 1: CT abdomen and pelvis without contrast, showing mild inflammation surrounding the sigmoid colon. Diverticulosis is present.

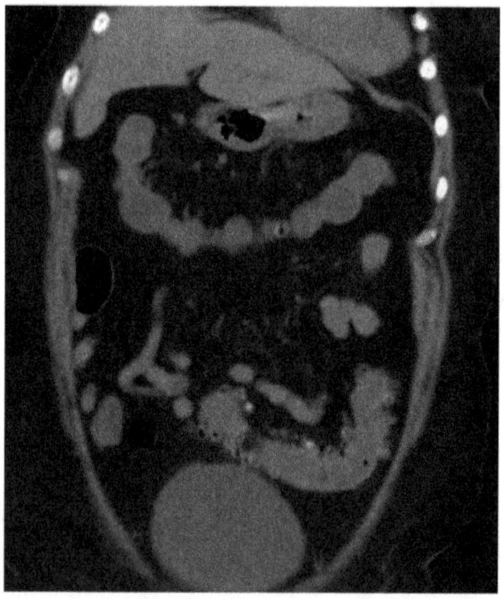

FIGURE 2: CT abdomen and pelvis without contrast, showing mild inflammation surrounding the sigmoid colon. Diverticulosis is present.

ischemic colitis, this would not explain the diarrhea or stool culture results.

Pseudomonas aeruginosa has been reported as a cause of enterocolitis in children and may affect healthy children [1]. Outbreaks in nurseries and infant wards have been reported [2, 3]. The most common risk factor is antibiotic use [1], though it also occurs in association with conditions that cause immunosuppression, including acute leukemia [4]. *Pseudomonas* enterocolitis in children may be severe, with bloody diarrhea, prolonged fever, markedly elevated inflammatory markers, and necrotizing enterocolitis, or mild with watery diarrhea in the absence of prolonged fever [1]. *Pseudomonas aeruginosa* has also been reported to colonize the gastrointestinal tract in patients with cystic fibrosis [5]. A combination of both host and pathogen factors likely contribute to this organisms' ability to cause overt infection [6].

Pseudomonas aeruginosa has been reported to cause rare cases of hospital-associated diarrhea in adults. A Korean study by Kim et al. described seven cases of nosocomial antibiotic-associated diarrhea due to *Pseudomonas aeruginosa*, as diagnosed by stool culture [7]. One patient was also diagnosed with *C. difficile* infection. All probable offending antibiotics were either carbapenems or cephalosporins, with an average duration of therapy of 13 days prior to onset of diarrhea and median onset at day 19 of hospitalization. Unlike our patient, fluoroquinolones were not implicated in this series. Sensitivity testing demonstrated that all strains of *Pseudomonas* were resistant to the previously administered antibiotics, suggesting a loss of competitive inhibition may have occurred. In one case series from a public hospital in Brazil, 14 patients admitted to the intensive care unit had a stool culture positive for *Pseudomonas aeruginosa*, although six of those patients also tested positive for *C. difficile* [8]. Alternative causes are important to consider, and patients with suspected *Pseudomonas* colitis should undergo testing for *C. difficile*.

An Australian study by Adlard et al. of 23 patients with diarrhea for more than 1 week found *Pseudomonas aeruginosa* in 20 cases without any other associated cause for diarrhea [9]. Of these patients, 19 were immunosuppressed due to age, comorbid illness, or medication therapy [3]. After pretreating rats with clindamycin, inoculation with *Pseudomonas aeruginosa* led to prolonged fecal shedding of the bacterium as well as ulceration and necrosis of the terminal ileum in 75 percent of the animals [9].

In cases of antibiotic-associated *Pseudomonas aeruginosa* enterocolitis, discontinuation of the antibiotic may be sufficient for clinical improvement. However, patients with ongoing clinically significant diarrhea would likely benefit from antimicrobial therapy, which may aid in recovery and facilitate restoration of normal bowel flora. Improvement has been reported with ciprofloxacin therapy [10]. However, the role for antimicrobial therapy in *Pseudomonas aeruginosa*-associated diarrhea has not been studied; further investigation is warranted.

To our knowledge, this is the first reported case of acute postantibiotic diarrhea caused by *Pseudomonas aeruginosa* in an immunocompetent ambulatory host in the United States. Previous reports of *Pseudomonas* colitis have primarily involved immunosuppressed or hospitalized patients and children. This pathogen may represent an important diagnostic consideration in patients presenting with diarrhea following antibiotics, with negative *C. difficile* stool testing. The role for antibiotic therapy in *Pseudomonas*-associated diarrhea warrants further research.

Disclosure

This case report was presented in abstract form as a poster presentation at the American College of Gastroenterology Annual Conference in San Antonio, Texas, in 2019.

Authors' Contributions

All authors participated in writing and reviewing the article. All authors approved the final manuscript.

References

[1] C.-H. Chuang, R. P. Janapatla, Y.-H. Wang et al., "*Pseudomonas aeruginosa*-associated diarrheal diseases in children," *The Pediatric Infectious Disease Journal*, vol. 36, no. 12, pp. 1119–1123, 2017.

[2] D. P. Falcão, C. P. Mendonca, A. Scrassolo et al., "Nursery outbreak of severe diarrhoea due to multiple strains of *Pseudomonas aeruginosa*," *Lancet*, vol. 300, no. 7766, pp. 38–40, 1972.

[3] A. L. Florman and N. Schifrin, "Observations on a small outbreak of infantile diarrhea associated with *Pseudomonas aeruginosa*," *The Journal of Pediatrics*, vol. 36, no. 6, pp. 758–766, 1950.

[4] A. De, H. Mathurkar, S. Baveja, and M. Manglani, "Pseudomonas diarrhea in a child suffering from acute lymphatic leukemia," *Indian Journal of Medical and Paediatric Oncology*, vol. 30, no. 4, pp. 147-148, 2009.

[5] G. Döring, H. Bareth, A. Gairing, C. Wolz, and K. Botzenhart, "Genotyping of *Pseudomonas aeruginosa*sputum and stool isolates from cystic fibrosis patients: evidence for intestinal colonization and spreading into toilets," *Epidemiology and Infection*, vol. 103, no. 3, pp. 555–564, 1989.

[6] C.-H. Chuang, Y.-H. Wang, H.-J. Chang et al., "Shanghai fever: a distinct *Pseudomonas aeruginosa*enteric disease," *Gut*, vol. 63, no. 5, pp. 736–743, 2014.

[7] S. W. Kim, K. R. Peck, S. I. Jung et al., "*Pseudomonas aeruginosa*as a potential cause of antibiotic-associated diarrhea," *Journal of Korean Medical Science*, vol. 16, no. 6, pp. 742–744, 2001.

[8] A. P. Marcon, M. A. Gamba, and L. A. C. Vianna, "Nosocomial diarrhea in the intensive care unit," *Brazilian Journal of Infectious Diseases*, vol. 10, no. 6, pp. 384–389, 2006.

[9] P. A. Adlard, S. M. Kirov, K. Sanderson, and G. E. Cox, "*Pseudomonas aeruginosa* as a cause of infectious diarrhoea," *Epidemiology and Infection*, vol. 121, no. 1, pp. 237–241, 1998.

[10] F. V. Porco and E. B. Visconte, "*Pseudomonas aeruginosa* as a cause of infectious diarrhea successfully treated with oral ciprofloxacin," *Annals of Pharmacotherapy*, vol. 29, no. 11, pp. 1122-1123, 1995.

29

Eosinophilic Gastritis in a Patient Previously Treated with Dupilumab

Masaya Iwamuro,[1] Toshi Murakami,[2] Takehiro Tanaka,[3] Shohei Oka,[1] Seiji Kawano,[1] Yoshiro Kawahara,[4] and Hiroyuki Okada[1]

[1]*Department of Gastroenterology and Hepatology, Okayama University Graduate School of Medicine, Dentistry and Pharmaceutical Sciences, Okayama 700-8558, Japan*
[2]*Satsuki Naika Clinic, Okayama 703-8258, Japan*
[3]*Department of Pathology, Okayama University Graduate School of Medicine, Dentistry and Pharmaceutical Sciences, Okayama 700-8558, Japan*
[4]*Department of Practical Gastrointestinal Endoscopy, Okayama University Hospital, Okayama 700-8558, Japan*

Correspondence should be addressed to Masaya Iwamuro; pr145h2k@okayama-u.ac.jp

Academic Editor: Haruhiko Sugimura

A 77-year-old Japanese man with bronchial asthma was treated with dupilumab. Dupilumab treatment was discontinued at the patient's request after two injections separated by a 2-week interval. The blood eosinophil count was elevated, and an esophagogastroduodenoscopy performed 3 months after dupilumab treatment revealed gastric ulcers; subsequently, eosinophilic gastritis was diagnosed from biopsy examinations. The gastric lesions were resolved by steroid administration. This case report underscores that eosinophil-associated gastrointestinal diseases should be considered in the differential diagnosis of gastric lesions occurring in patients who were treated with dupilumab.

1. Introduction

Dupilumab, a human monoclonal antibody against interleukin-4 (IL-4) and IL-13, is a subcutaneous injectable prescription medicine used for the treatment of asthma and atopic dermatitis [1, 2]. IL-4 and IL-13 initiate type 2 helper T-cell (Th2) mediated inflammatory processes, such as immunoglobulin *E* (IgE) production, smooth muscle contraction, mucus production, and innate cell recruitment to sites of inflammation, leading to allergic diseases [3]. As dupilumab inhibits both IL-4 and IL-13 signaling, it has beneficial effects in patients with asthma and atopic dermatitis. The efficacy, safety, and tolerability of dupilumab have been investigated and confirmed in clinical trials [4, 5]. However, a higher frequency of eosinophilia in dupilumab-treated patients has been reported both in clinical studies [6, 7] and a real-world study [8].

Herein, we have reported the case of a patient with asthma who developed eosinophilic gastritis after the administration of dupilumab, with a focus on the possible pathogenesis of eosinophil infiltration in the stomach.

2. Case Presentation

A 77-year-old Japanese man had visited a hospital with respiratory distress, cough, and sputum. The patient had hyperlipidemia, hypertension, atrophic rhinitis, duodenal ulcers, hyperuricemia, prostatic hypertrophy, and overactive bladder, for which he had been taking pravastatin, cilnidipine, trichlormethiazide, lansoprazole, febuxostat, silodosin, mirabegron, and a probiotic *Lactobacillus* preparation. He was a social drinker and an ex-smoker who smoked 30 cigarettes/day for 13 years. He had received

Helicobacter pylori eradication treatment at 68 years of age. Although the patient had a history of paranasal sinusitis and occasionally suffered from a cough, he had not previously been diagnosed with bronchial asthma.

His respiratory distress, cough, and sputum were improved by the temporary administration of formoterol inhaler and antibiotics. However, his symptoms reemerged after 3 months, and he visited a clinic. At that time, lung auscultation revealed a wheeze in both the lungs. His oxygen saturation was 89%–91%, his forced expiratory volume percentage in one second was 76.9%, his peak expiratory flow rate was 22.5%, and his exhaled nitric oxide level was 29–31 ppb. The laboratory tests showed increased values for C-reactive protein (1.53 mg/dL) and immunoglobulin *E* (740 IU/mL), whereas the number of white blood cells was within the normal range (6,900 μL). Radioallergosorbent tests were broadly positive for multiple allergens, such as house dust, mites, pollens, candida, and wheat. Fluticasone, formoterol, montelukast, and azithromycin were administered in addition to intravenous methylprednisolone. Although his medication was changed to vilanterol, fluticasone, and montelukast, his respiratory distress, cough, and sputum production were not completely resolved. Thus, dupilumab was administered twice separated by a 2-week interval. However, dupilumab treatment was discontinued at the patient's request because his symptoms were unchanged. Although his eosinophil count was within the normal range before the administration of dupilumab, it varied from 152 to 860 μL after dupilumab injections were initiated. The patient was subsequently treated with montelukast, bilastine, and zinc acetate.

The patient underwent an esophagogastroduodenoscopy 3 months after the dupilumab treatment for annual screening purposes. Esophagogastroduodenoscopy revealed gastric ulcers in the lesser curvature of the cardia (Figure 1(a)) and in the posterior wall of the gastric body (Figure 1(b)). Whitish mucosa was also observed in the lesser curvature of the gastric body (Figure 1(c)). Although the patient had undergone annual esophagogastroduodenoscopy for 9 years, gastric ulcers or whitish mucosa had not previously been identified. Biopsy of the gastric ulcers revealed more than 100 eosinophils per high-power field, which were infiltrating into the lamina propria and even the epithelium of the gastric mucosa (Figure 2); no neoplastic cells were noted. Consequently, a diagnosis of eosinophilic gastritis was made. The laboratory tests showed slightly increased values for C-reactive protein (0.33 mg/dL) and immunoglobulin *E* (366 IU/mL), whereas white blood cells (6,900 μL) and eosinophils (5.3%) were within the normal ranges. Computed tomography scanning showed no remarkable changes in the gastrointestinal tract. Consequently, 30 mg prednisone was administered to treat eosinophilic gastritis. Esophagogastroduodenoscopy performed 4 weeks after prednisone administration revealed the resolution of gastric ulcers (Figure 3). No eosinophils were identified in the biopsied specimens.

3. Discussion

Several randomized, placebo-controlled phase 3 trials revealed that dupilumab was effective for moderate-to-severe atopic dermatitis [9–11]. Alexis et al. performed post hoc analysis from three phase 3 trials assessing the efficacy and safety of dupilumab vs placebo and identified that serious adverse events occurred more frequently in the placebo groups [11]. However, a real-life study in a French multicenter adult cohort revealed a higher frequency of eosinophilia and conjunctivitis in patients with atopic dermatitis treated with dupilumab, compared with clinical trials [12].

Placebo-controlled phase 3 trials showed the efficacy of dupilumab for patients with moderate-to-severe or severe asthma [6, 7, 13]. In one phase 3 trial involving 1,902 patients with uncontrolled asthma [7], 52/1,264 patients in the dupilumab-treated group (4.1%) had eosinophilia, which was associated with symptoms such as the deterioration of chronic eosinophilic pneumonia and hypereosinophilia in four patients. Meanwhile, eosinophilia was observed in 4/638 patients in the placebo group (0.6%). Another phase 3 trial showed that transient blood eosinophilia was more frequently observed in the dupilumab group (14/103 patients, 13.6%) than in the placebo group (1/107 patients, 0.9%). These results indicated that dupilumab treatment may increase the blood eosinophil count in some patients with atopic dermatitis and/or asthma. As dupilumab is considered to inhibit the migration of eosinophils into tissues by blocking IL-4 and IL-13 signaling, it may transiently increase circulating blood eosinophil counts [7, 14]. Another possible mechanism of eosinophilia observed in clinical trials was the withdrawal of glucocorticoids in dupilumab-treated patients, which caused the elevation of blood eosinophils [6, 7].

Other adverse events reported in association with dupilumab included nasopharyngitis, bronchitis, sinusitis [15], injection-site reactions [6], headache [16], skin infections, cutaneous psoriatic lesions [17], alopecia [18, 19], and chronic eosinophilic pneumonia [20]. To the best of our knowledge, the development of gastrointestinal diseases in association with dupilumab use has not been reported previously. Thus, this report is the first to describe a patient with eosinophilic gastritis that occurred after the use of dupilumab.

In the present patient, dupilumab was administered twice separated by a 2-week interval for the treatment of asthma, and dupilumab treatment was discontinued thereafter. Esophagogastroduodenoscopy performed 3 months after dupilumab treatment revealed eosinophilic gastritis. There are several hypotheses regarding the occurrence of eosinophil infiltration in the present patient's stomach. First, the migration of eosinophil into organs was blocked by dupilumab administration, and the chemotaxis behavior may be altered when the migration was resumed after the withdrawal of dupilumab, resulting in stomach-predominant infiltration of eosinophils. Second, the stomach may escape the chemotaxis-sparing effect of dupilumab, and eosinophils converged in the gastric mucosa. Third, the patient was hyperallergic, which caused both asthma and eosinophilic gastritis. Eosinophilic gastroenteritis is frequently found in patients with atopic conditions [21]. Therefore, eosinophilic gastritis might occur coincidentally, independent of dupilumab treatment. However, these hypotheses are speculative and not substantiated by any

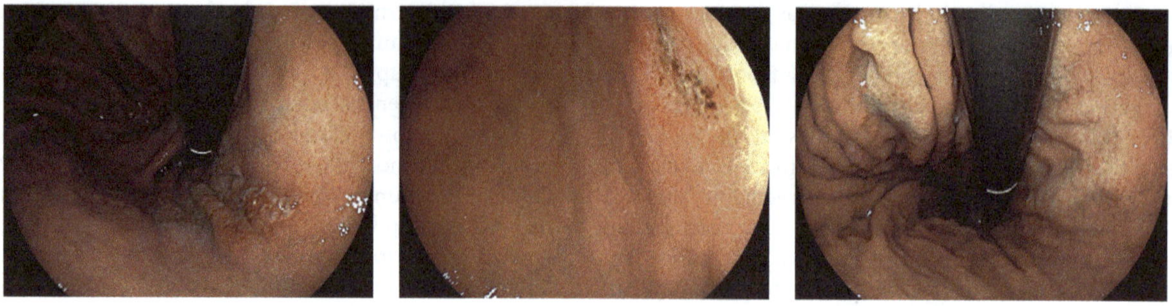

(a) (b) (c)

FIGURE 1: Esophagogastroduodenoscopy images. Esophagogastroduodenoscopy performed 3 months after dupilumab treatment revealed gastric ulcers in the lesser curvature of the cardia (a) and posterior wall of the gastric body (b). Whitish mucosa was also noted in the lesser curvature of the gastric body (c).

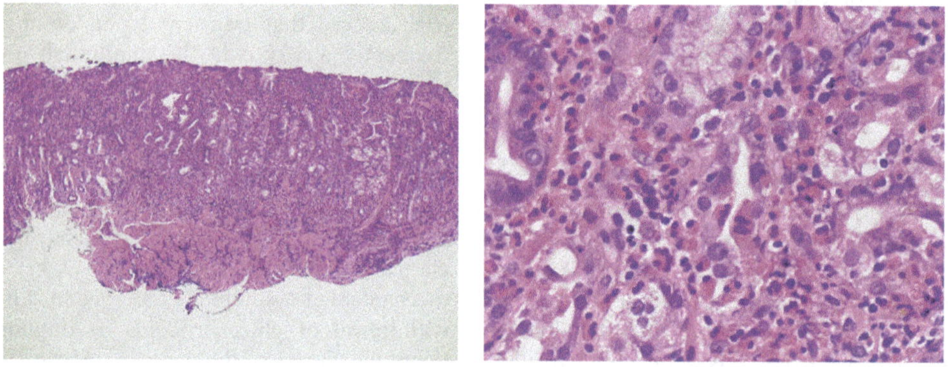

(a) (b)

FIGURE 2: Pathology images. Biopsy from the gastric ulcers showed the infiltration of eosinophils (a × 4; b × 40).

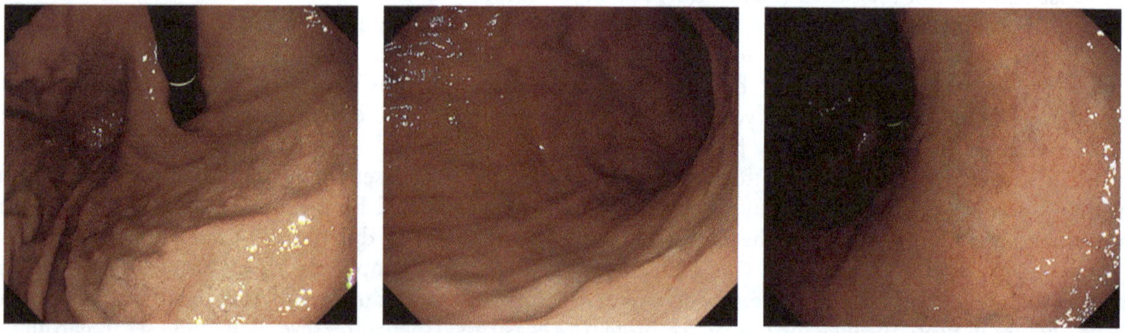

(a) (b) (c)

FIGURE 3: Esophagogastroduodenoscopy images. Endoscopy performed 4 weeks after prednisone administration revealed the resolution of gastric ulcers. No eosinophils were identified in the biopsied specimens.

supporting facts. Because this report includes only one patient with such a case, further investigation is required to clarify the relationship between eosinophilic gastritis and dupilumab use.

Menzella et al. reported a patient with chronic eosinophilic pneumonia that developed after the tenth injection of dupilumab [20]. Although a great improvement in asthma control was obtained, the patient manifested eosinophilia, fever, and bilateral pulmonary thickening. The authors described a progressive increase in blood eosinophil count after dupilumab injections were started, followed by the onset of chronic eosinophilic pneumonia. In the present patient, blood eosinophil count was also elevated after the administration of dupilumab. These results suggested that end-organ manifestations of eosinophilia may occur, regardless of whether the patient is receiving dupilumab treatment or treatment has been discontinued. It was also noteworthy that the patient had no gastrointestinal symptoms despite having multiple stomach ulcers secondary to eosinophil infiltration. Although screening esophagogastroduodenoscopy after administration of dupilumab may reveal asymptomatic gastrointestinal involvement—particularly in patients with eosinophilia—this concept needs further investigation. We hope this report will raise awareness of the potential for eosinophil-associated gastrointestinal disease following dupilumab use.

In conclusion, we encountered a patient with asthma who developed eosinophilic gastritis 3 months after dupilumab use. This case supports the consideration of eosinophilic gastritis in the differential diagnosis of gastric lesions emerging in patients who were treated with dupilumab.

References

[1] K. K. Rathinam, J. J. Abraham, and T. M. Vijayakumar, "Dupilumab in the treatment of moderate to severe asthma: an evidence-based review," *Current Therapeutic Research*, vol. 91, pp. 45–51, 2019.

[2] M. Kraft and M. Worm, "Dupilumab in the treatment of moderate-to-severe atopic dermatitis," *Expert Review of Clinical Immunology*, vol. 13, no. 4, pp. 301–310, 2017.

[3] K. Bao and R. L. Reinhardt, "The differential expression of IL-4 and IL-13 and its impact on type-2 immunity," *Cytokine*, vol. 75, no. 1, pp. 25–37, 2015.

[4] M. de Bruin-Weller, D. Thaçi, C. H. Smith et al., "Dupilumab with concomitant topical corticosteroid treatment in adults with atopic dermatitis with an inadequate response or intolerance to ciclosporin a or when this treatment is medically inadvisable: a placebo-controlled, randomized phase III clinical trial (LIBERTY AD CAFÉ)," *British Journal of Dermatology*, vol. 178, no. 5, pp. 1083–1101, 2018.

[5] A. Blauvelt, M. de Bruin-Weller, M. Gooderham et al., "Long-term management of moderate-to-severe atopic dermatitis with dupilumab and concomitant topical corticosteroids (LIBERTY AD CHRONOS): a 1-year, randomised, double-blinded, placebo-controlled, phase 3 trial," *The Lancet*, vol. 389, no. 10086, pp. 2287-2303, 2017.

[6] K. F. Rabe, P. Nair, G. Brusselle et al., "Efficacy and safety of dupilumab in glucocorticoid-dependent severe asthma," *New England Journal of Medicine*, vol. 378, no. 26, pp. 2475–2485, 2018.

[7] M. Castro, J. Corren, I. D. Pavord et al., "Dupilumab efficacy and safety in moderate-to-severe uncontrolled asthma," *New England Journal of Medicine*, vol. 378, no. 26, pp. 2486–2496, 2018.

[8] C. Wang, C. N. Kraus, K. G. Patel, A. K. Ganesan, and S. A. Grando, "Real-world experience of dupilumab treatment for atopic dermatitis in adults: a retrospective analysis of patients' records," *International Journal of Dermatology*, vol. 59, no. 2, pp. 253–256, 2020.

[9] M. J. Cork, D. Thaçi, L. F. Eichenfield et al., "Dupilumab in adolescents with uncontrolled moderate-to-severe atopic dermatitis: results from a phase IIa open-label trial and subsequent phase III open-label extension," *British Journal of Dermatology*, vol. 182, no. 1, pp. 85–96, 2020.

[10] C. Bachert, J. K. Han, M. Desrosiers et al., "Efficacy and safety of dupilumab in patients with severe chronic rhinosinusitis with nasal polyps (LIBERTY NP SINUS-24 and LIBERTY NP SINUS-52): results from two multicentre, randomised, double-blind, placebo-controlled, parallel-group phase 3 trials," *The Lancet*, vol. 394, no. 10209, pp. 1638–1650, 2019.

[11] A. F. Alexis, M. Rendon, J. I. Silverberg et al., "Efficacy of dupilumab in different racial subgroups of adults with moderate-to-severe atopic dermatitis in three randomized, placebo-controlled phase 3 trials," *Journal of Drugs in Dermatology*, vol. 18, no. 8, pp. 804–813, 2019.

[12] S. Faiz, J. Giovannelli, C. Podevin et al., "Effectiveness and safety of dupilumab for the treatment of atopic dermatitis in a real-life French multicenter adult cohort," *Journal of the American Academy of Dermatology*, vol. 81, no. 1, pp. 143–151, 2019.

[13] S. Wenzel, M. Castro, J. Corren et al., "Dupilumab efficacy and safety in adults with uncontrolled persistent asthma despite use of medium-to-high-dose inhaled corticosteroids plus a long-acting β_2 agonist: a randomised double-blind placebo-controlled pivotal phase 2b dose-ranging trial," *The Lancet*, vol. 388, no. 10039, pp. 31–44, 2016.

[14] P. C. Fulkerson and M. E. Rothenberg, "Targeting eosinophils in allergy, inflammation, and beyond," *Nature Reviews Drug Discovery*, vol. 12, no. 2, pp. 117–129, 2013.

[15] X. F. Xiong, M. Zhu, H. X. Wu, L. L. Fan, and D. Y. Cheng, "Efficacy and safety of dupilumab for the treatment of uncontrolled asthma: a meta-analysis of randomized clinical trials," *Respiratory Research*, vol. 20, no. 1, p. 108, 2019.

[16] Z. Ou, C. Chen, A. Chen, Y. Yang, and W. Zhou, "Adverse events of dupilumab in adults with moderate-to-severe atopic dermatitis: a meta-analysis," *International Immunopharmacology*, vol. 54, pp. 303–310, 2018.

[17] G. Safa and V. Paumier, "Psoriasis induced by dupilumab therapy," *Clinical and Experimental Dermatology*, vol. 44, no. 3, pp. e49–e50, 2019.

[18] I. Salgüero-Fernández, M. A. Gonzalez de Domingo, D. Suarez, and G. Roustan-Gullón, "Dermatitis and alopecia in a patient treated with dupilumab: a new adverse effect?" *Clinical and Experimental Dermatology*, vol. 44, no. 3, pp. e41–e43, 2019.

[19] B. Barroso-García, M. Rial, A. Molina, and J. Sastre, "Alopecia areata in severe atopic dermatitis treated with dupilumab," *Journal of Investigational Allergology and Clinical Immunology*, vol. 28, no. 6, pp. 420-421, 2018.

[20] F. Menzella, G. Montanari, G. Patricelli et al., "A case of chronic eosinophilic pneumonia in a patient treated with dupilumab," *Therapeutics and Clinical Risk Management*, vol. 15, pp. 869–875, 2019.

[21] Y. Kinoshita, S. Oouchi, and T. Fujisawa, "Eosinophilic gastrointestinal diseases–pathogenesis, diagnosis, and treatment," *Allergology International*, vol. 68, no. 4, pp. 420–429, 2019.

Megacystis-Microcolon-Intestinal Hypoperistalsis Syndrome (MMIHS): Series of 4 Cases Caused by Mutation of ACTG2 (Actin Gamma 2, Smooth Muscle) Gene

Katarzyna Ignasiak-Budzyńska, Mikołaj Danko, and Janusz Książyk

Department of Paediatrics, Nutrition and Metabolic Diseases, Children's Memorial Health Institute, Al. Dzieci Polskich 20, Warsaw 04-730, Poland

Correspondence should be addressed to Katarzyna Ignasiak-Budzyńska; katarzynaignasiak93@gmail.com

Academic Editor: Hirotada Akiho

MMIHS, also known as Berdon's syndrome, is a rare disease that belongs to primary causes of CIPOS (chronic intestinal pseudoobstruction syndrome). Clinical characteristics of MMIHS are differential, but we come across the following classic symptoms: disorders of intestinal peristalsis, microcolon, and megacystis. In this article, we present a series of 4 patients with Berdon's syndrome, in whom we managed to identify the genetic causes of MMIHS. All infants showed clinical features of bowel obstruction and dysfunction of the urinary system after birth. Two of them also manifested disorders from other systems. The prognosis for these patients is poor, but a constant betterment of management in MMIHS, in which the leading role plays TPN (total parental nutrition), causes improvement of patients' survival.

1. Introduction

Berdon's syndrome, also known as MMIHS (megacystis-microcolon-intestinal hypoperistalsis syndrome), is a rare motility disorder of gastrointestinal and urinary tract caused by primary dysfunction of the architecture of the smooth muscle cell membrane or intestinal nervous system. The clinical features of MMIHS are various, but we come across three classic symptoms: disorders of intestinal peristalsis, microcolon, and megacystis [1, 2]. The severity of MMIHS and conditions of other organ systems depend on differential variants of genetic mutations that have been identified as molecular causes of Berdon's syndrome. The following genes are known to be involved in pathogenesis of MMIHS: ACTG2 (the most frequent), MYH11 (myosin heavy chain 11), MYLK (myosin light chain kinase), LMOD1 (leiomodin 1), and MYL9 (myosin light chain 9) [3]. However, genetic causes have been identified in approximately 50% of Berdon's syndrome cases. Seven patients with MMIHS have been under treatment at Department of Paediatrics, Nutrition and Metabolic Diseases so far. Here we report a case series of 4 patients with detected ACTG2 gene mutations. The others are without ascertained genetic causes.

2. Case 1

A 3-month-old female infant weighing 3050 g with Apgar score of 9 and 8 at 1 min and 5 min was referred to our centre to enter Home Parenteral Nutrition Program (HPN). The girl was born to a non-consanguineous Polish couple and delivered by spontaneous labour at 35 weeks of pregnancy. There were no records of genetic diseases in the family tree. During the ultrasound scan at 22 weeks, megacystis has been noticed in the fetal pelvis with bilateral pelvicalyceal dilatation. At 24 weeks gestation, fetal magnetic resonance imaging (MRI) was performed which revealed a large cystic mass with a maximum diameter of 8 cm and moderate bilateral hydronephrosis. Because of lower urinary tract obstruction, fetal vesico-amniotic shunt (VAS) was implanted at 31 weeks. At birth, there was abdomen distension and absence of intestinal sounds. A few hours after birth, the patient presented food intolerance and gradually developed respiratory distress. The infant has not passed stool for the first 24 hours. Because of these symptoms, intestinal obstruction was suspected. The nasogastric tube for decompression of gastrointestinal tract was inserted, and the central line was implanted to apply total parental nutrition (TPN). Abdominal radiography showed gastric distention and multiple dilated loops of small bowel (Figure 1). Contrast study of upper gastrointestinal tract excluded the mechanical bowel obstruction. Microcolon was detected in the barium enema (Figure 2). The infant underwent exploratory laparotomy on 2nd day of life, in which markedly enlarged intestinal loops extending to 20 cm from Bauhin's valve were discovered. A full-thickness biopsy was taken and ileostomy was performed.

The histological findings were nonspecific (smooth muscle cell vacuolization and insignificant disorders of cytoskeletal architecture). Alpha-smooth muscle actin (alpha-SMA) immunoreactivity was maintained. After surgery, the patient still presented oral feeding intolerance. Stoma has not passed intestinal content, and retention in the nasogastric tube was observed. The rectal biopsy was performed to exclude long-segment Hirschsprung's disease. The histological picture showed normal ganglion cells, and acetylcholinesterase (AChE) activity was normal. Because of persistent motility disorders and oral feeding intolerance, the patient was qualified to decompress gastrostomy tube, and the long-term central venous access (Broviac type) was implanted. Except for gastrointestinal disturbances, the patient was anuric and required protracted catheterization. Ultrasonography (USG) and abdomen MRI showed diminished corticomedullary differentiation, bilateral hydronephrosis, and tortuous ureters (Figure 3). Urodynamics testing revealed hypotonic bladder and detrusor-sphincter dyssynergia. The patient required intermittent catheterization every 3 hours during daytime and night interruption. MMIHS was suspected. The diagnosis was confirmed in genetic tests. Heterozygous de novo missense mutation (c.533G>A/p.Arg178His) was identified in the 5th exon of ACTG2 gene. At present, the girl is one-year-old and has satisfying nutritional status.

She had repeated catheter-related bloodstream infections and one episode of urosepsis.

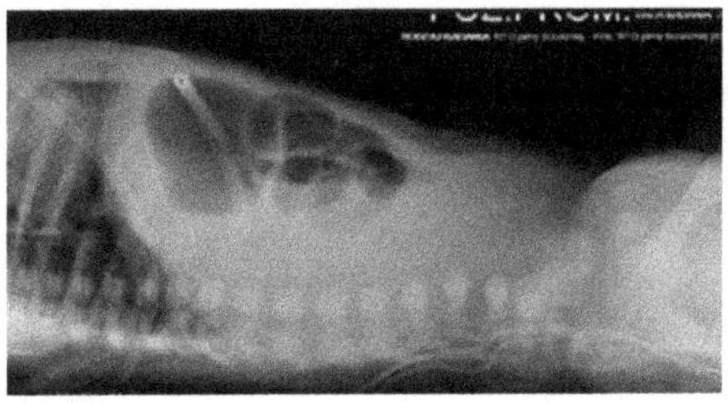

Figure 1: Abdominal X-ray on the first day of life—dilated stomach and bowel loops.

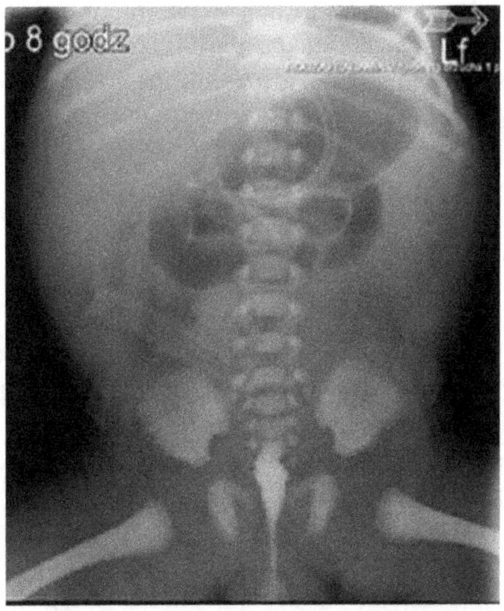

Figure 2: Barium enema revealed microcolon.

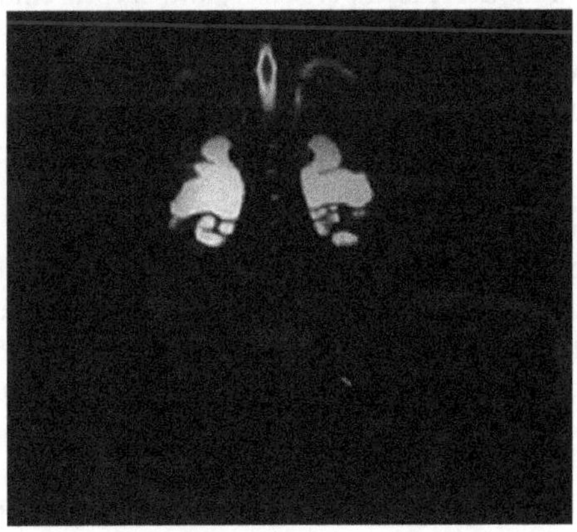

Figure 3: MRI showed bilateral pelvicalyceal dilation and tortuous ureters.

3. Case 2

A 5-month-old female infant with a history of abdominal distension was admitted to our Clinic to continue treatment. The girl was delivered by spontaneous labour at 36 weeks of gestation with a birth weight of 2600 g and Apgar scores of 10 at 1 min and 5 min. This patient was born to a 25-year-old gravida three of a non-consanguineous marriage, with no relevant family history. A second-trimester ultrasound scan showed abdominal cystic structure, moderate bilateral hydronephrosis, and umbilical cord hernia. At 30 weeks of pregnancy, VAS was performed. Initial physical examination disclosed massively distended abdomen and hypoactive bowel sounds. The patient required urinary bladder catheterization. Exploratory laparotomy showed a segment of ileum in which meconium was arrested, but no organic obstruction was found. The umbilical hernia was placed back into the abdominal cavity. Abdominal radiography revealed dilated stomach and nonmajor gas in the distal bowel segments. Because of persistent oral intake intolerance, a central venous catheter was placed into the right internal jugular vein to administer TPN. The infant subsequently developed

Enterococcus faecalis sepsis and required antibiotic therapy. Because of duodenal obstruction, the patient was operated on 26 days after birth. Ladd's bands and abdominal adhesions were resected, and Santulli stoma was made. Histological findings of the intestinal biopsy revealed vacuolar degeneration of smooth muscle cells. Pathological evaluation of rectal biopsy revealed normal ganglion cells. Percutaneous endoscopic gastrostomy was performed to decompress the stomach. The urodynamics disclosed post-void residual urine, bilateral hydronephrosis, and detrusor-sphincter dyssynergia. The urologists recommended intermittent catheterization and persistent antibiotic prophylaxis.

Genetic testing was performed on the patients and their parents. De novo missense mutation (c.533G>A/ p.Arg178His) was identified in the ACTG2 gene in the infant that confirmed MMIHS. At present, the girl is 1.5-year-old, and her growth and development are normal.

She had repeated catheter-related bloodstream infections.

4. Case 3

A 9-week-old male infant (2500 g birth weight and with Apgar scores of 6 at 1 min and 5 min after birth) with abdominal distension was referred to our Department to start advanced diagnostic procedures. He was born to healthy non-consanguineous parents and delivered by caesarean section in the 33rd week of pregnancy. The couple did not have the history of hereditary diseases in their family. The boy was delivered by caesarean section in the 33rd week of pregnancy. Prenatal ultrasound studies imaged bilateral obstructive uropathy at 13 weeks, and VAS was implanted at 30 weeks. After birth, the infant presented with a lax abdominal wall, decreased peristalsis, and cryptorchidism. He had poor feeding and bilious vomiting. Conservative treatment (nasogastric tube, intermittent catheterization) and TPN were administered. Abdominal X-ray showed features of small bowel obstruction and a small amount of free gas under the diaphragm.

Because of unresolved intestinal obstruction, surgical intervention (laparotomy) was performed of the 5th day of life. Intraoperative findings revealed vesicointestinal fistula, microcolon, and flaccid bladder. The ileostomy 25 cm far from the ileocaecal valve was performed, and biopsy specimens were taken. Hirschsprung's disease has also been ruled out. The trophic feeding was started to stimulate the sucking and swallowing. The gastrostomy tube for persistent gastric decompression was implanted.

Elevated conjugated bilirubin levels were observed during the first weeks of TPN treatment. After fish oil-based lipid emulsion implementation, the cholestasis was reversed.

Urodynamics testing revealed hypotonic bladder, functional micturition disorders, and vesicoureteral reflux grade 3. Because of this, it was decided to create a vesicostomy.

Patent foramen ovale (PFO) was detected in the echocardiography.

Heterozygous de novo missense mutation (c.188G>A/ p.Arg63Gln) was identified in the ACTG2 gene, and the diagnosis of Berdon's syndrome was obtained. At present, the patient is 2.5-year-old and has satisfying nutritional status. He has not developed long-term TPN-associated complications so far.

5. Case 4

A 6-week-old girl was referred to our Clinic to continue treatment. She was a preterm baby (delivered by caesarean section at 34 weeks of pregnancy with 2500 g birth weighting and with Apgar scores 10 at 1 min and 5 min). The patient was patient was born to a 35-year-old gravida four of a non-consanguineous Polish marriage. The other siblings were healthy, and there were no signs of hereditary diseases in their family tree. During an ultrasound scan at 22 weeks, megacystis with bilateral pyelocalyceal dilation had been noticed. At 29 weeks of pregnancy, VAS was implanted. On initial examination, abdominal distension, abdominal flaccidity, and hyporeactive peristalsis were present. Oral intake induced vomiting. The patient was also anuric. After insertion of the Foley catheter and a nasogastric tube, the urinary bladder and the stomach were decompressed. The obstruction of the gastrointestinal tract was suspected. A central venous catheter was implanted and TPN was started. Upper gastrointestinal tract X-ray examination showed dilated bowel loops and delay in the passage of contrast. The patient was operated on 72 hours after birth. Intestinal malrotation and microcolon with small bowel dilatation up to terminal ileum were seen on laparotomy. The Bishop Koop stoma 15 cm far from the ileocaecal valve was performed, and a full-thickness intestinal biopsy was taken. Voiding cystourethrogram (VCUG) showed a large, distended bladder with bilateral vesicoureteral reflux (Figure 4). The patient has required intermittent catheterization.

Because of the suspicion of deafness, the auditory brainstem response (ABR) was performed. Conductive hearing loss was ascertained.

Heterozygous de novo missense mutation (c.188G>A/ p.Arg63Gln) was identified in the ACTG2 gene, which confirmed MMIHS. At present, the patient is 14-month-old and had recurrent urinary tract infection.

We observed cholestasis with elevated transaminases in all patients during the first weeks of TPN (Table 1). However, after the introduction of trophic feedings and modification of TPN by the implementation of fish oil-based intravenous lipid emulsion, direct bilirubin levels have been normalized. Moreover, the patients (especially patient number 3) have begun to tolerate increased quantities of feeding in the following months, which is not characteristic for patients with Berdon's syndrome.

The prognosis is poor, and all our patients with ACTG2 mutations survive probably to their early adulthood. The life expectancy also depends on occurrence of long-term TPN-associated complications and repeated urosepsis.

6. Other Patients with MMIHS

Three of our patients with MMIHS are without ascertained genetic causes. They showed all characteristic symptoms for

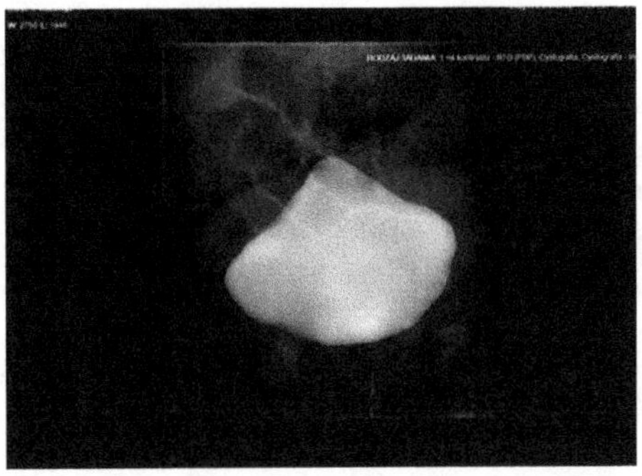

FIGURE 4: Cystography showed enlarged, hypotonic urinary bladder.

TABLE 1: Characteristics of the patients.

Number of patient	The current age (number of months)	The current weight (kg)	The highest level of conjugated bilirubin (mg/dl)	Percentile of weight-for-height	Calories in oral intake (kcal/kg)	Calories in TPN (kcal/kg)
1	11	7.6	1.89	3–10	16.3	88
2	30	11	4.11	3–10	8	86
3	33	15.4	5.56	75–90	84	43
4	9	6.8	11.91	10	15	73

Berdon's syndrome: disorders of intestinal peristalsis, microcolon, and dilated urinary bladder. However, they have less severe presentation of intestinal dysmotility than patients with detected ACTG2 gene mutations. They tolerated larger portions of enteral feeding, and urinary tract infections occurred sporadically in these patients. However, life expectancy of patients with diagnosed MMIHS is similar, regardless of the gene mutation.

7. Discussion

Berdon's syndrome is a rare disease that belongs to the primary causes of CIPOS. According to current literature (in the period 1976–2019), 450 patients with MMIHS were reported. Because of the severity and broad spectrum of possible clinical presentations that accompany cardinal symptoms, management of Berdon's syndrome is complicated. Some of them have been noted in our patients (deafness, blindness, congenital heart defect (PFO), cryptorchidism, and prune belly syndrome). This ambiguousness stems from differential missense or nonsense mutations of genes that code for ingredients of cytoskeletal and play a leading role in smooth muscle contraction [4, 5].

The most frequent disorders are detected in the ACTG2 gene, whose mutations are responsible for 44.1% of cases with known genetic aetiology. The c.533G>A (p.Arg178His) missense alteration of ACTG2 gene, which was in two of our patients, correlates with the most severe presentation of MMIHS (6). The mutation of the following genes: MYH11, MYLK, LMOD1, and MYL9, is also involved in the pathogenesis of Berdon's syndrome in individual cases. However, 50% of patients with MMIHS are without established genetic causes [6–8]. Characteristic prenatal ultrasonography images can suggest MMIHS. The prenatal USG showed megacystis in 88% of the fetus with MMIHS, pelvicalyceal dilation in 66% of prenatally diagnosed cases, or hydramnios [9, 10]. After birth, the newborn presented symptoms of gastrointestinal obstruction and urinary tract dysfunction. Because of this, the initial diagnosis is based on imaging findings, in which microcolon, nonmechanical intestinal obstruction, and dilated urinary bladder are revealed. Despite nonspecific histological changes (vacuolar degeneration of smooth muscle cells, the variability of the number and shape of the ganglion cells in the submucosa and the myenteric plexus, abnormal distribution, or increased connective tissue), the histopathology analysis is also crucial to exclude other possible primary causes of CIPOS.

Berdon's syndrome used to have a fatal prognosis. In the beginning, the mortality rate was approximately 80%, and about 90% of infants died in their first year of life [11]. However, long-term survival rates have increased to 55.6%, respectively (for patients diagnosed with MMIHS in 2004–2011) [12]. It is associated with the improvement of the management of MMIHS and enhanced treatment standards, in which TPN plays a key role. The current evidence confirmed that TPN has a significant impact on prolongation of survival in patients. Unfortunately, individuals develop complications from TPN, including infections, liver failure, thrombosis, etc., which are the main causes of deaths at a later time [13].

The alternative approach is isolated intestinal transplantation or in combination with liver graft. In 1999, Masetti et al. reported the first three patients with MMIHS, who underwent multivisceral transplantation. The patients were alive 17 and 24 months after surgery. One of them died on day 44 of multiple organ failure [14]. The subsequent reports were more promising. In 2013, Huang et al. noticed the case of an eight-year-old boy who was completely off

TPN after isolated intestinal transplantation at 4 years of age [15]. Moreover, in 2005, Loinaz et al. described 12 patients with CIPOS (6 with Berdon's syndrome), and 6 of them survived from 2 to 7 years after transplantation. They have begun enteral feeding (after strenuous dietary rehabilitation) and have not required TPN [16]. The analysis of survival after transplantation is hopeful but distant from being satisfying. Because of this, the TPN is currently the most important part of the treatment of MMIHS and would be still a crucial element in the next coming years.

8. Conclusions

To sum up, the prognosis of MMIHS is poor, but slow upswing of patients' survival is observed. The management of Berdon's syndrome should be based on improving the quality of nutritional care. At present, the clinician's priority is to avoid long-term TPN-associated complications. Because of unknown molecular causes in most cases, it is a good practice to offer genetic counselling to families with a history of Berdon's syndrome.

Disclosure

This study was performed as part of the employment of the authors at Children's Memorial Health Institute, Warsaw, Poland. The funder had no role in the manuscript writing, editing, approval, or decision to publish.

Authors' Contributions

All authors participated in writing and reviewing the article. All authors approved the final manuscript.

Acknowledgments

The photos were taken with the consent of Department of Radiology of the Children's Health Institute.

References

[1] E. López-Muñoz, A. Hernández-Zarco, A. Polanco-Ortiz, J. Villa-Morales, and L. Mateos-Sánchez, "Megacystis-microcolon-intestinal hypoperistalsis syndrome (MMIHS): report of a case with prolonged survival and literature review," *Journal of Pediatric Urology*, vol. 9, no. 1, pp. e12–e18, 2013.

[2] P. Puri and M. Shinkai, "Megacystis microcolon intestinal hypoperistalsis syndrome," *Seminars in Pediatric Surgery* vol. 14, no. 1, pp. 58–63, 2005.

[3] L. Ambartsumyan, "Megacystis-microcolon-intestinal hypoperistalsis syndrome overview," in *GeneReviews® [Internet]* M. P. Adam, H. H. Ardinger, R. A. Pagon et al., Eds., pp. 1993–2020, University of Washington, Seattle, WA, USA, 2019, https://www.ncbi.nlm.nih.gov/books/NBK540960/.

[4] U. Rolle, S. O'Briain, R. H. Pearl, and P. Puri, "Megacystis-microcolon-intestinal hypoperistalsis syndrome: evidence of intestinal myopathy," *Pediatric Surgery International*, vol. 18, no. 1, pp. 2–5, 2002.

[5] A. P. Piotrowska, U. Rolle, B. Chertin, D. De Caluwé, A. Bianchi, and P. Puri, "Alterations in smooth muscle contractile and cytoskeleton proteins and interstitial cells of Cajal in megacystis microcolon intestinal hypoperistalsis syndrome," *Journal of Pediatric Surgery*, vol. 38, no. 5, pp. 749–755, 2003.

[6] N. Assia Batzir, P. Kishor Bhagwat, A. Larson et al., "Recurrent arginine substitutions in the ACTG2 gene are the primary driver of disease burden and severity in visceral myopathy," *Human Mutation*, vol. 41, no. 3, pp. 641–654, 2020.

[7] H. Nakamura, A. M. O'Donnell, and P. Puri, "Consanguinity and its relevance for the incidence of megacystis microcolon intestinal hypoperistalsis syndrome (MMIHS): systematic review," *Pediatric Surgery International*, vol. 35, no. 2, pp. 175–180, 2019.

[8] D. Halim, R. M. W. Hofstra, L. Signorile et al., "ACTG2-variants impair actin polymerization in sporadic megacystis microcolon intestinal hypoperistalsis syndrome," *Human Molecular Genetics*, vol. 25, no. 3, pp. 571–583, 2016.

[9] J. R. Whittington, A. T. Poole, E. H. Dutta, and M. B. Munn, "A novel mutation in ACTG2 gene in mother with chronic intestinal pseudoobstruction and fetus with megacystis microcolon intestinal hypoperistalsis syndrome," *Case Reports in Genetics*, vol. 2017, 3 pages, Article ID 9146507, 2017.

[10] L. Tuzovic, K. Anyane-Yeboa, A. Mills, K. Glassberg, and R. Miller, "Megacystis-microcolon-intestinal hypoperistalsis syndrome: case report and review of prenatal ultrasonographic findings," *Fetal Diagnosis and Therapy*, vol. 36, no. 1, pp. 74–80, 2014.

[11] M. Mantan, G. Sethi, K. Singhal, and S. Aggarwal, "Megacystis, microcolon, intestinal hypoperistalsis syndrome and bilateral streak gonads," *Indian Journal of Nephrology*, vol. 21, no. 3, pp. 212–214, 2011.

[12] H. Soh, M. Fukuzawa, A. Kubota, H. Kawahara, T. Ueno, and T. Taguchi, "Megacystis microcolon intestinal hypoperistalsis syndrome: a report of a nationwide survey in Japan," *Journal of Pediatric Surgery*, vol. 50, no. 12, pp. 2048–2050, 2015.

[13] M. F. Wangler, C. Gonzaga-Jauregui, T. Gambin et al., "Heterozygous de novo and inherited mutations in the smooth muscle actin (ACTG2) gene underlie megacystis-microcolon-intestinal hypoperistalsis syndrome," *PLoS Genetics*, vol. 10, no. 3, Article ID e1004258, 2014.

[14] M. Masetti, M. M. Rodriguez, J. F. Thompson et al., "Multivisceral transplantation for megacystis microcolon intestinal hypoperistalsis syndrome," *Transplantation*, vol. 68, no. 2, pp. 228–232, 1999.

[15] C.-M. Huang, S.-H. Tseng, C.-C. Weng, and Y. Chen, "Isolated intestinal transplantation for megacystis microcolon intestinal hypoperistalsis syndrome: case report," *Pediatric Transplantation*, vol. 17, no. 1, pp. E4–E8, 2013.

[16] C. Loinaz, M. M. Rodríguez, T. Kato et al., "Intestinal and multivisceral transplantation in children with severe gastrointestinal dysmotility," *Journal of Pediatric Surgery*, vol. 40, no. 10, pp. 1598–1604, 2005.

31

Debilitating Manifestation of a Disease with Multiple Names: A Severe Case of Sclerosing Mesenteritis

Valeriia Klymenko, Reba Varughese, Katherine A Woolley, Joseph M Wetherell, Haritha Mopuru, Edward Mensah, and Imran Siddiqui

Department of Medicine, St. Vincent's Medical Center, Bridgeport, CT, USA

Correspondence should be addressed to Joseph M Wetherell; joseph.wetherell@quinnipiac.edu

Academic Editor: Hirotada Akiho

Sclerosing mesenteritis (SM) is a rare inflammatory condition with unknown etiology that affects the mesenteric adipose tissue. We present a case of a 49-year-old male with severe abdominal pain who underwent abdominal biopsy confirming the presence of adipose inflammation and necrosis. The diagnosis of SM was made, and the patient was treated with prednisone and tamoxifen. As this condition is rare, there are no standard guidelines for management. This case aims to outline a possible treatment plan.

1. Introduction

Sclerosing mesenteritis (SM) is a rare, idiopathic disorder involving inflammation and fibrosis of the mesenteric adipose tissue [1]. SM is noted to be poorly understood and difficult to classify as it has a wide range of definitions and terminology. It was first described in 1924 and named retractile mesenteritis [2]. The term sclerosing mesenteritis is used to encompass many similar conditions including mesenteric panniculitis, mesenteric fibrosis, retractile mesenteritis, mesenteric lipodystrophy, and misty mesentery which are all distinguished histologically [2]. A pathologic predominance of fibrosis as opposed to inflammation is found in mesenteric fibrosis, whereas inflammation predominance indicates mesenteric panniculitis, with fat necrosis indicating mesenteric lipodystrophy [3]. With an estimated prevalence ranging from >1%–1.26%, this rare condition may lead to a wide array of nonspecific symptoms such as abdominal pain, weight loss, change in bowel habits, nausea and vomiting, anorexia, and fever [1, 2]. On a review of 92 cases of SM, 51 patients (51%) had a normal abdominal exam, 22 (24%) had tenderness, 14 (15%) had an abdominal mass, and 13 (14%) had chylous ascites [4]. The nondescript physical exam findings with a majority of patients having a normal physical exam make this condition difficult to recognize. The etiology remains largely unknown with cases suggesting association with trauma, autoimmune conditions, infection, and malignancy [1]. Computed tomography (CT) is the diagnostic imaging of choice, while biopsy is utilized to rule out malignancy. SM is often an incidental finding on abdominal imaging, and since this condition is extremely rare, there are insufficient data about the clinical course and therefore no standard guidelines for management. We present a case of SM treated with prednisone and tamoxifen to contribute to the existing knowledge base on SM.

2. Case Presentation

A 49-year-old male with a past medical history of hypertension, hyperlipidemia, posttraumatic stress disorder, and depression presented to the emergency department with complaints of diffuse abdominal pain, diarrhea, weight loss, night sweats, and subjective fever.

One month prior to admission, the patient suddenly developed diffuse, sharp abdominal pain, which was associated with nonbloody diarrhea, nausea, and night sweats; it was aggravated by eating. History was notable for a 40 lb unintentional weight loss prior to the onset of symptoms. The patient's surgical history was insignificant. Family

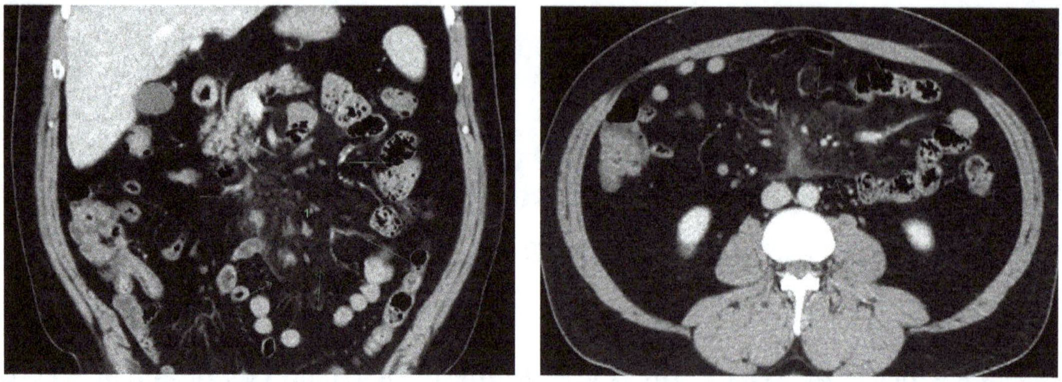

(a) (b)

FIGURE 1: CT abdomen w/contrast: there is moderate "misty" infiltration of the root of the small bowel mesentery (arrows), where an increased number of subcentimeter normal-size mesenteric lymph nodes are also identified. (a) Coronal view. (b) Axial view.

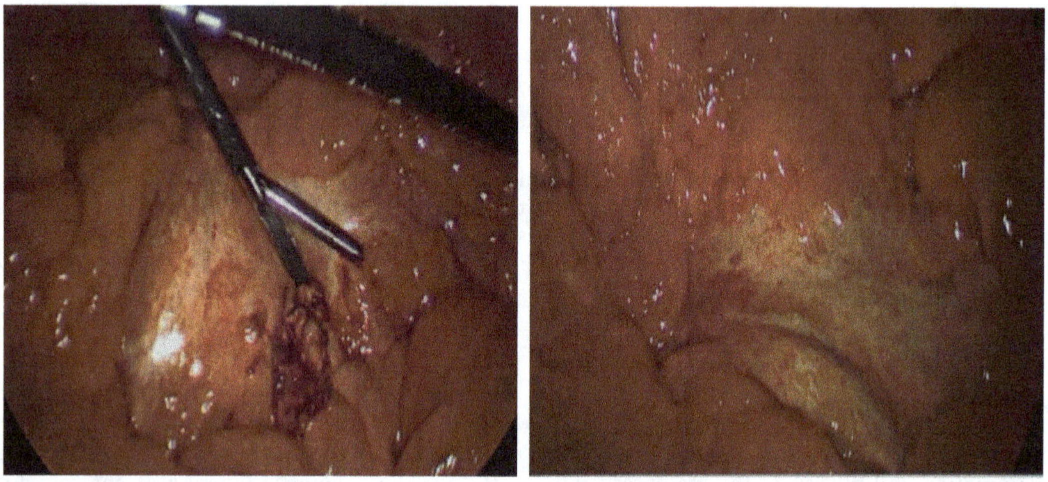

FIGURE 2: Mosaic white stranding of the mesentery in the proximal aspect in the areas involved on CT imaging. The bowel was hyperemic but obviously viable.

history was notable for lymphoma in a first-degree relative and an uncle who died from colon cancer at the age of 62.

On examination, vital signs were unremarkable. Physical examination revealed diffuse abdominal tenderness without rebound tenderness or guarding. Rectal exam was normal, and the stool occult was negative for blood. Laboratory studies were notable for leukocytosis 12.2×10^3/mcL with left-sided shift, erythrocyte sedimentation rate 20 mm/hr, and mild transaminitis; electrolytes, creatinine, lipase, C-reactive protein, lactic acid, lithium levels, ANA, and rheumatoid factor were all within normal limits. Stool examination revealed no ova or parasites, and C. diff toxin and culture were also negative.

CT scan of abdomen and pelvis with contrast was done demonstrating hazy infiltration with subcentimeter lymph nodes, slightly more prominent in the right abdomen, which was concerning for sclerosing mesenteritis and mild splenomegaly (Figure 1). The hospital course was complicated by severe pain and vomiting requiring intravenous opiates. Diagnostic laparoscopy was pursued which revealed mosaic white stranding of the proximal mesentery in the areas involved (Figure 2). Biopsy of small bowel mesentery showed mature adipose tissue with patchy chronic inflammation and fat necrosis; thus, the diagnosis of SM was established (Figure 3). The patient was initially treated with tamoxifen 10 mg BID and prednisone 40 mg with no improvement within 3 months of therapy. This patient was not able to tolerate an oral diet, suffering abdominal pain and watery diarrhea after each meal. Overall, he had 60 lbs of weight loss. In the next phase of treatment following steroid/tamoxifen resistance, the patient was started on total parenteral nutrition (TPN), adalimumab 80 mg subcutaneously every 14 days and pentoxifylline 400 mg PO TID, while steroids were tapered off in an appropriate manner. Four months after treating the patient with adalimumab/pentoxifylline therapy, he started feeling better, and he was taken off TPN, able to tolerate 1 meal/day, and maintained weight.

Meanwhile, the patient was still experiencing night sweats periodically. Since SM is associated with various malignancies, including GI adenocarcinoma, the patient underwent an extensive workup. Esophagoduodenoscopy/

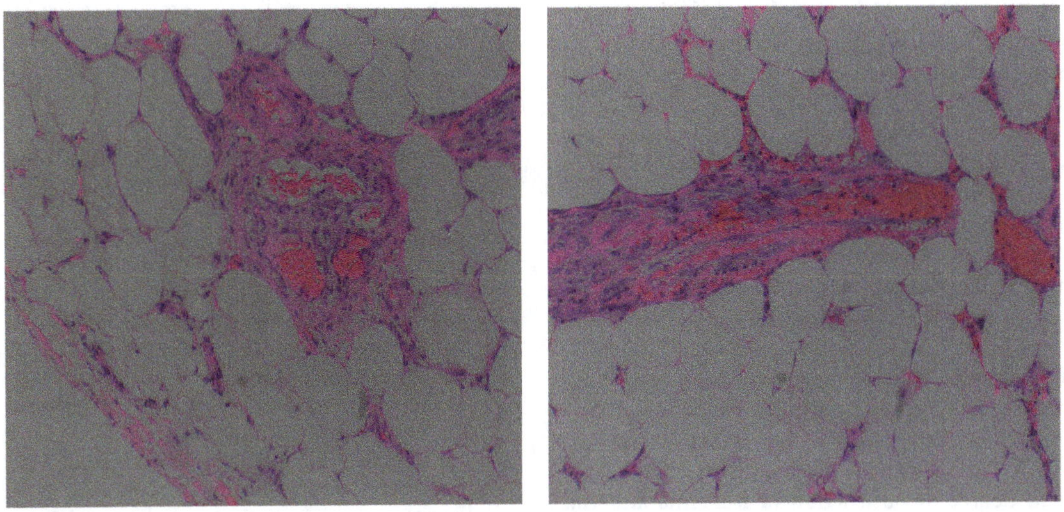

(a) (b)

FIGURE 3: Histopathologic findings of (a) Soft tissue, small bowel mesentery, biopsy: mature adipose tissue with patchy chronic inflammation and fat necrosis; (b) soft tissue, epiploic appendage, biopsy: mature adipose tissue with focal acute and chronic inflammation. Focal small vessel vasculitis and foci of microthrombi.

colonoscopy was done and did not reveal any significant abnormality. PET scan was also performed and did not demonstrate any lymphadenopathy or abnormal FDG activity within the mesentery. Liver, gallbladder, adrenal glands, spleen, and pancreas had normal appearance as well.

3. Discussion

Sclerosing mesenteritis is a diagnosis of exclusion, as conditions such as lymphoma, carcinoid tumor, and carcinomatosis could present in a similar fashion. On CT, the most specific features for SM are the "fat ring sign" and tumor pseudocapsule surrounding the inflammation. SM could also present as a soft tissue homogeneous/heterogeneous mass, sometimes with calcifications from fat necrosis or as an increased attenuation of mesenteric fat without mass, which is called "misty mesentery" [1]. As this condition is extremely rare and multiple nomenclature were used in the past, we have limited understanding of its etiology, pathophysiology, and clinical course. It has been postulated to be associated with a history of abdominal surgery; autoimmune conditions such as lupus and rheumatoid arthritis; infectious agents such as tuberculosis, cryptococcus, schistosomiasis, HIV, and cholera; medications including paroxetine and pergolide; and malignancy [1]. However, it remains controversial as multiple case-control studies have brought these associations into questions. Two studies failed to show any association between SM and prior abdominal trauma, surgery, comorbidities such as diabetes mellitus, or malignancy [5, 6]. While the pathophysiology remains unclear, histological analysis appears to suggest a chronic progression of fat necrosis to inflammation to fibrosis, resultant from an initial proinflammatory cytokine response [7].

Management of SM and treatment regimens is based on case reports and other fibrosing diseases, such as sclerosing encapsulating peritonitis [8]. The most commonly cited treatment regimen includes the combination of 40 mg daily prednisone and 10 mg twice daily tamoxifen [1]. This is continued for 3 months, followed by a gradual prednisone taper if there is symptomatic improvement. Tamoxifen is recommended to continue indefinitely due to the high rate of relapse seen in other fibrotic diseases when tamoxifen is discontinued [1]. Other agents have been explored as well, including the angiogenesis inhibitor thalidomide. One small, open-label pilot study looked at 5 patients with symptomatic SM who were treated with 200 mg thalidomide nightly for 3 months, with 4 reporting clinical response and 1 complete remission. As thalidomide is known for adverse effects including peripheral neuropathy and teratogenicity, it is recommended only in those who either failed or who have contraindications to corticosteroid/tamoxifen therapy [9].

There are a few case reports written about successful SM treatment with TNF-alpha inhibitors, such as infliximab and adalimumab. Rothlein et al. described a case report about a patient with sacroiliitis and similar presentation of SM with debilitating paroxysmal abdominal pain, who was successfully treated with significant improvement in abdominal symptoms with infliximab treatment [10]. In another study, Nyberg et al. presented 27 patients with SM. In this group, for one patient, despite therapy with prednisone and methotrexate, treatment was initiated with the TNF-alpha inhibitor adalimumab for a psoriatic arthritis flare, which resulted in decreased abdominal pain [11].

Sharma et al. in a systematic review of 192 patients with SM reported that, in terms of medical treatment, the majority of patients ($n = 56$, 83.5%) received steroids. TNF-alpha inhibitor, infliximab, was given to only 2.9% of participants ($n = 2$) with other treatment options reported as well—colchicine, tamoxifen, 6-mercaptopurine, antibiotics, azathioprine, methotrexate, cyclophosphamide, IVIG, and D-penicillamine. Since there was an overlap between the various agents of medical treatment, it was not possible to address their efficacy in this particular study but again showed a potential role for biologic therapy in SM [3].

The role of pentoxifylline therapy in SM is also not yet well established. Kapsoritakis et al. described a case report of retractile mesenteritis with malabsorption syndrome, which was successfully treated with pentoxifylline therapy (800 to 1200 mg/day). An exact mechanism of pentoxifylline anti-fibrotic/anti-inflammatory activity is unknown. In some studies, it is reported that pentoxifylline could act on the synthesis of proinflammatory cytokines—TNF-α, intercellular adhesion molecule-1, IL-1β, IL-6— and activation of lymphocytes [12].

Surgical therapy is indicated for those who do not respond to medical management and have evidence of persistent mechanical obstruction or bowel ischemia. Specific procedures performed vary according to involvement of the mesentery and degree of obstruction or ischemia and can include bowel resection, mass resection, or palliative bypass [1].

4. Conclusion

SM is a rare disease, and therefore sufficient data are unavailable regarding clinical course and treatment. For this reason, it is vital that physicians have a broad differential diagnosis when patients come with abdominal pain into the emergency room. Since a gold standard treatment of patients with SM has not yet been clearly established, our clinical case of steroid/tamoxifen-resistant SM with a good response to TNF-alpha inhibitors/pentoxifylline may represent an important clinical interest for consideration in future patients.

Disclosure

This case was presented as a Poster Presentation at the 2020 Scientific Meeting of the American College of Physicians.

References

[1] C. J. Danford, S. C. Lin, and J. L. Wolf, "Sclerosing Mesenteritis," *The American Journal of Gastroenterology*, vol. 114, no. 6, pp. 867–873, 2019.

[2] M. S. Green, R. Chhabra, and H. Goyal, "Sclerosing mesenteritis: a comprehensive clinical review," *Annals of Translational Medicine*, vol. 6, no. 17, p. 336, 2018.

[3] P. Sharma, S. Yadav, C. M. Needham, and P. Feuerstadt, "Sclerosing mesenteritis: a systematic review of 192 cases," *Clinical Journal of Gastroenterology*, vol. 10, no. 2, pp. 103–111, 2017.

[4] S. Akram, D. S. Pardi, J. A. Schaffner, and T. C. Smyrk, "Sclerosing mesenteritis: clinical features, treatment, and outcome in ninety-two patients," *Clinical Gastroenterology and Hepatology*, vol. 5, no. 5, pp. 589–596, 2007.

[5] L. Protin-Catteau, G. . Thiéfin, C. Barbe, D. Jolly, P. Soyer, and C. Hoeffel, "Mesenteric panniculitis: review of consecutive abdominal MDCT examinations with a matched-pair analysis," *Acta Radiologica (Stockholm, Sweden*, vol. 57, pp. 1438–1444, 1987.

[6] G. D. Cherayil, K. S. Scaria, G. T. Hensley, and W. H. Elliott, "Abnormal lipid composition of fat tissue in human mesenteric panniculitis," *Lipids*, vol. 16, no. 3, pp. 199–202, 1981.

[7] K. Endo, R. Moroi, M. Sugimura et al., "Refractory sclerosing mesenteritis involving the small intestinal mesentery: a case report and literature review," *Internal Medicine*, vol. 53, no. 13, pp. 1419–1427, 2014.

[8] C. J. Danford, S. C. Lin, M. P. Smith, and J. L. Wolf, "Encapsulating peritoneal sclerosis," *World Journal of Gastroenterology*, vol. 24, no. 28, pp. 3101–3111, 2018.

[9] P. M. Ginsburg and E. D. Ehrenpreis, "A pilot study of thalidomide for patients with symptomatic mesenteric panniculitis," *Alimentary Pharmacology & Therapeutics*, vol. 16, no. 12, pp. 2115–2122, 2002.

[10] L. R. Rothlein, A. W. Shaheen, J. P. Vavalle et al., "Sclerosing mesenteritis successfully treated with a TNF antagonist," *Case Reports*, vol. 2010, no. 1, Article ID bcr0720103145, 2010.

[11] L. Nyberg, J. Björk, P. Björkdahl, O. Ekberg, K. Sjöberg, and L. Vigren, "Sclerosing mesenteritis and mesenteric panniculitis – clinical experience and radiological features," *BMC Gastroenterology*, vol. 17, Article ID 75, 2017.

[12] A. N. Kapsoritakis, C. D. Rizos, S. Delikoukos, D. Kyriakou, G. K. Koukoulis, and S. P. Potamianos, "Retractile mesenteritis presenting with malabsorption syndrome. Successful treatment with oral pentoxifylline," *Journal of Gastrointestinal and Liver Diseases: JGLD*, vol. 17, no. 1, pp. 91–94, 2008, PMID: 18392253.

Gastrointestinal Bleeding Secondary to Metastatic Duodenal Choriocarcinoma in a Patient with Concomitant Peptic Ulcer Disease

Ahmed Elfiky,[1] Asmaa Mokhtar,[1] Mira Alsheikh,[2] Hassan Almoussawi,[2] and Stephen Mulrooney[2]

[1] *Department of Internal Medicine, Staten Island University Hospital-Northwell Health, New York, NY, USA*
[2] *Department of Gastroenterology, Staten Island University Hospital-Northwell Health, New York, NY, USA*

Correspondence should be addressed to Ahmed Elfiky; aelfiky1@northwell.edu

Academic Editor: Haruhiko Sugimura

Testicular tumors are one of the most common solid tumors in young males. Choriocarcinoma usually presents as metastatic disease. Gastrointestinal tract involvement is rare. We report a case of a 40-year-old male presenting to our hospital with a three-day history of dyspnea on exertion and black stool after recent diagnosis of testicular choriocarcinoma. Urgent EGD performed revealed small clean-based fundal ulcer and an antral ulcer without the stigma of recent bleeding. Capsule endoscopy was performed and revealed a bleeding ill-defined mass in the proximal duodenum. A subsequent push enteroscopy showed an ulcerated bleeding mass in the third part of the duodenum that was treated with a hemospray with adequate hemostasis. Pathology was consistent with pure choriocarcinoma. The patient received a cisplatin-based chemotherapy regimen. The patient tolerated the chemotherapy regimen well and was discharged for outpatient follow-up. At the three-month follow-up, the patient did not show evidence of recurrent gastrointestinal bleeding.

1. Introduction

Testicular tumors are one of the most common solid tumors in males aged 15–35 years, with germ cell tumors being the most common type [1]. Choriocarcinoma, the most aggressive subtype, usually presents with metastasis owing to the frequent hematogenous and lymphatic spread. The most common sites of metastasis are the lungs, liver, brain, and bone [2]. Gastrointestinal tract involvement is rare. We report a case of a 40-year-old male presenting with upper gastrointestinal bleed secondary to metastatic duodenal choriocarcinoma.

2. Case Description

A 40-year-old male presented to the hospital with a three-day history of dyspnea on exertion and black stool. He was recently diagnosed with testicular choriocarcinoma and lung metastasis. He underwent left radical orchiectomy ten days prior to admission. The pathology revealed choriocarcinoma with immunopathological stain positive for human chorionic gonadotropin. The patient was in the process of evaluation for chemotherapy at the time of the presentation. Vital signs upon presentation were notable for a heart rate of 122/minute, otherwise stable. Physical exam was significant for mild epigastric tenderness and melena on the digital rectal exam. Initial blood work revealed acute microcytic anemia with a hemoglobin of 8.4 g/dL. Hemoglobin three weeks before the presentation was 14 g/dL. Upper gastrointestinal bleeding was suspected; the patient was resuscitated and started on pantoprazole infusion. Urgent esophagogastroduodenoscopy (EGD) performed after 10 hours of presentation with the finding of one small clean based fundic ulcer and a 2 cm antral ulcer without the stigma of recent bleeding.

Because of persistent melena and a drop in the hemoglobin level requiring transfusion of 2 pRBCs, colonoscopy was performed with unremarkable finding. Capsule endoscopy was pursued to look for other possible etiologies. It revealed a bleeding ill-defined mass within 3 minutes from the first duodenal image consistent with proximal small bowel bleed.

A subsequent push enteroscopy revealed a friable ulcerated bleeding mass in the third portion of the duodenum that was treated with a hemospray with adequate hemostasis (Figure 1).

The patient received a total of 8 units of packed RBCs during the hospital stay of 10 days. Pathology from enteroscopy was consistent with pure choriocarcinoma, and the immunohistochemical stain is positive for human chorionic gonadotropin (Figures 2 and 3).

Laboratory tests revealed serum human chorionic gonadotropin 516139 mIU/ml [<1, mIU/ml] and alpha-fetoprotein 1.83 ng/ml [<8.3 ng/ml]. The patient started a chemotherapy regimen with etoposide, ifosfamide, and cisplatin. Bleeding was controlled acutely by hemospray and completely ceased after beginning chemotherapy. The patient tolerated the chemotherapy regimen well and was discharged for outpatient follow-up. At the three-month follow-up, the patient did not show evidence of recurrent gastrointestinal bleeding.

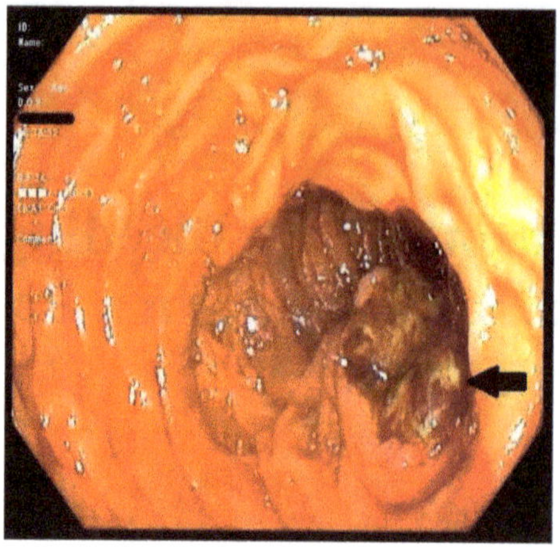

FIGURE 1: Arrow pointing at a friable ulcerated mass in the third portion of the duodenum.

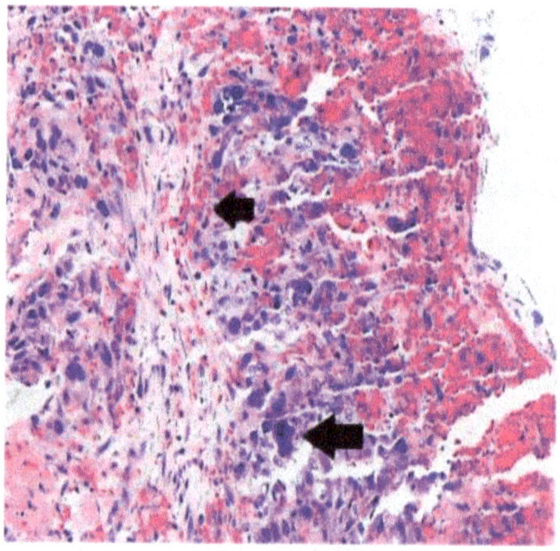

FIGURE 2: Upper arrow: clusters of cytotrophoblast and hemorrhage; lower arrow: syncytiotrophoblast.

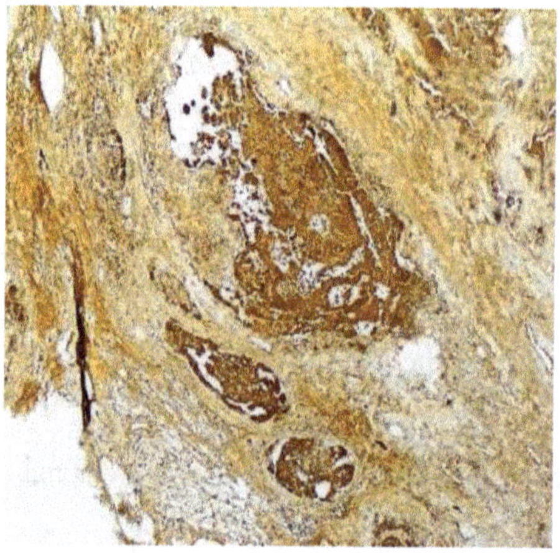

FIGURE 3: Human chorionic gonadotropin-positive immunohistochemical stain.

3. Discussion

Germ cell tumor is the most common testicular cancer. The most aggressive and least common type of germ cell tumor is choriocarcinoma [3]. Less than 8% of testicular germ cell tumors contain a component of choriocarcinoma, and less than 1% of the primary testicular germ cell tumors are pure choriocarcinoma [4].

Testicular tumors usually present as painless testicular mass or swelling. However, in choriocarcinoma, widespread hematogenous dissemination occurs early, and many patients present with metastatic disease [5]. Measurement of serum tumor markers human chorionic gonadotropin and alpha-fetoprotein can be helpful as they are elevated in roughly 80% of choriocarcinoma cases.

A definite diagnosis of choriocarcinoma requires a radical inguinal orchiectomy. The determination of metastatic choriocarcinoma can be challenging as extensive tissue sampling and careful microscopic examination are essential. The most important pathologic characteristic of choriocarcinoma is the coexistence of both syncytiotrophoblast and cytotrophoblast cells, which distinguishes this tumor from other germ cell tumors with only scattered syncytiotrophoblast. Tumor markers can be of great help in establishing the diagnosis. GATA3 is a transcription factor emerging as a sensitive immune marker for choriocarcinoma [6].

Gastrointestinal tract metastasis occurred in 5% of germ cell tumors. The small intestine, most commonly the duodenum, is the most frequent site for metastasis (72%) followed by the esophagus, stomach, and colon [7]. Small bowel involvement manifests as intestinal obstruction or gastrointestinal bleeding, as choriocarcinoma is a highly vascular tumor. Rosenblatt et al. described the first case of severe upper gastrointestinal bleed secondary to metastatic testicular tumor [8].

Treatment of testicular choriocarcinoma depends on the disease stage. Radical orchiectomy of the affected testis and dissection of the affected lymph nodes are the treatment of early-stage disease. Metastatic disease is usually treated with cisplatin-based chemotherapy. The serum level of human chorionic gonadotropin is used to monitor response to treatment [9].

Acute treatment modalities of the bleeding gastrointestinal metastasis are similar to other bleeding etiologies and include endoscopic intervention, embolization, or surgical resection. Bain et al. presented a case of bleeding duodenal choriocarcinoma that was treated with angiography and embolization [10]. Iglesias Gasrcia et al. also presented another case that required surgical intervention for achieving hemostasis after failure of endoscopic injection with adrenaline and arogon plasma coagulation [11]. Bleeding control is usually consolidated by chemotherapy. In our case, despite finding two ulcers on the EGD, high clinical suspicion for separate pathology was required to pursue capsule endoscopy. Despite being a rare presentation, the metastatic bleeding tumor should be considered in a patient with testicular tumors presenting with gastrointestinal bleeding.

Disclosure

This case has been presented as a poster in the annual meeting of American College of Gastroenterology (ACG) 2020.

Acknowledgments

The authors would like to thank Dr. Mesut Toprak for his help in obtaining pathology figures.

References

[1] A. Bleyer, A. Ferrari, J. Whelan, and R. D. Barr, "Global assessment of cancer incidence and survival in adolescents and young adults," *Pediatric Blood & Cancer*, vol. 64, no. 9, p. e26497, 2017.

[2] J. J. Bredael, D. Vugrin, and W. F. Whitmore Jr, "Autopsy findings in 154 patients with germ cell tumors of the testis," *Cancer*, vol. 50, no. 3, pp. 548–51, 1982.

[3] H.-J. Schmoll, "Extragonadal germ cell tumors," *Annals of Oncology*, vol. 13, no. Suppl 4, pp. 265–272, 2002.

[4] H. J. Schmoll, R. Souchon, S. Krege et al., "European consensus on diagnosis and treatment of germ cell cancer: a report of the European Germ Cell Cancer Consensus Group (EGCCCG)," *Annals of Oncology*, vol. 15, no. 9, pp. 1377–1399, 2004.

[5] S.-C. Lee, K. H. Kim, S. H. Kim, N. S. Lee, H. S. Park, and J.-H. Won, "Mixed testicular germ cell tumor presenting as metastatic pure choriocarcinoma involving multiple lung metastases that was effectively treated with high-dose chemotherapy," *Cancer Research and Treatment*, vol. 41, no. 4, pp. 229–232, 2009.

[6] M. Miettinen, P. A. McCue, M. Sarlomo-Rikala et al., "GATA3: a multispecific but potentially useful marker in surgical pathology: a systematic analysis of 2500 epithelial and nonepithelial tumors," *American Journal of Surgical Pathology*, vol. 38, no. 1, pp. 13–22, 2014.

[7] M. M. Chait, R. C. Kurtz, and S. I. Hajdu, "Gastrointestinal tract metastasis in patients with germ-cell tumor of the testis," *The American Journal of Digestive Diseases*, vol. 23, no. 10, pp. 925–928, 1978.

[8] G. S. Rosenblatt, C. J. Walsh, and S. Chung, "Metastatic testis tumor presenting as gastrointestinal hemorrhage," *The Journal of Urology*, vol. 164, no. 5, p. 1655, 2000.

[9] M. J. Reilley and L. C. Pagliaro, "Testicular choriocarcinoma: a rare variant that requires a unique treatment approach," *Current Oncology Reports*, vol. 17, no. 2, p. 2, 2015.

[10] A. J. Bain, D. J. Owens, and T. J. Savides, "Image of the month. upper gastrointestinal bleeding caused by metastatic testicular choriocarcinoma," *Clinical Gastroenterology and Hepatology*, vol. 8, no. 4, p. A22, 2010.

[11] J. Iglesias García, E. López García, F. Macías García et al., "Severe gastrointestinal bleeding secondary to duodenal metastasis from a choriocarcinoma," *Revista Española de Enfermedades Digestivas*, vol. 101, no. 10, pp. 720–722, Oct 2009.

Brown Bowel Syndrome is a Rare and Commonly Missed Disease: A Case Report and Literature Review

Joaquin Ponce-Zepeda,[1] Wenchang Guo,[1] Giorgioni Carmen,[1] Daniel Moon Kim,[2] Gregory C. Albers,[2] Vishal Suresh Chandan,[1] and Xiaodong Li[1]

[1]*Department of Pathology and Laboratory Medicine, University of California-Irvine, Irvine, CA, USA*
[2]*Department of Internal Medicine, Gastroenterology, University of California-Irvine, Irvine, CA, USA*

Correspondence should be addressed to Xiaodong Li; xiaodol4@uci.edu

Academic Editor: Daniel C. Damin

Background. Brown bowel syndrome (BBS) is a rare gastrointestinal condition, and vitamin E deficiency has been considered to be a main contributor. However, vitamin E deficiency has been found in only a few patients throughout the published literature studies and its cutoff lab value for diagnosis is not entirely clarified. *Case Presentation.* A 56-year-old female patient with a history of congenital bowel obstruction (repaired at birth) presented with bloating, abdominal pain, and chronic diarrhea. Endoscopy identified unremarkable gastrointestinal mucosa except a few small polyps in the colon. A partial obstruction was detected by a small bowel follow-through series and then confirmed by CT scan. The resected small bowel was significantly dilated with a thickened brown wall and extensive serosal adhesion. Microscopic examination revealed unremarkable mucosa, but dense granular brown pigments were identified in the cytoplasm of the smooth muscle cells in the muscularis propria. These deposits resulted to be lipofuscin, and BBS was diagnosed. The patient was asymptomatic at 9-month follow-up after surgery without vitamin E supplement. *Conclusion.* Mitochondrial damage with lipofuscin deposition is at the root of BBS pathogenesis. Any etiology associated with mitochondrial damage can cause this disease, and vitamin E deficiency is just one of them. Dysmotility from extensive serosal adhesion could be a possible etiology for this patient. Due to overlapping symptoms, lipofuscin deposition primarily in the muscularis propria, and unclear serum value of vitamin E, this syndrome is often missed in routine clinical practice from the superficial biopsy. A transmural biopsy is necessary for a definite diagnosis.

1. Introduction

Brown discoloration accumulating in the human intestinal wall secondary to lipofuscin was first observed by Wagner in 1861 [1], and the terminology of brown bowel syndrome (BBS) was formally introduced by Toffler in 1963 [2]. BBS is a rare gastrointestinal condition, and less than 70 cases have been reported in the literature. Since this syndrome usually occurred in patients with underlying conditions causing chronic long-term or severe malabsorption, vitamin E deficiency has been accordingly considered to be a main contributor. However, vitamin E deficiency has been confirmed in only a few patients throughout these literature studies, and its cutoff lab value for diagnosis is not still clarified.

2. Case Presentation

A 56-year-old female presented with bloating, abdominal pain, and chronic diarrhea for one year and weight loss of 20 pounds. As per the patient, she had a congenital bowel obstruction repaired at birth; however, the official details were not documented in a formal medical report. Her family history included diverticulitis, colitis, and colon cancer on her maternal side. Endoscopic examination showed unremarkable mucosa of both stomach and duodenum; colonoscopy identified two small polyps in the distal transverse colon and proximal descending colon. A small bowel follow-through was further conducted and revealed relatively high-grade partial mechanical bowel obstruction. The following

CT scan confirmed the small bowel obstruction along with marked hepatic steatosis.

An open exploration revealed a segment of small bowel with marked dilation and extensive adhesions to the abdominal wall. A resected segment of the small bowel (35.5 cm in length) showed an extensive fibrotic and adhesive serosal surface, which was significantly dilated at the proximal end (11.0 cm in greatest diameter). Upon sectioning, the small bowel mucosa was unremarkable, and the wall of the small bowel was distinctly thickened (measuring 0.6–0.8 cm) and appeared dark brown (Figure 1(a)). Microscopic examinations revealed prominent hypertrophy of the muscularis propria with normal small bowel mucosa. However, the fine granular brown pigments were identified to be confined in the cytoplasm of the smooth muscle cells in the muscularis propria, not in muscular mucosae (Figures 1(b) and 1(c)). Special stains were performed, and these granular deposits were negative for iron and trichrome, strongly positive for periodic acid-Schiff (PASD) (Figure 1(d)), and patchy positive for Fontana-Masson in both smooth muscle cells in the muscularis propria (Figure 1(e)) and blood vessels (Figure 1(f)). These granular deposits resulted to be lipofuscin by these special stains. The immunohistochemistry (IHC) for CD117, calretinin, and S100 revealed normal interstitial cells of Cajal, nerve cells, and ganglion cells and ruled out neuropathic disease. An infection process has also been ruled out by both normal mucosa morphology and negative specific stains for Gomori methenamine silver (GMS), PAS, and acid-fast bacilli (AFB). Celiac disease and inflammatory bowel disease (IBD) have been excluded based on both normal endoscopic and histologic mucosa. Severe malnutrition is unlikely due to normal hemoglobin (11.8 G/DL) and albumin (4.2 G/DL). Ultimately, BBS was the final diagnosis, and the patient was discharged without vitamin E supplement. She was closely followed up and remained asymptomatic as of the date of this manuscript writing.

3. Discussion

3.1. Pathogenesis. BBS is histologically characterized by pathologic lipofuscin accumulation in the cytoplasm of smooth muscle cells in the gastrointestinal wall [3]. Lipofuscin is a lysosomal degradation product of damaged mitochondria due to oxidative stress (an imbalance between antioxidant defenses and reactive oxygen species) [4]. In BBS patients, lipofuscin is confined in smooth muscle cells primarily in the muscularis propria, but also can be seen in the muscular mucosae and blood vessel wall. The remaining cells of the intestine including epithelial cells are not affected [5]. This accumulation can be seen in any part of the gastrointestinal wall including the appendix and gallbladder [3]; however, it shows the propensity to the small intestine.

Vitamin E deficiency has been considered to be a main contributor for the pathogenesis of BBS based on the following three major facts: First, vitamin E has antioxidative property and its deficiency has been proved to cause damage to the phospholipid layer of the mitochondrial membrane [6], which in turn leads to the pathologic accumulation of lipofuscin [7, 8]. Secondly, BBS usually occurs in patients with malabsorptive disorders that may cause vitamin E deficiency: celiac disease [9, 10], IBD [11], cystic fibrosis [12], liver disease [12, 13], chronic pancreatitis [10], motility disorders [14–16], and postoperative conditions (obesity/bypass surgery) [6, 12, 17]. Third, some BBS patients were identified to have deficient vitamin E levels and showed an improvement in clinical symptoms after vitamin E supplementation [1, 12, 15, 18]. However, these findings have been reported in only a few cases [1, 12, 15, 18] (for example, only one out of six patients in a recently published study [12]) and there is no literature to define the cutoff value of vitamin E for diagnosis and therapy. Other antioxidants, such as glutathione peroxidase, have been also found depleted in a patient with BBS [15]. Therefore, a large prospective study to clarify the oxidative stress, not only limited to vitamin E, is necessary for the understanding of this disease.

Mitochondrial damage with lipofuscin deposition is the core of the pathogenesis of BBS. In this literature review, the emphasis is placed on a positive and continuous feedback loop between oxidative stress, damaged mitochondria, and lipofuscin deposition. Lipofuscin deposition, as a product of damaged mitochondria, also inhibits the effective degradation of oxidatively modified proteins [4]. Lipofuscin in smooth muscle cells further disrupts the muscle fiber architecture by interrupting the contractile myofibrils and finally causes dysmotility and eventually muscularis propria hypertrophy [19]. The resulting dysmotility in the bowel increases oxidative stress and further causes mitochondrial dysfunction. The patient in this report did not show obvious malnutrition, and the underlying disorders causing malnutrition, such as IBD, celiac disease, and chronic pancreatitis, have been excluded. The liposuction is primarily deposited in the adhesive small bowel segment, not the whole intestine. It was intestinal dysmotility that initiated this positive feedback loop of pathogenesis (shown in Figure 2).

3.2. Clinical Symptoms. Besides symptoms from the underlying disorders, BBS patients, like this case report, usually present with intestinal motility disorders (e.g., intestinal dilation, volvulus, and intussusception) [14, 20, 21]. Intestinal bleeding, an uncommon but fatal symptom, is another symptom secondary to lipofuscin in vascular walls [14]. Some patients may also present with extraintestinal manifestations of the syndrome including myopathy and neuromuscular dysfunction [1]. Only a few cases of carcinoma have been reported in BBS patients [22–24]. These occasional reports of carcinoma are most likely a concurrent carcinoma arising from underlying disorders (such as celiac disease and IBD) because carcinoma arises from epithelial cells, but the lipofuscin coalesces in the smooth muscle cells (not the epithelial cells) [5].

3.3. Diagnosis. BBS has been often missed or ignored due to several reasons. First, the incidence of the disease is rare (the level of suspicion is accordingly low). Second, the clinical

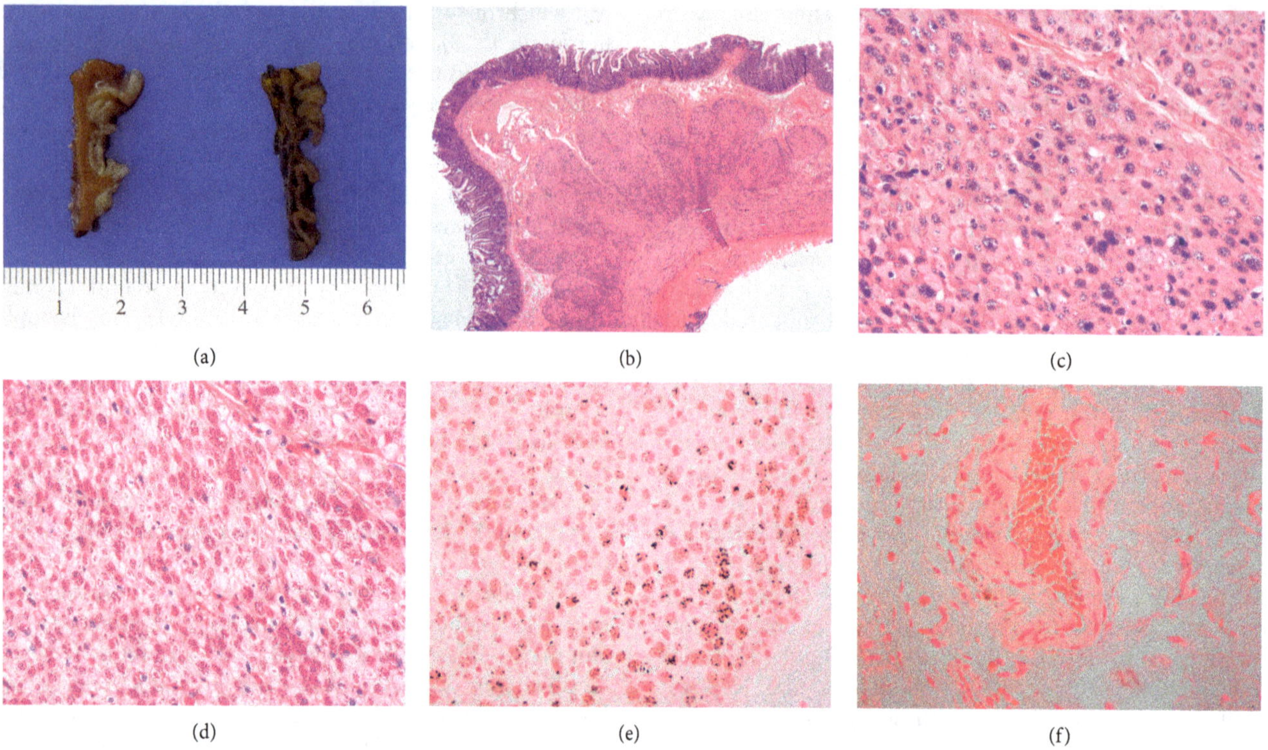

Figure 1: (a) Gross photos of small bowel from BBS (left) and from trauma patient as control (right). The wall is thicker and brown in comparison with the right. (b) H&E stain (x2) showing brown deposits in the muscularis propria. (c) H&E stain (x40) showing brown deposits in smooth muscle cells of the muscularis propria. (d) PASD stain (x40) highlighting brown deposits in the cytoplasm of smooth muscle cells. (e) Fontana-Masson stain (x40) highlighting brown deposits in the cytoplasm of smooth muscle cells. (f) Fontana-Masson stain (x40) highlighting brown deposits in smooth muscle cells of the blood vessel.

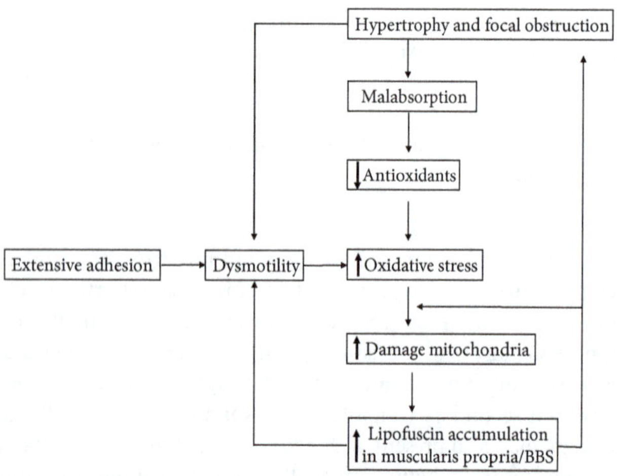

Figure 2: The positive feedback loop of the pathogenesis of BBS in this patient.

symptoms are not specific (BBS can be secondary to and coexist with the underlying diseases). Third, besides underlying disease, the endoscopic findings are unremarkable since lipofuscin accumulations are mainly in the muscularis propria which are not usually biopsied. Fourth, vitamin E cutoff value for diagnosis has not been established though its deficiency has been overestimated. Therefore, the transmural nature of the biopsy is critical for a definitive diagnosis. The key features for differential diagnosis are shown in Table 1.

3.4. Therapy and Prognosis. The treatment of BBS depends on the causes and the severity of symptoms. The patient with severe acute complications, such as bleeding or acute obstruction, usually requires immediate surgical intervention [1]. If BBS is found early or incidentally, the therapy is primarily conservative and includes treating the underlying malabsorption. Vitamin E supplementation usually takes months to show the benefits [1, 12, 17], and caution must be taken because high doses can surpass its antioxidant properties and begin to work as a pro-oxidant [25, 26]. The application of MitoTEMPO [4] or melatonin [27] has been also shown to prevent the accumulation of the lipofuscin protein aggregate and may be a potential novel therapy of targeting antioxidants to mitochondria. The prognosis of BBS is not clear due to rare cases reported; however, in a recent study [12], only one of eight patients died due to encephalitis with a mean clinical follow-up of 208 weeks (range: 10 to 770).

There is no definite proof of malnutrition, and dysmotility has been considered as the main cause in this BBS patient. The treatment for this patient included surgical procedure and close follow-up; however, vitamin E supplement was not provided. The patients did not show any

TABLE 1: The key features of BBS for differential diagnosis.

Brown bowel syndrome
(1) Normal mucosa detected by endoscopy and histology (if no overlapping disease)
(2) PAS-positive pigments in smooth muscle cells of the muscularis propria
(3) EM: osmophilic pigments
Infection (Whipple disease and mycobacterium)
(1) Traveling or close contacting history
(2) Abnormal endoscopic findings
(3) PAS-positive granules in macrophages in lamina propria
(4) IHC for microorganism
(5) Normal muscularis propria
(6) EM: bacteria
Melanosis coli or duodeni
(1) Usually no clinical symptoms
(2) History of usage of anthraquinone laxatives or renal disease
(3) Dark endoscopic mucosa
(4) PAS-positive granules in macrophages in lamina propria
Celiac disease
(1) Inflamed duodenum detected by an endoscopy: scalloping or flattening of duodenal folds, fissuring over the folds, and a mosaic pattern of mucosa of folds
(2) Destruction of mucosa by intraepithelial lymphocytes
(3) Positive serology: antitransglutaminase antibodies, antiendomysial antibodies, and antigliadin antibodies
(4) Response to gluten-free products
Inflammatory bowel disease
(1) Bloody diarrhea
(2) Abnormal endoscopic findings: inflammation, ulcer, and loss of vascularity
(3) Active and chronic inflammation in mucosa or granuloma and transmural inflammation (Crohn's disease)
(4) No pigments seen

symptoms up to the date of this manuscript writing. The motility test (small bowel follow-through) and the detection of antioxidants such as thiamine and vitamins A and E have been suggested as additional studies in the evaluation of this patient.

4. Conclusion

BBS is a rare gastrointestinal disease usually associated with various chronic underlying diseases. Mitochondrial damage with lipofuscin deposition due to oxidative stress is the main process occurring in the pathogenesis of BBS. There are many factors at play in the pathogenesis of BBS, and any one of these factors, if involved, can cause BBS, whereas vitamin E deficiency is simply one of these factors. In this case, the dysmotility from extensive serosal adhesion could be a possible etiology.

Due to overlapping symptoms and deposits of lipofuscin within the muscularis propria, this disease has often been missed. BBS patients usually present with intestinal motility disorders, and a transmural biopsy is necessary to make a definitive diagnosis.

Authors' Contributions

All authors were involved in concept, design, writing, or revision of the manuscript.

References

[1] R. Parente, M. Pinamonti, and S. Martina, "Brown bowel syndrome in a middle-aged woman with chronic idiopathic malabsorption," *Case Reports in Surgery*, vol. 2019, Article ID 4706592, 2019.

[2] A. H. Toffler, P. B. Hukill, and H. M. Spiro, "Brown bowel syndrome," *Annals of Internal Medicine*, vol. 58, no. 5, pp. 872–877, 1963.

[3] G. A. Herrera, E. A. Turbat-Herrera, and V. G. Lockard, "Unusual pigmented vesical lesion in a middle-aged woman," *Ultrastructural Pathology*, vol. 14, no. 6, pp. 529–535, 1990.

[4] J. König, C. Ott, M. Hugo et al., "Mitochondrial contribution to lipofuscin formation," *Redox Biology*, vol. 11, pp. 673–681, 2017.

[5] E. Kaiserling, R. Schäffer, and J. Weckermann, "Brown bowel syndrome with manifestation in the gastrointestinal tract and thyroid gland," *Pathology-Research and Practice*, vol. 183, no. 1, pp. 65–74, 1988.

[6] H. Lee, A. M. Carlin, A. H. Ormsby, and M. W. Lee, "Brown bowel syndrome secondary to jejunoileal bypass: the first case report," *Obesity Surgery*, vol. 19, no. 8, pp. 1176–1179, 2009.

[7] Vitamin E, "Deficiency in dogs," *Canadian Journal of Comparative Medicine and Veterinary Science*, vol. 4, no. 4, p. 117, 1940.

[8] D. O. Cordes and A. H. Mosher, "Brown pigmentation (lipofuscinosis) of canine intestinal muscularis," *The Journal of Pathology and Bacteriology*, vol. 92, no. 1, pp. 197–206, 1966.

[9] C. E. Connolly, M. Kennedy, F. M. Stevens, and C. F. McCarthy, "Brown bowel syndrome occurring in coeliac

disease in the west of Ireland," *Scandinavian Journal of Gastroenterology*, vol. 29, no. 1, pp. 91–94, 1994.
[10] H. Reynaert, S. Debeuckelaere, B. De Waele, M. Meysman, A. Goossens, and G. Devis, "The Brown bowel syndrome and gastrointestinal adenocarcinoma," *Journal of Clinical Gastroenterology*, vol. 16, no. 1, pp. 48–51, 1993.
[11] J. R. Lambert, S. C. Luk, and K. P. Pritzker, "Brown bowel syndrome in Crohn's disease," *Archives of Pathology & Laboratory Medicine*, vol. 104, no. 4, pp. 201–205, 1980.
[12] C. A. Arnold, A. P. Burke, E. Calomeni et al., "Brown bowel syndrome," *American Journal of Surgical Pathology*, vol. 44, no. 6, pp. 834–837, 2020.
[13] C. N. Lin, A. H. Huang, S. I Hsu et al., "Brown bowel syndrome: report of two cases," *Journal of the Formosan Medical Association = Taiwan Yi Zhi*, vol. 92, no. 12, pp. 1090–1094, 1993.
[14] C. Ruchti, S. Eisele, and M. Kaufmann, "Fatal intestinal pseudo-obstruction in brown bowel syndrome," *Archives of Pathology & Laboratory Medicine*, vol. 114, no. 1, pp. 76–80, 1990.
[15] H. C. Ward, J. Leake, P. J. Milla, and L. Spitz, "Brown bowel syndrome: a late complication of intestinal atresia," *Journal of Pediatric Surgery*, vol. 27, no. 12, pp. 1593–1595, 1992.
[16] G. Oberhuber, R. Pointner, E. Lauer, P. Waldenberger, and T. Radaszkiewicz, ""Brown bowel" syndrome--lipofuscinosis of the intestine as a cause of atonia," *Leber Magen Darm*, vol. 19, no. 5, pp. 270–274, 1989.
[17] P. F. D. C. Soares, R. B. de Carvalho, E. A. Chaim, and E. Cazzo, "Brown bowel syndrome: a rare malnutrition-related complication of bariatric surgery," *Nutricion Hospitalaria*, vol. 36, no. 3, pp. 743–747, 2019.
[18] S. P. Lee and G. I. Nicholson, "Ceroid enteropathy and vitamin E deficiency," *The New Zealand Medical Journal*, vol. 83, no. 563, pp. 318–320, 1976.
[19] E. J. Feeney, S. Austin, and Y. H. Chien, "The value of muscle biopsies in Pompe disease: identifying lipofuscin inclusions in juvenile-and adult-onset patients," *Acta Neuropathologica Communications*, vol. 2, p. 2, 2014.
[20] A. Anand and B. M. Jaffe, "Brown bowel syndrome: case report and review," *Journal of Louisiana State Medical Society*, vol. 157, no. 6, pp. 338–340, 2005.
[21] C. S. Foster, "The brown bowel syndrome: a possible smooth muscle mitochondrial myopathy?" *Histopathology*, vol. 3, no. 1, pp. 1–17, 1979.
[22] M. Raithel, T. T. Rau, and A. F. Hagel, "Jejunitis and brown bowel syndrome with multifocal carcinogenesis of the small bowel," *World Journal of Gastroenterology*, vol. 21, no. 36, pp. 10461–10467, 2015.
[23] M. Shiller, I. Cohen, M. Munichor, N. Loberant, A. Bickel, and R. Reshef, "The "brown bowel syndrome" associated with jejunal carcinoma," *American Journal of Gastroenterology*, vol. 88, no. 10, pp. 1788-1789, 1993.
[24] H. Reynaert and G. Devis, "The brown bowel syndrome and gastrointestinal adenocarcinoma," *The American Journal of Gastroenterology*, vol. 89, no. 5, pp. 812-813, 1994.
[25] G. Bjelakovic, D. Nikolova, and C. Gluud, "Antioxidant supplements to prevent mortality," *JAMA*, vol. 310, no. 11, pp. 1178-1179, 2013.
[26] E. Jansen, D. Viezeliene, P. Beekhof, E. Gremmer, and L. Ivanov, "Tissue-specific effects of vitamin e supplementation," *International Journal of Molecular Sciences*, vol. 17, no. 7, 2016.
[27] F. E. Martin-Cano, C. Camello-Almaraz, D. Acuña-Castroviejo, M. J. Pozo, and P. J. Camello, "Age-related changes in mitochondrial function of mouse colonic smooth muscle: beneficial effects of melatonin," *Journal of Pineal Research*, vol. 56, no. 2, pp. 163–174, 2014.

34

Gastroduodenal Ulcerative Colitis in Association with Ulcerative Pancolitis

Khin San Aye [1] **Lin Lin Htun,** [2] **Thet Mar Win,** [1] **Mya Thida Aye,** [1] **Drmyothettin Tin,** [3] **and Than Than Aye** [1]

[1] *Department of Gastroenterology, University of Medicine 2, Yangon, Myanmar*
[2] *Department of Pathology, Thingangyun General Hospital, Yangon, Myanmar*
[3] *Yangon General Hospital, Yangon, Myanmar*

Correspondence should be addressed to Khin San Aye; ksaye.08@gmail.com

Academic Editor: Hirotada Akiho

Ulcerative colitis (UC) is a chronic inflammatory bowel disease, traditionally regarded as being limited to the colorectum. Although several gastroduodenal lesions have been reported in cases of UC, in general, duodenal lesions in UC are believed to be uncommon and gastric lesions in UC are a rare presentation. In this report, we presented a 66-year-old lady with upper GI presentation with gastroduodenal ulcerative colitis accompanying pancolonic UC.

1. Introduction

Ulcerative colitis (UC) is a chronic inflammatory bowel disease (IBD) of the colon that has an unknown etiology. UC is localized to the colon and spares the upper gastrointestinal (GI) tract. This disease usually begins in the rectum and extends proximally for a variable distance [1]. The annual incidence of UC is 10.4 to 12/100,000 people, and the prevalence is 35 to 100/100,000 people in the USA [2]. Prevalence is lower in Asia [3]. In IBD demographics in a Southern Asia study, a total of 10400 patients were found in 15 countries of South Asia, South East Asia, and the Middle East. A total of 248 IBD patients from Myanmar were included in this study [4]. Although UC is known to have various extracolonic manifestations, the upper GI tract is not generally considered a target organ. The concept of gastroduodenal UC (GDUC) was first proposed by Hori et al., but the diagnosis standard is not rigorous enough due to the scanty reports. Extensive colitis and a lower dose of prednisolone administration might be the main risk factors for GDUC [5]. Several case reports describing upper GI involvement in UC have been published. These reports described gastritis or diffuse duodenitis that resembled colonic lesions of UC in both the endoscopic and pathological findings [6–9]. In a study from Japan, only 4.7% (15 out of 322) of patients had ulcerative gastroduodenal lesions (UGDL) accompanied by pancolitis or after proctocolectomy [10]. There are no RCT and observational studies although several case reports were published because of less number of cases all over the world.

The aim of this report is to present a rare occurrence of the typical UC apparently localized not only to the whole colon but also the upper GI tract, stomach, and duodenum.

2. Case Presentation

A 66-year-old previously healthy woman, without UC family history, started to complain of diffuse abdominal pain and decreased appetite since 3 months ago. She also complained of loose motions almost containing mucous and, sometimes, blood more than 10 times per day for 3 months of duration. She also noted significant weight loss of about 10 kg. No other comorbid disease was there except hypertension for 20 years which was controlled with antihypertensive treatment. She underwent colonoscopy in her early onset of symptoms. Colonoscopy finding was multiple polyps throughout the colon, and her doctor advised surgery. However, she refused to undergo surgery and went abroad and sought further management. She underwent upper and lower endoscopy again there, and tissue biopsy was performed from both the GI tract and colon. Biopsy results showed chronic inflammation only and were not conclusive of ulcerative colitis. She was diagnosed as ulcerative colitis based on the endoscopic findings. She received mesalazine 1500 mg twice a day and prednisolone 5 mg twice a day since after diagnosed. Symptoms were improved after treatment. She continued taking medicine without a follow-up visit again.

Two months later, she developed similar episodes of abdominal pain and bloody diarrhea despite taking medicines. She looked pale and had generalized edema. Her heart rate was 112/min, and the blood pressure (110/70 mmHg) and respiratory rate (24/min) were normal. The abdomen was soft; mild tenderness was present in the lower abdomen, but there was no guarding.

Blood investigation showed pancytopenia, hemoglobin 9.2 gm /dl, WBC count 2.75×10^3/ul, and platelet 44×10^3/ul, and hypokalaemia, 2.8 mmol/L. The creatinine level was low (10 umol/L) likely due to low muscle bulk and low serum protein although there were no liver diseases. Low blood calcium level (1.6 mmol/L), low serum phosphate level (0.5 mmol/L), normal magnesium level (0.8 mmol/L), and low serum albumin level (2.1 gm/dl) were found. The blood sugar level was normal. High inflammatory makers such as CRP 447 mg/L, ESR 90 mm/hr, and fecal calprotectin level 827 ug/g were found. Procalcitonin was normal. Serologic testing for antineutrophil cytoplasmic antibodies (ANCA) and antisaccharomyces cerevisiae (ASCA) antibodies were negative in this patient. Stool microscopy showed numerous RBC and pus cells. Blood, stool, and urine culture were negative. Due to previous exposure with steroid hormonal therapy, stool test for CMV and stool test for *Clostridium difficile* for toxin A and B were negative.

CXR showed mild cardiomegaly and small bilateral effusion. CT abdomen remarked as diffuse mucosa-wall thickening throughout the stomach and the first part of the duodenum. Enhancement was noted at the contrast study. The imaging report considered MALT lymphoma. Small amount of ascites were noted in the abdomen and pelvis. Small bilateral effusion was also noted.

Upper and lower endoscopy and biopsy were repeated for the reason of recurrent symptoms, inconclusive of previous histological results although treated as UC and to exclude other differential diagnosis, especially MALT lymphoma.

Esophagogastroduodenoscopy findings were mucosa granularity, friability with rough and eroded ulcers, multiple inflammatory polyps, and complete obliteration of the vascular pattern diffusely involving the entire GI tract and duodenum. These gastroduodenal findings were similar to that we found in ulcerative lesions of ulcerative colitis in the colon (Figure 1). The rapid urease test for *Helicobacter pylori* infection was negative. Tissue biopsies were taken from the stomach and duodenum separately.

Colonoscopy findings were mucosa granularity, friability with multiple inflammatory polyps throughout the colon (from the rectum to caecum) with patchy obliteration of the vascular pattern. Inflammations more marked at caecum and ileo-cecal valve. Diffuse mucosal inflammation with obliteration of the vascular pattern shown in terminal ileum is likely backwash ileitis (Figure 2). As the ulcerative colitis endoscopic index of severity (UCEIS) was 9 by 11 and as the Mayo scoring system for assessment of UC activity was 9 by 12 in this patient, it showed severe disease activity since admission.

2.1. Histopathologic Report. Both gastric and duodenum mucosa are severely inflamed with edematous lamina propria and architecture changes. Histological findings are consistent with ulcerative colitis with upper GI involvement. The gastric mucosa shows ulcerations, architecture changes with loss of foveolar pits, basal intense mixed inflammations, and edematous laminopropria. Superficial plasmacytosis are also noted. The glands are cystically dilated and filled with secretions (Figure 3). Microabscesses are appreciated. Granulomas are not seen. The duodenum mucosa shows villous atrophy, architecture changes, edematous lamina propria, and infiltration by lymphocytes and plasma cells (Figure 4). However, neither intraepithelial lymphocytosis nor lesions are appreciated. Epitheloid granulomas are not seen. The histological findings are consistent with inflammatory bowel disease (ulcerativecolitis) with upper GI involvement.

The colonic biopsy result was consistent with ulcerative colitis with superimposed bacterial infection. All pieces of colonic polyps showed architecture changes, crypt dropout with edematous stroma and severely inflamed mucosa, and mild diffuse mononuclear infiltrates in the lamina propria. Some crypts are lined by columnar cells with reactive changes. Few bacilli are seen in the crypt lumen. Dysplasia and features of malignancy are not seen. No features of MALT lymphoma were seen (Figure 5).

During hospital stay, she developed many significant events. Right calf muscle pain due to deep vein thrombosis was proved with a vascular Doppler and received anticoagulant, subcutaneous LMW heparin. Fast atrial fibrillation was controlled with amiodarone by the cardiologist. Hypokalaemia, hypomagnesemia, and hypoalbuminemia were replaced according the results. The patient developed refeeding syndrome and was fed according to the nutritionist's advice. The patient could not take oral feeding due to abdominal pain and reduced appetite, which is why parenteral nutrition was given. Pancytopenia was corrected under hematologist guidance. Although there was a clinical association between UC and myelodysplastic syndromes and aplastic anemia, no bone marrow biopsy was performed in this patient. Broad-spectrum antibiotics were prescribed.

The treatment of UGDL is similar to that of UC, so the patient was treated with mesalazine and steroid hormones. Pantoprazole was given concomitant along with intravenous corticosteroid injection. Diarrhea was controlled after 10 days of treatment. Her appetite was improved, and she started to tolerate liquid diet. Oral prednisolone was changed, and it was tried to tail off the drug. Pancytopenia

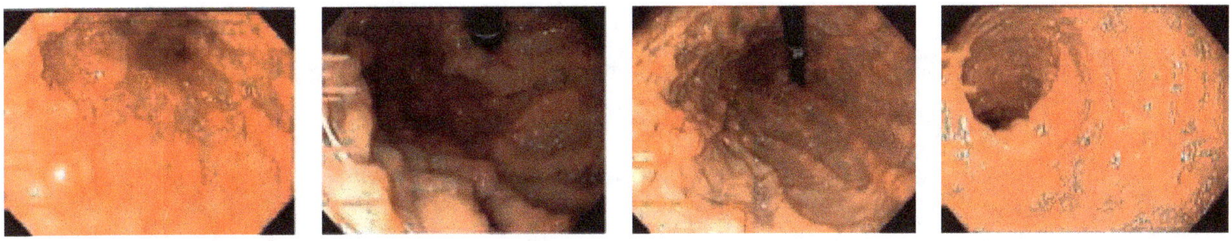

(a) (b) (c) (d)

Figure 1: EGD scopy findings; panulcerative gastritis and ulcerative duodenitis. (a) Antrum, (b) fundus, (c) proximal body stomach, and (d) descending part of the duodenum.

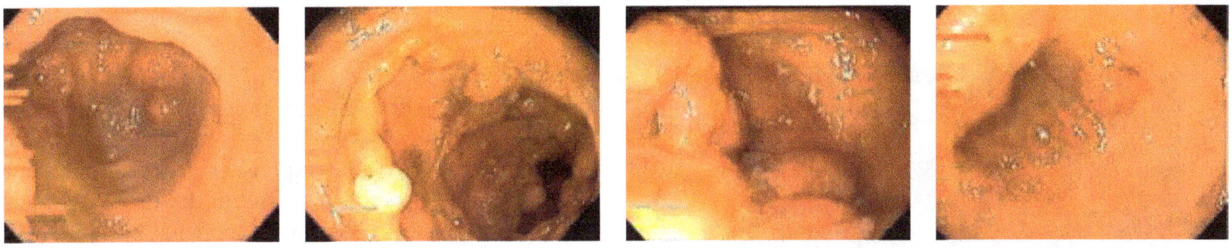

(a) (b) (c) (d)

Figure 2: Colonoscopy findings; pancolitis with inflammatory polyps. (a) Rectum, (b) ascending colon, (c) caecum, and (d) terminal ileum.

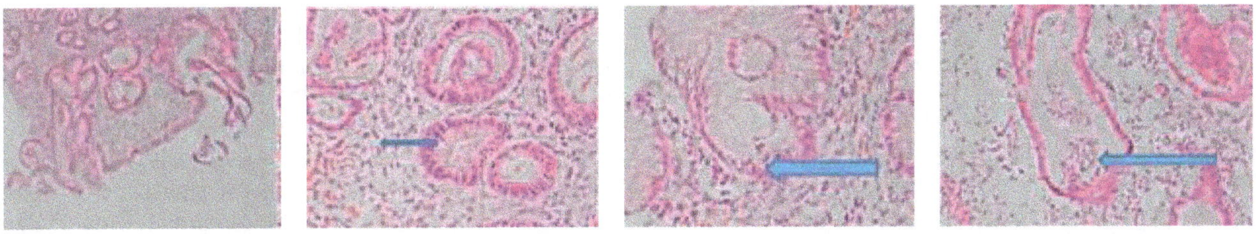

(a) (b) (c) (d)

Figure 3: Histologic findings of gastric biopsy; the gastric mucosa shows (a) severe inflammation, ulcerations, and architecture changes, (b) plasmacytosis in the lamina propria, (c) inflammation in the gastric foveolar epithelium, and (d) microabscess formations.

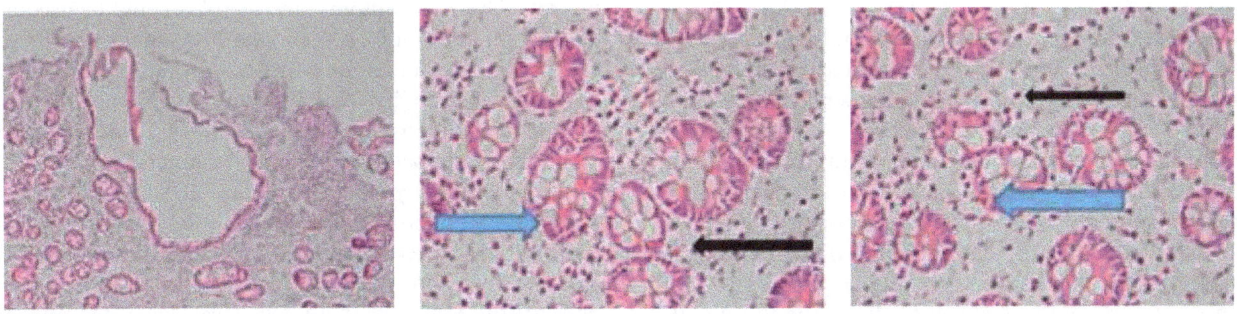

(a) (b) (c)

Figure 4: Histologic findings of duodenal biopsy; the duodenum mucosa shows (a) villous atrophy, architecture changes, and edematous lamina propria, (b) plasma cells (black arrow), and (c) cryptitis (blue arrow) in the lamina propria.

was improved (Hb 9.8 g/dl, WBC 3.8×10^3/ul, and platelet 100×10^3/ul). Serum potassium raised to near normal 3.3 mmol/l. Serum albumin was raised to 3.2 g/dl.

On her 3rd week of treatment, diarrhea recurred and cardiac arrhythmias worsened. She was kept in an intensive care unit. Two days later, the patient suddenly developed severe pain in the right shoulder and right upper limb. In plain X-ray abdomen, gas was found under the diaphragm (Figure 6), and she was urgently referred to a surgeon for intestinal perforation. Unfortunately, her blood pressure

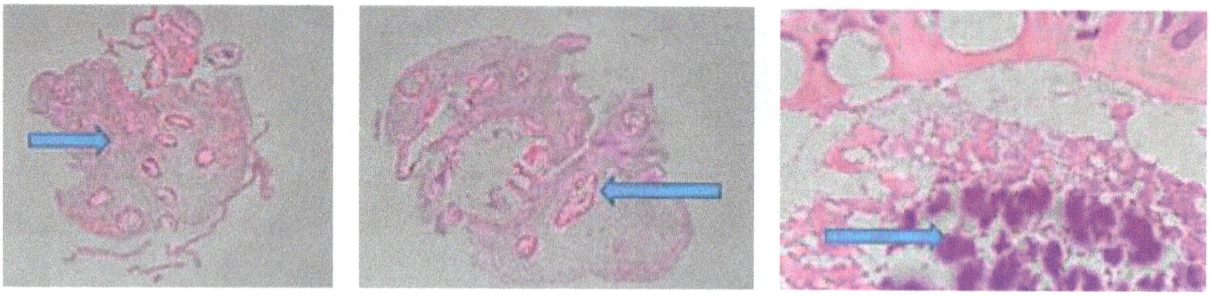

(a) (b) (c)

Figure 5: Histologic findings of colon biopsy; all pieces of the colonic polyps show (a) edematous lamina propria, crypt dropout, and mononuclear infiltrates, (b) crypts lined by reactive columnar cells, and (c) bacterial colonies.

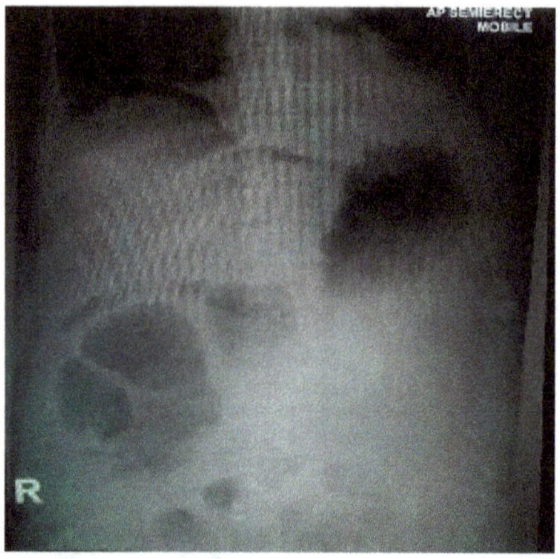

Figure 6: Plain X-ray abdomen; gas under diaphragm positive, gas-filled distended stomach, and some bowel loops.

and respiratory function were unstable, and we lost the patient before identifying the site of perforation in operation.

3. Discussion

The typical endoscopic findings in patients with UC include edematous mucosa, erythema, loss of vascular markings, and mucosal friability [11]. More severe cases may be associated with erosions, ulcers, and spontaneous bleeding. Luminal narrowing and pseudopolyps may occur due to chronic inflammation, which results in mucosal atrophy [12]. Although inflammation in UC patients is mostly limited to the colon, ileal inflammation (backwash ileitis) may infrequently be observed [13]. In this study, pseudopolyps present in both the upper GI tract and colon may be due to the chronicity of disease although the symptoms were there for 3 months only, and terminal ileum inflammation may be the backwash ileitis.

UC complicated with upper GI tract lesions is rare. An earlier study reported that two patients with UC developed duodenitis after total colectomy [14]. Subsequently, other studies have reported the same complication [7, 15–18]. The concept of GDUC was first proposed by Hori et al., but the diagnosis standard is not rigorous enough due to the scanty reports. More extensive colitis and a lower dose of prednisolone administration might be the main risk factors for GDUC [4]. Although the etiology of GDUC is unclear, several studies have revealed that it may be associated with the imbalance of immune response of genetically susceptible hosts to bacterial antigens, resulting in an excessive autoimmune response to the gastroduodenal epithelium [10]. The diagnostic criteria are lesions that do not respond to standard treatment for ulcers, such as H2 blockers and proton pump inhibitors, and lesions that are sensitive to medication used to treat UC, such as steroids and mesalazine [19].

Ulcerative gastroduodenal lesion (UGDL) and UC have similar histologic features, and previous reports have shown that many patients with UGDL, especially those with mild symptoms, respond positively to the treatment of UC with drugs such as sulfasalazine or mesalazine [9, 20]. For some patients with severe UGDL, either sulfasalazine or steroid hormones could not control the condition effectively, and the tumor necrosis factor (TNF) antagonist infliximab (IFX) or a calcineurin antagonist could be more effective in preventing the condition from deteriorating [20, 21]. To date, it is considered that early diagnosis with application of sulfasalazine or mesalazine is a quick and effective way to improve UGDL symptoms, and steroids could be used as a 2nd-line therapy for UGDL and the TNF antagonist IFX or a calcineurin antagonist for patients with rapid progress and hormone insensitivity. With the increasing number of upper GI mucosal lesions in patients with UC, we should pay attention to the pathogenesis and treatment of UGDL.

There are many evidences about GDUC which may be associated with progressing UC or total colitis, may have occurred in postcolectomy patients of UC, and may be associated with long-time lower dose of prednisolone. The present study suggests that GDUC was diagnosed since the diagnosis of UC. There were similar endoscopic findings and histological findings in both the upper GI tract and colon. This report may be the first case of synchronous UC of gastroduodenal and colonic lesion which is not reported yet.

The intestinal perforation represents the most serious complication in UC and is usually associated with instrumentation (colonoscopy) or with the presence of toxic megacolon and delay in diagnosis, due to the consequent presence of perforation [22]. In this study, perforation may represent the serious complication of UC and history of having taken low dose prednisolone for two months of duration. The patient did not start rescue therapy (IFX or cyclosporine) as she developed many clinical events such as cardiac arrhythmia, pancytopenia, and refeeding syndrome during periods, and bowel symptom was improved with mesalasine and steroid therapy.

4. Conclusions

UC may not be restricted to the large intestine; it is important to examine the upper gastrointestinal tract to confirm whether GDUC exists. Many case series and studies described that GDUC involvement in UC may be more frequent than previously estimated. The synchronous finding of UC in both gastroduodenal and colonic lesion may happen rarely. As for further studies involving a large number of adult patients, it needs to be clarified whether the upper gastrointestinal tract is a target organ in UC to better understanding the etiology and pathogenesis of UC.

References

[1] A. B. Grossman, R. N. Baldassano, R. M. Kligman et al., *Chronic Ulcerative Colitis Nelson Textbook of Pediatrics*, W B Saunders, Philadelphia, PA, USA, 19th edition, 2011.

[2] E. S. Jang, D. H. Lee, J. Kim et al., "Age as a clinical predictor of relapse after induction therapy in ulcerative colitis," *Hepatogastro-Enterology*, vol. 56, no. 94-95, pp. 1304–1309, 2009.

[3] K. A. Diefenback and C. K. Breuer, "Pediatric inflammatory bowel disease," *World Journal of Gastroenterology*, vol. 12, pp. 3204–3212, 2006.

[4] R. Banerjee, P. Pal, I. Hilmi et al., *IBD demographics in Southern Asia*, IBD-ENC, Hyderabad, Telangana, 2019.

[5] K. Hori, H. Ikeuchi, H. Nakano et al., "Gastroduodenitis associated with ulcerative colitis," *Journal of Gastroenterology*, vol. 43, no. 3, pp. 193–201, 2008.

[6] R. Valdez, H. D. Appelman, M. P. Bronner, and J. K. Greenson, "Diffuse duodenitis associated with ulcerative colitis," *The American Journal of Surgical Pathology*, vol. 24, no. 10, pp. 1407–1413, 2000.

[7] H. Ikeuchi, K. Hori, T. Nishigami et al., "Diffuse gastroduodenitis and pouchitis associated with ulcerative colitis," *World Journal of Gastroenterology*, vol. 12, no. 36, pp. 5913–5915, 2006.

[8] S. Terashima, Y. Hoshino, N. Kanzaki, M. Kogure, and M. Gotoh, "Ulcerative duodenitis accompanying ulcerative colitis," *Journal of Clinical Gastroenterology*, vol. 32, no. 2, pp. 172–175, 2001.

[9] H. Mitomi, E. Atari, H. Uesugi et al., "Distinctive diffuse duodenitis associated with ulcerative colitis," *Digestive Diseases and Sciences*, vol. 42, no. 3, pp. 684–693, 1997.

[10] T. Hisabe, T. Matsui, M. Miyaoka et al., "Diagnosis and clinical course of ulcerative gastroduodenal lesion associated with ulcerative colitis: possible relationship with pouchitis," *Digestive Endoscopy*, vol. 22, no. 4, pp. 268–274, 2010.

[11] C. H. Choi, S. A. Jung, B. I. Lee et al., "Diagnostic guideline of ulcerative colitis," *Korean Journal of Gastroenterology*, vol. 53, no. 3, pp. 145–160, 2009.

[12] J. D. Waye, "Endoscopy in inflammatory bowel disease: indications and differential diagnosis," *Medical Clinics of North America*, vol. 74, no. 1, pp. 51–65, 1990.

[13] H. Haskell, C. W. Andrews Jr, S. I. Reddy et al., "Pathologic features and clinical significance of ??? Backwash??? ileitis in ulcerative colitis," *The American Journal of Surgical Pathology*, vol. 29, no. 11, pp. 1472–1481, 2005.

[14] R. Kato, M. Iwamuro, S. Hiraoka et al., "Evaluation of the upper gastrointestinal tract in ulcerative colitis patients," *Acta Med Okayama*, vol. 72, no. 2, pp. 105–113, 2018.

[15] G. Rosenfeld, H. J. Freeman, M. Brown, and U. P. Steinbrecher, "Severe and extensive enteritis following colectomy for ulcerative colitis," *Canadian Journal of Gastroenterology*, vol. 26, no. 12, pp. 866-867, 2012.

[16] I. R. Gooding, R. Springall, I. C. Talbot, and D. B. A. Silk, "Idiopathic small-intestinal inflammation after colectomy for ulcerative colitis," *Clinical Gastroenterology and Hepatology*, vol. 6, no. 6, pp. 707–709, 2008.

[17] M. Danelius, Å. Öst, and A. B. Lapidus, "Inflammatory bowel disease-related lesions in the duodenal and gastric mucosa," *Scandinavian Journal of Gastroenterology*, vol. 44, no. 4, pp. 441–445, 2009.

[18] J. Rubenstein, A. Sherif, H. Appelman, and W. D. Chey, "Ulcerative colitis associated enteritis," *Journal of Clinical Gastroenterology*, vol. 38, no. 1, pp. 46–51, 2004.

[19] M. D. C. GarcíaGavilán, M. C. López Vega, and I. M. Sánchez, "Ulcerative colitis with gastric and duodenal involvement," *Rev Esp Enferm Dig*, vol. 109, no. 7, pp. 535-536, 2017.

[20] S. Corporaal, A. Karrenbeld, K. Van der Linde, J. H. Voskuil, J. H. Kleibeuker, and G. Dijkstra, "Diffuse enteritis after colectomy for ulcerative colitis: two case reports and review of the literature," *European Journal of Gastroenterology & Hepatology*, vol. 21, no. 6, pp. 710–715, 2009.

[21] M. Chiba, I. Ono, H. Wakamatsu, I. Wada, and K. Suzuki, "Diffuse gastroduodenitis associated with ulcerative colitis: treatment by infliximab," *Digestive Endoscopy*, vol. 25, no. 6, pp. 622–625, 2013.

[22] M. Uchino, H. Ikeuchi, A. Sugita et al., "Pouch functional outcomes after restorative proctocolectomy with ileal-pouch reconstruction in patients with ulcerative colitis: Japanese multi-center nationwide cohort study," *Journal of Gastroenterology*, vol. 53, no. 5, pp. 642–651, 2017.

35

Increased Risk of Liver Cirrhosis during Azathioprine Therapy for Crohn's Disease

Jenny Roselli, Tommaso Innocenti, Erica Nicola Lynch, Laura Parisio, Giuseppe Macrì, Monica Milla, Tommaso Mello, Andrea Galli, Stefano Milani, and Mirko Tarocchi

Department of Experimental and Clinical Biomedical Sciences "Mario Serio", University of Florence, Florence, Italy

Correspondence should be addressed to Tommaso Innocenti; tommaso.innocenti@unifi.it

Academic Editor: Yoshihiro Moriwaki

Azathioprine is a cornerstone of the therapy of Crohn's disease. Unfortunately, infections and malignancies are relatively common adverse effects related to this drug; however, cirrhosis is exceptionally reported as a side effect. We report the case of a 49-year-old male patient with ileocolonic steno-penetrating Crohn's disease who developed hepatic cirrhosis while treated with azathioprine. After taking azathioprine for 3 years with regular follow-up, he developed pancytopenia, and liver cirrhosis was diagnosed with ultrasound, abdomen computed tomography scan, transient elastography, and liver biopsy. As all other causes of liver damage were excluded, azathioprine was believed to be the cause of liver injury and therefore was interrupted.

1. Introduction

Thiopurines (azathioprine AZA and 6-mercaptopurine 6-MP) are the gold standard for the treatment of steroid-dependent ileocolonic Crohn's disease with moderate-to-severe disease activity [1].

There are numerous adverse events related to these drugs, such as nonmelanoma skin cancer (NMSC) [2–5], lymphoma, infections, and pancreatic and liver injury [6]. In most cases (5–15% of all patients on thiopurine therapy [6]), elevated liver enzymes (glutamate oxaloacetate transaminase (GOT) and glutamate pyruvate transaminase (GPT)) detect the presence of liver damage, although patients generally remain asymptomatic. The liver function test usually normalizes after reducing or stopping treatment [3, 6, 7]. Less commonly, thiopurines can cause cholestatic hepatitis, and in rare cases, they can be associated with noncirrhotic portal hypertension, caused by nodular regenerative hyperplasia or by hepatic veno-occlusive disease [3, 6, 8].

In this report, we present the case of a patient with Crohn's disease who developed hepatic cirrhosis while treated with AZA.

2. Case Report

A 49-year-old male Italian patient was diagnosed with ileocolonic steno-penetrating Crohn's disease in 1997. He was initially treated with oral steroids and achieved disease remission. He was then treated with mesalazine alone for many years. The patient was referred to our center in September 2014 for a disease relapse. He underwent a colonoscopy and a digestive MRI that showed wall thickening of the last 35 cm of the ileum and of the descending colon; thus, we proposed a step-up therapy with azathioprine 2 mg/kg/day, which the patient started in October 2014. The patient regularly attended follow-up visits every three months, and routine blood tests revealed normal complete blood count, C-reactive protein, and pancreatic and hepatic enzymes until December 2017, when they gave the following results: pancytopenia (WBC 2200 cells/mm^3, RBC 2500 cells/mm^3, and PLT 108000 cells/mm^3), high levels of bilirubin (total 2.2 mg/dL and direct 0.77 mg/dL), and normal levels of GOT, GPT, and γGT (respectively, 41, 26, and 59 U/L). The patient was diagnosed with liver cirrhosis with ultrasound, abdomen computed tomography scan, transient elastography, and a liver biopsy. Ultrasound showed signs of liver cirrhosis, like hypertrophy of the left lobe of the liver, ragged edges, and slightly increased liver echogenicity; portal vein Doppler ultrasound showed a portal diameter of 1 cm, hepatopetal portal venous circulation with a venal flow of 16 cm/sec, thin suprahepatic veins, and splenic enlargement (17 cm). The abdomen CT scan is shown in Figure 1. Transient elastography results were as follows: stiffness 21.6 kPa, IQR 3.4 kPa, and controlled attenuation parameter (CAP) 246 dB/m. The liver biopsy (Figure 2) showed signs of liver cirrhosis, excluding nodular regenerative hyperplasia, veno-occlusive hepatic disease, or a biliary tract disease. The gastroscopy showed congestive gastropathy. Research of possible viral liver damage (HAV, HBV, HCV, HEV, EBV, and CMV) came out negative. There were no laboratory signs of dyslipidemia, insulin resistance, or diabetes mellitus. Laboratory tests for autoimmune liver diseases (research of antinuclear antibodies (*ANA*), antineutrophil cytoplasmic antibodies (*ANCA*), anti-soluble liver antigen antibodies (*anti-SLA*), anti-smooth muscle antibodies (*ASMA*), anti-SP100 antibodies, anti-liver kidney microsome antibodies (*anti-LKM*), antimitochondrial antibodies (*AMA*), anti-mitochondrial M2 antibodies (*AMA-M2*), anti-GP210 antibodies, and anti-liver cytosol type 1 antibodies (*anti-LC1*)) were all negative. Specific tests were performed to exclude iron and copper overload. As all other causes of liver damage were excluded, AZA therapy was believed to be the cause of liver injury and therefore was interrupted. Six months after discontinuation of AZA treatment, ultrasound and CT scans revealed similar results, whereas white cells and platelet count gradually normalized. The patient was Child-Pugh class A during the whole follow-up period. The patient was monitored every 6 months with abdomen ultrasound and serum alpha-fetoprotein. The patient is currently treated with mesalazine alone and regularly attends follow-up visits at our center.

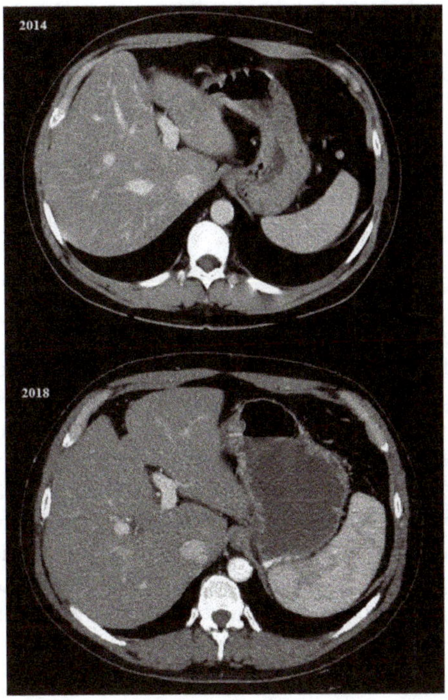

Figure 1: Comparison between arterial-phase abdomen CT scans from 2014 (before AZA therapy) and 2018 (after AZA therapy).

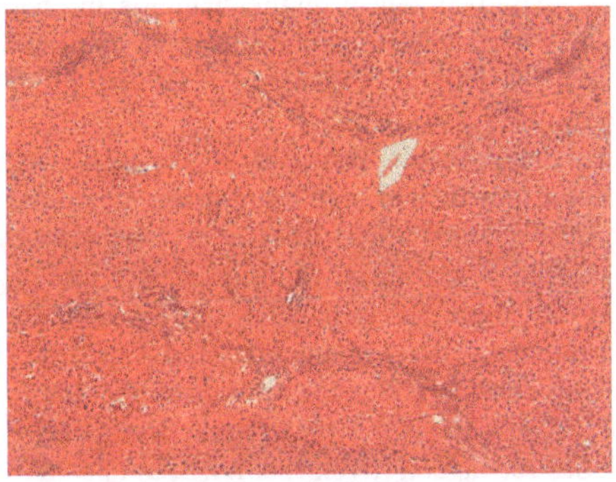

Figure 2: Findings of histology: marked bridging with regenerative nodules; hematoxylin and eosin stain.

3. Discussion

3.1. Review of Literature. There are only two other reported cases of thiopurine-induced liver cirrhosis. Trabelsi et al. described the case of an ileocolonic steno-penetrating Crohn's disease patient who was diagnosed with liver cirrhosis during a surgical treatment for an intestinal stenosis. The patient had been treated with AZA therapy for four years, and no alterations of liver enzymes have been detected before [9]. In the second case, which was presented by De Boer et al., liver cirrhosis was discovered as further investigations were made for a new-onset thrombocytopenia, which arose after three years of therapy with azathioprine. In both cases, a liver biopsy was used to diagnose liver cirrhosis, so as to exclude noncirrhotic causes of portal hypertension (veno-occlusive disease, nodular regenerative hyperplasia, hepatic peliosis, etc.) [10].

3.2. What Is the Cause of Thiopurine-Induced Liver Damage? Liver damage induced by AZA seems to be related to an accumulation of its methylated metabolites [11, 12]. Azathioprine is converted to 6-mercaptopurine (6-MP) by glutathione-S-transferase (GST). 6-MP is then converted to 6-thioguanine nucleotides (6-TGN) by the enzymes hypoxanthine-guanine phosphoribosyltransferase (HGPRT), inosine-5′-monophosphate dehydrogenase (IMPDH), and guanosine monophosphate synthetase (GMPS). 6-MP can also be converted to 6-methylmercaptopurine (6-MeMP) by thiopurine methyltransferase (TPMT) [13, 14]. Meijer et al. showed that the liver damage induced by thiopurine is twice as frequent in the patient with higher levels of 6-MeMP ($>5700\,\text{pmol}/8\times10^8$ RBC) than patients with levels of 6-MeMP in range [11].

3.3. Genetic Mutations of TPMT: Is There a Predictive Test for Thiopurine-Induced Liver Damage? Mutations of TPMT can lead to a modified ability to convert 6-MP in 6-MeMP. Thus, patients with modified TPMT activity, who are treated with standard doses of thiopurine (AZA 2-2, 5 mg/kg/day and 6-MP 1-1, 5 mg/kg/day), have higher levels of 6-MeMP and therefore have an increased risk of thiopurine-induced toxicity [15]. Screening for variants in TPMT may allow the identification of patients with a high risk of thiopurine-induced toxicity, to whom drugs should be administered in reduced doses [16].

4. Conclusions

Liver cirrhosis is a rare but possible adverse event of AZA therapy for Crohn's disease; hence, we suggest adding the routine platelet count and upper abdomen US in Crohn's disease patients who receive thiopurine treatment. If thrombocytopenia arises during AZA therapy, further investigations should be performed. Furthermore, for preventive purposes, screening for variants in TPMT should be carried out in all patients before initiating thiopurine therapy, in order to adjust the dose of the drug, reduce the risk of complications, and avoid wasting a valid therapeutic option.

References

[1] F. Gomollón, A. Dignass, V. Annese et al., "3rd European evidence-based consensus on the diagnosis and management of crohn's disease 2016: part 1: diagnosis and medical management," *Journal of Crohn's and Colitis*, vol. 11, no. 1, pp. 3–25, 2017.

[2] S.-Z. Huang, Z.-C. Liu, W.-X. Liao et al., "Risk of skin cancers in thiopurines-treated and thiopurines-untreated patients with inflammatory bowel disease: a systematic review and meta-analysis," *Journal of Gastroenterology and Hepatology*, vol. 34, no. 3, pp. 507–516, 2019.

[3] S. B. Hanauer, W. J. Sandborn, and G. R. Lichtenstein, "Evolving considerations for thiopurine therapy for inflammatory bowel diseases-a clinical practice update: commentary," *Gastroenterology*, vol. 156, no. 1, pp. 36–42, 2019.

[4] J. Ariyaratnam and V. Subramanian, "Association between thiopurine use and nonmelanoma skin cancers in patients with inflammatory bowel disease: a meta-analysis," *American Journal of Gastroenterology*, vol. 109, no. 2, pp. 163–169, 2014.

[5] D. S. Kotlyar, J. D. Lewis, L. Beaugerie et al., "Risk of lymphoma in patients with inflammatory bowel disease treated with azathioprine and 6-mercaptopurine: a meta-analysis," *Clinical Gastroenterology and Hepatology*, vol. 13, no. 5, pp. 847–858, 2015.

[6] E. S. Björnsson, J. Gu, D. E. Kleiner, N. Chalasani, P. H. Hayashi, and J. H. Hoofnagle, "Azathioprine and 6-mercaptopurine-induced liver injury," *Journal of Clinical Gastroenterology*, vol. 51, no. 1, pp. 63–69, 2017.

[7] R. B. Gearry, M. L. Barclay, M. J. Burt, J. A. Collett, and B. A. Chapman, "Thiopurine drug adverse effects in a population of New Zealand patients with inflammatory bowel disease," *Pharmacoepidemiology and Drug Safety*, vol. 13, no. 8, pp. 563–567, 2004.

[8] C. Suárez Ferrer, E. Llop Herrera, M. Calvo Moya et al., "Idiopathic portal hypertension regarding thiopurine treatment in patients with inflammatory bowel disease," *Revista espanola de enfermedades digestivas: organo oficial de la Sociedad Espanola de Patologia Digestiva*, vol. 108, no. 108, pp. 79–83, 2016.

[9] A. B. E. S. Trabelsi, E. Hamami, A. Souguir et al., "Suspected azathioprine induced liver cirrhosis: an unusual side effect," *Pan African Medical Journal*, vol. 7, no. 17, p. 174, 2014.

[10] N. K. H. de Boer, C. J. J. Mulder, and A. A. van Bodegraven, "Myelotoxicity and hepatotoxicity during azathioprine therapy," *The Netherlands Journal of Medicine*, vol. 63, no. 11, pp. 444–446, 2005.

[11] B. Meijer, A. J. Wilhelm, C. J. J. Mulder, G. Bouma, A. A. van Bodegraven, and N. K. H. de Boer, "Pharmacology of thiopurine therapy in inflammatory bowel disease and complete blood cell count outcomes," *Therapeutic Drug Monitoring*, vol. 39, no. 4, pp. 399–405, 2017.

[12] K. Kiefer and W. El-Matary, "6-Mercaptopurine as an alternative to azathioprine in azathioprine-induced hepatoxicity," *Inflammatory Bowel Diseases*, vol. 15, no. 2, pp. 318-319, 2009.

[13] D. Van Asseldonk, N. de Boer, G. Peters, A. Veldkamp, C. Mulder, and A. Van Bodegraven, "On therapeutic drug monitoring of thiopurines in inflammatory bowel disease; pharmacology, pharmacogenomics, drug intolerance and clinical relevance," *Current Drug Metabolism*, vol. 10, no. 9, pp. 981–997, 2009.

[14] J. Y. Chang and J. H. Cheon, "Thiopurine therapy in patients with inflammatory bowel disease: a Focus on Metabolism and Pharmacogenetics," *Digestive Diseases and Sciences*, vol. 64, no. 9, pp. 2395–2403, 2019.

[15] C. Asadov, G. Aliyeva, and K. Mustafayeva, "Thiopurine S-methyltransferase as a pharmacogenetic biomarker: significance of testing and review of major methods," *Cardiovascular & Hematological Agents in Medicinal Chemistry*, vol. 15, no. 1, 2017.

[16] L. T. Ford and J. D. Berg, "Thiopurine S-methyltransferase (TPMT) assessment prior to starting thiopurine drug treatment; a pharmacogenomic test whose time has come," *Journal of Clinical Pathology*, vol. 63, no. 4, pp. 288–295, 2010.

36

Recurrent Ileal Variceal Bleeding as a Diagnostic and Therapeutic Challenge

Marek Cingel, Jakub Benko, Matej Samoš, and Marián Mokáň

Clinic of Internal Medicine I of University Hospital Martin, Jessenius Faculty of Medicine, Comenius University, Bratislava, Slovakia

Correspondence should be addressed to Jakub Benko; benko36@uniba.sk

Academic Editor: Yoshihiro Moriwaki

Introduction. Massive ileal variceal bleeding is a rare intricate condition that needs rapid management and treatment. The absence of randomized clinical trials in this field leads to a lack of evidence-based diagnostic and therapeutical approaches. We present a case report describing imaging, endoscopic, and surgical procedures leading to the diagnosis and resolution of severe ileal variceal bleeding. *Case Report.* We admitted a 63-year-old patient for recurrent anemia and ongoing bleeding from the gastrointestinal tract presenting as enterorrhagia. We were not able to elucidate the source by endoscopic, angiographic, or nuclear imaging methods. As a last resort, we carried out a surgical procedure with peroperative enteroscopy and subsequent resection of the affected part of the intestine. *Conclusion.* We present a patient with a case of ileal variceal bleeding, which required extensive diagnostic and therapeutic effort with a unique peroperative enteroscopic approach.

1. Introduction

Bleeding from the varices of the gastrointestinal tract is a relatively common complication associated with long-term portal hypertension. This condition is associated with high mortality due to the usually intense blood loss [1]. The incidence of varices in other parts of the digestive tract is significantly lower. Bleeding from ectopic varices accounts for 1–5% of all variceal bleedings [2]. Varicose veins that are not located at predilection sites accessible by standard gastrofibroscopy or colonoscopy can cause a significant diagnostic problem. Ectopic varices have a four-fold higher risk of bleeding compared to esophageal varices and can have a mortality of up to 40% [3]. To date, several cases of ileal varices have been reported, but management and therapy have varied from case to case. This is caused by the absence of randomized studies to guide the management and treatment of such patients. We report a case of recurrent, hemodynamically significant bleeding from an ileal varix in a 63-year-old patient, which was diagnosed with an exploratory laparotomy using perioperative enteroscopy and treated by partial resection of the small intestine.

2. Case Presentation

We admitted to our department a 63-year-old patient with obesity grade 3 (BMI = 53.36 kg/m^2), type 2 diabetes mellitus, and liver cirrhosis (Child–Pugh B) caused by nonalcoholic steatohepatitis because of gastrointestinal bleeding with a high risk of needing interventions and transfusions (Glasgow–Blatchford score 4 points). One year before, the patient was examined for anemia identifying diverticulosis as the source of bleeding. In the past, the patient also underwent an open surgery of the right ovary, cholecystectomy, and a hernioplasty but without the complete resolution of the umbilical hernia. Splenomegaly was also present. We proceeded by performing gastroscopy and colonoscopy without finding a source of bleeding but with obvious signs of gastrointestinal origin of the anemia as digested blood was present in the ileum and colon. The patient required repeated high amounts of transfusions of erythrocytes, and we were unable to stop the bleeding by conservative treatment. A control gastroscopy ruled out the esophagus, stomach, and duodenum as the site of bleeding. The jejunum was examined by single balloon-assisted enteroscopy. However, we

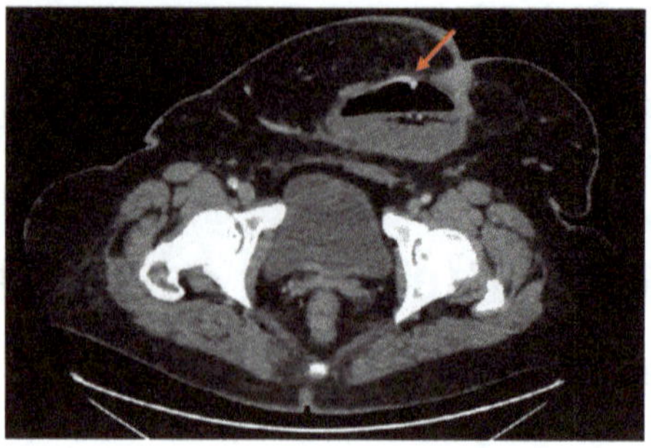

FIGURE 1: CT angiography showing a varix in the sac of the umbilical hernia.

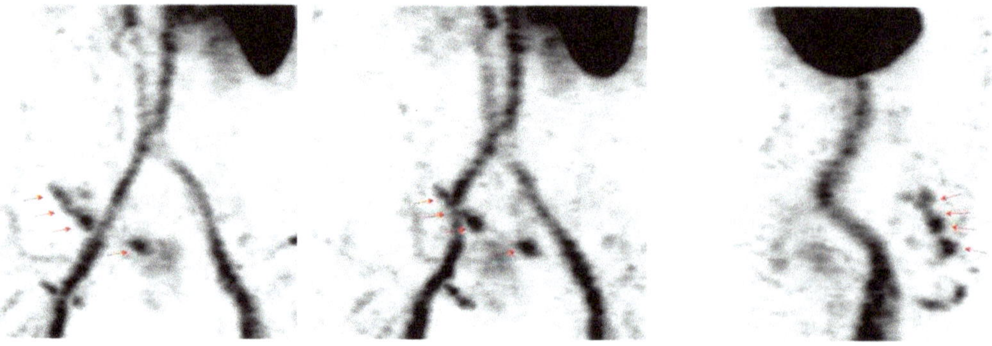

FIGURE 2: Red blood cell nuclear scan showing variceal vessels in the area of the hernia.

could not reach the ileum as the patient's habitus, and several adhesions prevented the safe advance of the endoscope. CT angiography and red blood cell nuclear scan were unable to identify any leak into the gastrointestinal system but described variceal vessels in the sac of the umbilical hernia and perigastric and perisplenic area (shown in Figures 1 and 2). The patient's state progressed, and as all endoscopic and imaging methods were unsuccessful, we carried out an explorative laparotomy to find a 5 mm thick varix in the ileum without active bleeding during the time of surgery (Figure 3). We confirmed the varix as the culprit lesion by peroperative enteroscopy showing typical signs of recent bleeding (Figure 4). A resection of the affected part of the ileum was performed without significant early complications (Figure 5). The histological examination found erosions of the mucous membrane with edema and variceal vessels in the submucosal and subserosal layers (Figure 6). The patient was, after the operation, stabilized without any signs of bleeding. Four months after the surgery, a wound dehiscence occurred, needing further treatment.

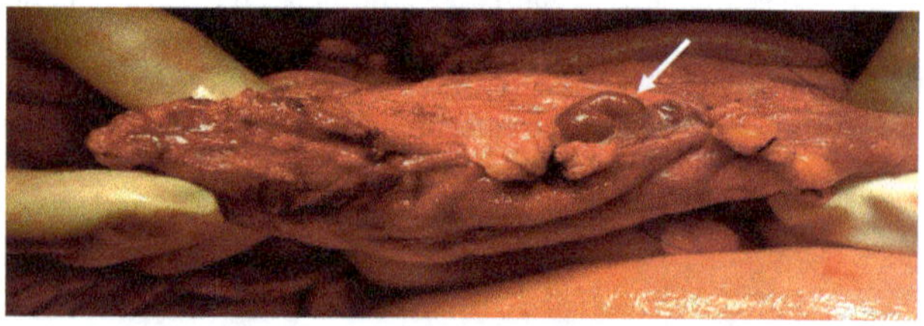

FIGURE 3: The ileum with the identified varix.

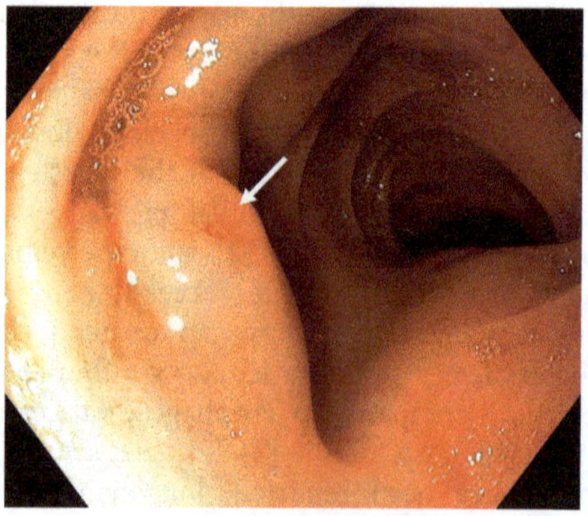

FIGURE 4: Enteroscopy showing the nipple sign at the site of the varix.

3. Discussion

Massive bleeding from an ileal varix is a rare but serious condition with high mortality rates. The mechanism of the formation of ectopic varices is not entirely understood. Several risk factors for incidence are recognized, e.g., liver cirrhosis, portal hypertension, primary biliary cholangitis, hepatic vein thrombosis, chronic intraperitoneal inflammation, past surgery, and intraabdominal adhesions. The most common ileal shunting occurs through the gonadal veins. Hence, a past intervention in the lesser pelvis is another recognized factor. Currently, no guidelines for the treatment of ileal variceal bleeding are available as we still lack any randomized clinical studies concerning this condition. The diagnostic and therapeutical approach is derived from case reports and small retrospective studies [3]. Minowa et al. in 2017 summarized 21 published cases of ileal

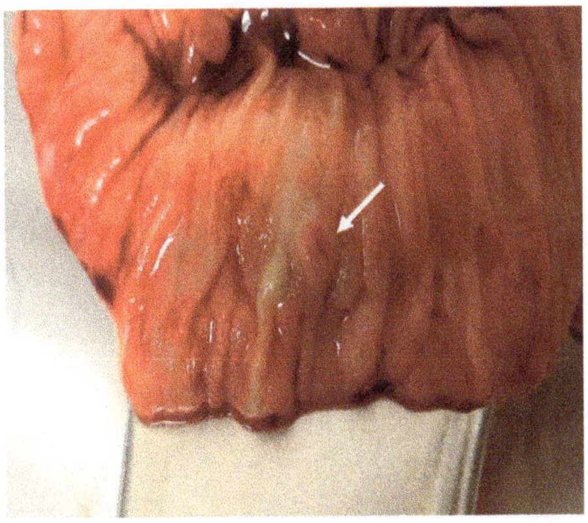

Figure 5: The resected part of the ileum.

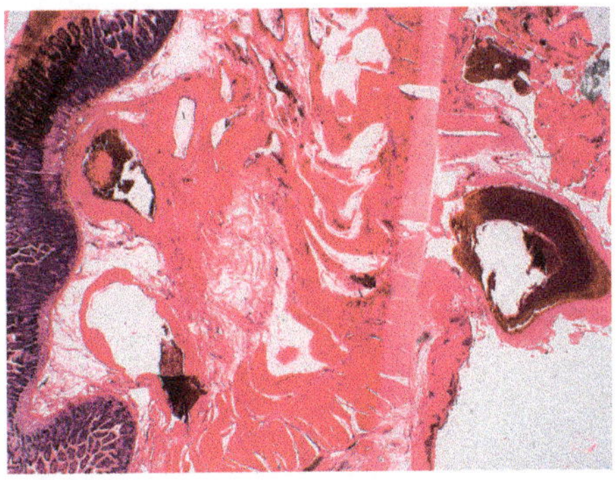

Figure 6: Histological examination of the resected part of the ileum.

variceal bleeding. The most common diagnostic procedure was a form of angiography or multidetector computed tomography [4]. In 3 cases, capsule endoscopy was the diagnostic tool, and an enteroscopy was used just in one case [5, 6]. Abdominal surgery with the resection of the affected part of the intestine was a general approach [5]. We present a patient where a combined surgical and endoscopic management was realized as other methods of diagnosis and treatment failed in a timely fashion. Our patient presented with several risk factors of ileal variceal bleeding, as mentioned before. An essential factor that led to diagnostic uncertainties was the intermittent nature of the bleeding. Therefore, no leak of contrast on a CT scan or marked corpuscles on the red blood cell nuclear scan was recognized, even though these could diagnose the varix by itself. As bleeding did not occur even at the time of the surgery, we needed to ensure that the varix was the culprit lesion. Consequently, an intraoperative enteroscopy through a small incision in the ileum was performed with a typical finding of recent bleeding at the site of the varix. In the end, the affected part of the intestine and the place of insertion of the endoscope were resected. The whole procedure was being complicated by extreme obesity and comorbidities, nevertheless, it went uneventful. In the late postoperative period, dehiscence at the incision site of the abdominal wall evolved. After the surgery, the bleeding resolved, and an increase in the hemoglobin concentration was documented. Nonselective beta-blockers were introduced in our patient in the postoperative period but had to be withdrawn as hypotension evolved. TIPS is another recognized treatment choice but with a relatively high recurrence rate of bleeding [7]. We did not carry out the TIPS procedure during the acute state as we were not certain of variceal bleeding at the time. Capsule endoscopy was considered during the whole diagnostic process, but the limited availability of the examination and the worsening state of the patient precluded the execution. The risk of rebleeding after an acute episode of variceal bleeding is around 60%, but this data is mainly derived from esophageal variceal bleeding studies [8]. It can be theorized that even though the ileal varix was resected, portal hypertension still drives the process of varix development, and future variceal bleeding should be anticipated.

4. Conclusion

We present a case of ectopic variceal bleeding, which after extensive diagnostic effort, required an explorative laparotomy with peroperative enteroscopy to confirm the diagnosis. Resection of the affected part of the ileum was the definite treatment with a satisfactory outcome.

References

[1] A. I. Sharara and D. C. Rockey, "Gastroesophageal variceal hemorrhage," *New England Journal of Medicine*, vol. 345, no. 9, pp. 669–681, 2001.

[2] I. D. Norton, J. C. Andrews, and P. S. Kamath, "Management of ectopic varices," *Hepatology*, vol. 28, no. 4, pp. 1154–1158, 1998.

[3] W. E. A. Saad, A. Lippert, N. E. Saad, and S. Caldwell, "Ectopic varices: anatomical classification, hemodynamic classification, and hemodynamic-based management," *Techniques in Vascular and Interventional Radiology*, vol. 16, no. 2, pp. 108–125, 2013.

[4] K. Minowa, S. Komatsu, K. Takashina et al., "Ectopic gastrointestinal variceal bleeding with portal hypertension," *World Journal of Gastrointestinal Surgery*, vol. 9, no. 12, pp. 288–292, 2017.

[5] G. D. De Palma, M. Rega, S. Masone et al., "Mucosal abnormalities of the small bowel in patients with cirrhosis and portal hypertension: a capsule endoscopy study," *Gastrointestinal Endoscopy*, vol. 62, no. 4, pp. 529–534, 2005.

[6] M. Traina, I. Tarantino, L. Barresi, and F. Mocciaro, "Variceal bleeding from ileum identified and treated by single balloon enteroscopy," *World Journal of Gastroenterology*, vol. 15, no. 15, pp. 1904-1905, 2009.

[7] V. Vidal, L. Joly, P. Perreault, L. Bouchard, M. Lafortune, and G. Pomier-Layrargues, "Usefulness of transjugular

intrahepatic portosystemic shunt in the management of bleeding ectopic varices in cirrhotic patients," *CardioVascular and Interventional Radiology*, vol. 29, no. 2, pp. 216–219, 2006.

[8] K. Bari and G. Garcia-Tsao, "Treatment of portal hypertension," *World Journal of Gastroenterology*, vol. 18, no. 11, pp. 1166–1175, 2012.

37

Importance of Extraintestinal Manifestations in Early Diagnosis of Gardner Syndrome

Bruno Besteiro,[1] **Filipa Gomes**,[1] **Cláudia Costa**,[2] **Raquel Portugal**,[3] **Isabel Garrido**,[4] **and Jorge Almeida**[1]

[1]*Internal Medicine Department, Centro Hospitalar e Universitário de São João, Oporto, Portugal*
[2]*Oncology Department, Instituto Português de Oncologia de Coimbra, Coimbra, Portugal*
[3]*Pathology Department, Centro Hospitalar e Universitário de São João, Oporto, Portugal*
[4]*Gastrenterology Department, Centro Hospitalar e Universitário de São João, Oporto, Portugal*

Correspondence should be addressed to Bruno Besteiro; bruno.besteiro4@gmail.com

Academic Editor: Haruhiko Sugimura

Gardner's syndrome is an autosomal dominant disease caused by a mutation in the *APC* gene with 20–30% of cases presenting de novo. This entity is a variant of familial adenomatous polyposis, with a prevalence of 3/100,000 habitants. It may present as early as 2 months of age with a variety of both colonic and extracolonic symptoms. We report a case of a 21-year-old man, without any known family history, presenting with microcytic hypochromic anemia and constitutional symptoms for two months. Ultimately, after the etiological study, Gardner syndrome diagnosis was established as an index primary familiar case. Gardner syndrome is a clinical challenge which requires a prompt suspicion in order to reach its diagnosis. Given the malignant evolution of adenomas in 100% of untreated patients, early identification of extraintestinal manifestations (identifiable prior to colonic symptoms) is of the essence. A consequent endoscopic study to confirm gastrointestinal involvement is essential for a more favorable prognosis.

1. Introduction

Gardner syndrome (GS) represents a phenotypic variant of familial adenomatous polyposis (FAP), caused by mutations of the *APC* tumor suppressor gene, which is inherited in autosomal dominant fashion [1].

In most cases, a family history of GS is present, although 20% to 30% appear to be new mutations of the *APC* gene [2].

It may present at any age with a variety of symptoms, either colonic or extracolonic [1].

The clinical spectrum of disease presentation is variable, and its diagnosis is frequently delayed, despite the presence of clues from early on. Once GS may involve different organs, it is usually quite hard to treat [3].

2. Case Report

We report the case of a 21-year-old white male, with a history of excision during childhood of paravertebral neurofibroma, nuchal fibroma and epidermoid cysts, never having met the childhood neurofibromatosis diagnostic criteria. He had no relevant familiar history.

He was admitted in the Internal Medicine Department with a two-month history of constitutional symptoms. The patient also recalled a unique episode of hematochezia which had been attributed to hemorrhoids. He had no other associated symptoms.

On admission, he presented noticeably pale. Physical examination revealed mild hepatomegaly. No other signs were present.

Laboratory test results unveiled microcytic hypochromic anemia (hemoglobin: 8.5 g/dL) with iron deficiency (serum iron < 10 μg/dL and ferritin of 12.3 ng/mL), leukocytosis (14,720/μL), thrombocytosis ($6.44 \times 10^4/\mu$L), elevated lactate dehydrogenase (2802 IU/L), mild C-reactive protein elevation (16.7 mg/L), mild hypoalbuminemia (36.6 g/dL), and mild erythrocyte sedimentation rate elevation (34 mm/1 h). Serologic markers for the human immunodeficiency virus and hepatitis B and C virus were negative.

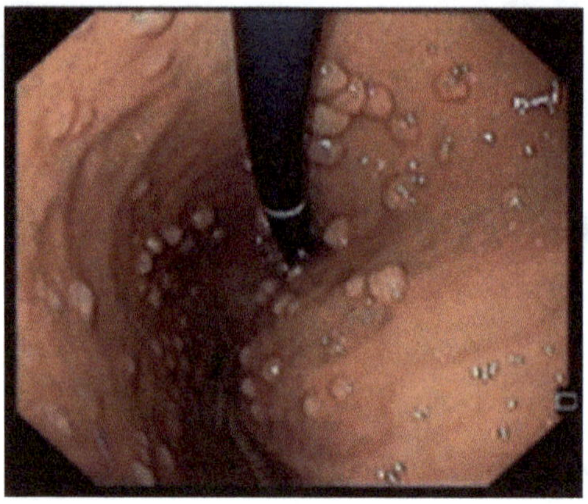

Figure 1: Gastric fundus with nodular aspect and numerous delineated polyps.

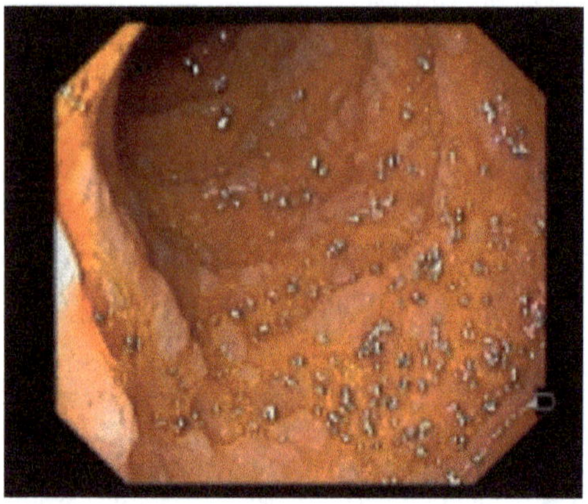

Figure 2: Duodenum with bulbous mucosa and the second duodenal portion with micronodular aspect.

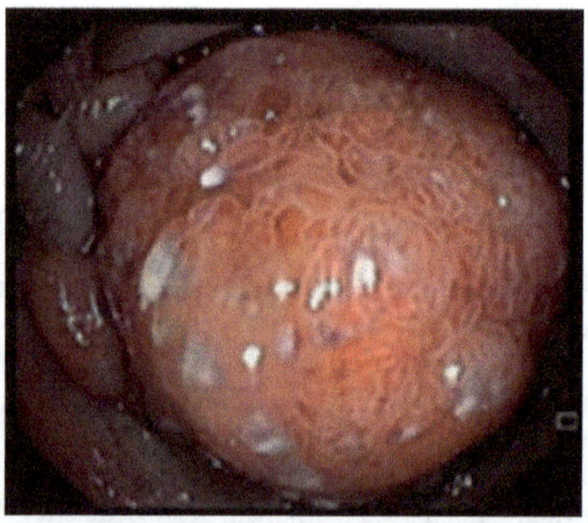

Figure 3: Vegetative lesion of the descending colon.

A computed tomography angiography was performed, and it revealed multiple hepatic nodules with neoplastic etiology suspicion and a right adrenal gland nodule.

Upper endoscopy displayed numerous delineated polyps, entirely carpeting the stomach and duodenum, consistent with the diagnosis of FAP (Figure 1). Moreover, other abnormal macroscopic findings included the duodenum with bulbous mucosa and the second duodenal portion with micronodular aspect (Figure 2).

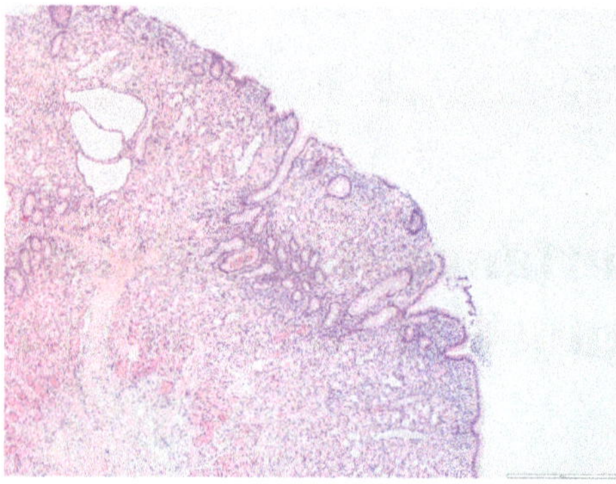

Figure 4: Gastric fundic gland polyp.

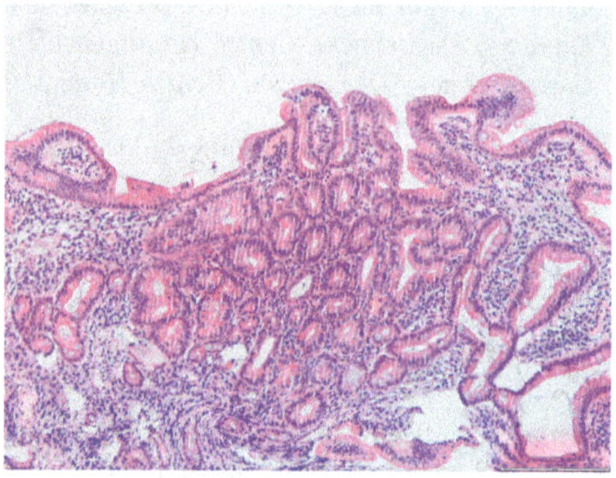

Figure 5: Duodenal mucosa with focal low-grade dysplasia.

Lower endoscopy documented nodularity of the terminal ileum, exuberant colic polyposis (>100), and a vegetative lesion of the descending colon (Figure 3).

Biopsies were taken on both of these exams. Histopathological examination showed fundic glands' polyps (gastric polyps) (Figure 4) and duodenal mucosa with focal low-grade dysplasia (Figure 5). The vegetating colon lesion biopsy revealed adenoma with low-grade dysplasia and a necrosing area in one of the fragments, leading to consideration of a peripheric lesion biopsy.

A liver biopsy was performed resulting in adenocarcinoma of a probable gastrointestinal origin (Figure 6).

The functional study of the adrenal nodule was compatible with the benign adenoma.

The association between intestinal adenomas, gastric fundic gland polyps, adrenal nodule, epidermoid cysts, and fibromas raised the suspicion of GS.

Once the most likely diagnosis was FAP, the patient underwent a thyroid ultrasound due to FAP's association with thyroid carcinoma which did not divulge any abnormality.

The diagnosis was later on confirmed through sequencing of the *APC* gene revealing a pathologic heterozygotic c.4612_4613delGA p.(Glu1538Ilefs*5) variant.

On discharge, all first-degree family members were referred to oncogenetics in order to be evaluated for FAP

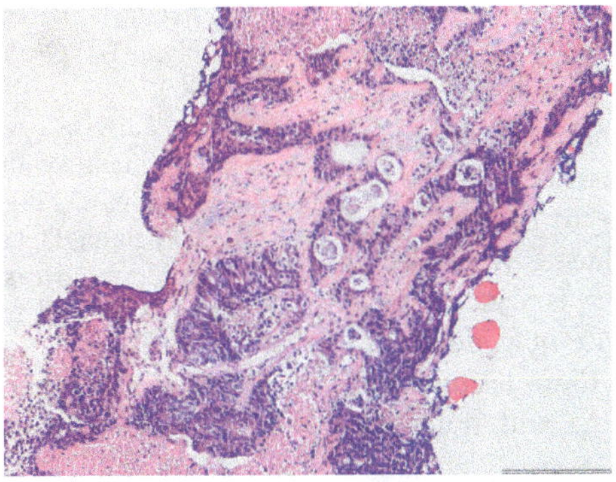

FIGURE 6: Liver biopsy-adenocarcinoma with necrosis, consistent with gastrointestinal origin.

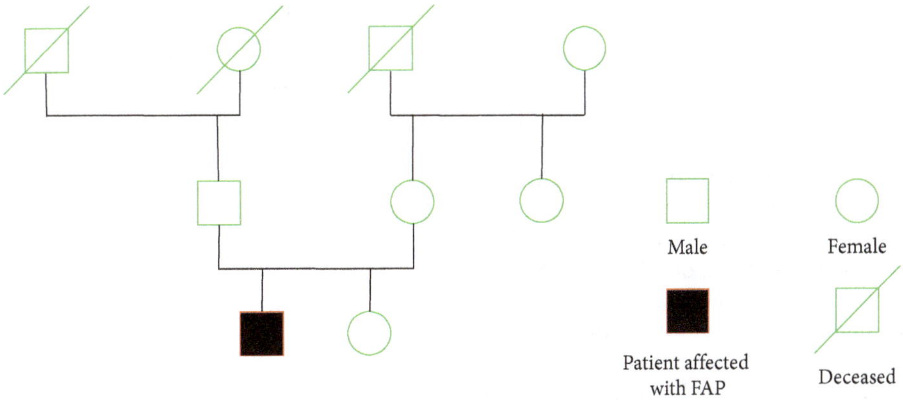

FIGURE 7: Family pedigree chart.

(Figure 7). His sister had negative lower endoscopy and genetic testing. His mother did not show any abnormality in colonoscopy, and his father refused to perform the same study. However, the father had a lower endoscopy performed in the previous 5 years without any changes.

At a cancer group meeting, colectomy and chemotherapy were decided with a palliative purpose.

3. Discussion

GS is characterized by a constellation of intestinal findings of PAF along with extraintestinal manifestations, including cutaneous lesions and adrenal adenoma, among others [3].

The diagnosis of FAP and GS can be attained through genetic testing for gene mutations or demonstration of multiple colonic polyps. Genetic testing is the most effective method for demonstrating a mutated *APC* gene [1].

This case is significant due to a germline pathogenic mutation c.4612_4613delGA p.(Glu1538Ilefs*5) in the *APC* gene which is absent in population databases (gnomAD, ExAC, and 1000 Genomes), showcasing the allele's low frequency. The gene is altered by a frameshift mutation due to deletion on the 5q22.2 region which potentially originates a nonfunctional truncated protein, therefore being classified as a pathogenic variant.

This case supports that this de novo variation of the *APC* gene should be documented in the literature as it results in a GS phenotype with multiple extracolonic symptoms occurring early in life. Until now, this variation had not been documented as causing this clinical presentation. The location of the mutation within the *APC* gene has been associated with the severity of colonic polyposis, degree of cancer risk, age of cancer onset, survival, and frequency of extracolonic manifestations.

In 1993, an English study which considered APC mutations in FAP families in England had already reported two patients with a severe Gardner's phenotype, both with a deletion in codon 1538 [4].

Although the current data are scarce, we may be facing a more aggressive fast-acting pathologic variant once the average age for cancer diagnosis in individuals with untreated FAP is 39 years. Generally, cancers start to develop a decade after the appearance of the polyps, and if the colon is intact, the majority of patients with FAP will develop colorectal cancer (CRC) by the fifth decade [5].

Hence, dissemination of the information gathered from this case and other similar instances of young patients with FAP and GS will better anticipate further testing and knowledge in order to attain better therapeutic weapons.

In what concerns to extraintestinal symptoms, epidermoid cysts are the most common benign skin lesions in GS [6] and occur most frequently on the face, extremities, and scalp. They show up most often during puberty [7].

In this particular clinical case, the patient presented with paravertebral neurofibroma, nuchal fibroma, and epidermoid cysts as early as an infant which probably then indicated extraintestinal manifestations since this age. Once GS is not typically diagnosed by the presence of these cutaneous lesions, clinicians must be able to recognize the distinct lesions of GS, and they must exclude PAF in a child with fibromas even when the family history is negative since 25% of GS patients can present with a new dominant mutation. Therefore, early detection of these lesions may lead to appropriate further investigations and treatment which might be lifesaving.

Patients with GS are at increased risk of several extracolonic malignancies such as duodenal/periampullary (3–5%), thyroid (2%), pancreatic (2%), hepatoblastoma (1.6%), central nervous system (<1%), gastric (<1%), and adrenal (<1%) [8].

In our patient, all the extracolonic malignancies were excluded.

The thyroid cancer risk is increased approximately 150-fold compared with the general population. Hence, and according to the literature, all patients diagnosed with GS should be screened periodically through physical examination and undergo an ultrasound annually [9].

Adrenal adenomas have been reported in 7% of GS. Despite malignancy of the adrenal incidentaloma is rare in this entity, the functional study should be done once the odds are greater compared with the general population [10].

Though screening guidelines for pediatric population at risk of classic FAP exist, there is no unified approach for any of the extracolonic manifestations. Such methods would be imperative once many early age cases present with these manifestations.

As the syndrome is genetically inherited, diagnosis may also have implications for other family members. Therefore, genetic testing of parents and siblings is a critical part of the evaluation process [1].

This case illustrates a genetic variant of GS rarely reported in the literature and highlights the need for not only a holistic view of sign and symptoms but also an individualized approach to treatment.

References

[1] C. Fotiadis, D. K. Tsekouras, Antonakis et al., "Gardner's syndrome: a case report and review of the literature," *World Journal of Gastroenterology*, vol. 11, no. 34, pp. 5408–5411, 2005.

[2] B. W. Neville, D. B. Damm, C. M. Allen et al., "Bone pathology," *Color Atlas of Oral and Maxillofacial Diseases*, Elsevier, Amsterdam, Netherlands, 1st edition, 2019.

[3] G.-L. Gu, S.-L. Wang, X.-M. Wei et al., "Desmoid tumor in Gardner's Syndrome presented as acute abdómen," *World Journal of Surgical Oncology*, vol. 4, p. 18, 2006.

[4] J. G. Armstrong, D. R. Davies, S. P. Guy, I. M. Frayling, and D. G. R. Evans, "APC mutations in familial adenomatous polyposis families in the northwest of England," *Human Mutation*, vol. 10, no. 5, pp. 376–380, 1997.

[5] E. Half, D. Bercovich, and P. Rozen, "Familial adenomatous polyposis," *Orphanet Journal of Rare Diseases*, vol. 4, p. 22, 2009.

[6] S. Panjwani, A. Bagewadi, V. Keluskar, and S. Arora, "Gardner's syndrome," *Journal of Clinical Imaging Science*, vol. 1, p. 65, 2011.

[7] U. Wollina, D. Langner, G. Tchernev, K. França, and T. Lotti, "Epidermoid cysts-a wide spectrum of clinical presentation and successful treatment by surgery: a retrospective 10-year analysis and literature review," *Open Access Macedonian Journal of Medical Sciences*, vol. 6, no. 1, pp. 28–30, 2018.

[8] R. D. Burt, "Gardner syndrome," 2018, http://www.uptodate.com.

[9] S. B. Punatar, V Notonha, A. Joshi, S. Punatar et al., "Thyroid cancer in Gardner's syndrome: case report and review of literature," *South Asian Journal of Cancer*, vol. 1, no. 1, pp. 43–47, 2012.

[10] N. M. Rekik, S. B. Salah, N. Kallel et al., "Adrenocortical secreting mass in a patient with Gardner's syndrome: a case report," *Case Reports in Medicine*, vol. 2010, Article ID 682081, 4 pages, 2010.

38

Wilkie's Syndrome following Chemotherapy: A Case Report and a Review of Literature

Nicholas J. Corsi,[1] **Ahmad A. Abu-Heija**,[1,2] **Anand Kumar Ravi**,[1,2] **Matthew P. Corsi**,[1] **and Murray N. Ehrinpreis**[1]

[1]*Wayne State University School of Medicine, Detroit, MI, USA*
[2]*John D. Dingell V.A. Medical Center, Detroit Medical Center, Wayne State University, Detroit, MI, USA*

Correspondence should be addressed to Nicholas J. Corsi; fv9108@wayne.edu

Academic Editor: Yoshiro Kawahara

Superior mesenteric artery (SMA) syndrome is a rare etiology of upper gastrointestinal obstruction. The measured angle between the SMA and the aorta is typically between 38 and 65° and maintained by mesenteric fat. Excessive fat loss can lead to intestinal obstruction due to an exaggerated acute angularity of the SMA, compressing the third part of the duodenum. We present a 22-year-old female with a history of aplastic anemia, status post bone-marrow transplant, who presented with intractable nausea and had confirmed SMA syndrome on CT angiography. Subsequently, the patient underwent nasogastric decompression and successful laparoscopic duodenojejunostomy.

1. Introduction

Superior mesenteric artery (SMA) syndrome, or Wilkie's syndrome, is a rare etiology of upper gastrointestinal obstruction, with potentially nonspecific symptoms on initial presentation. The prevalence of SMA syndrome in the general population is estimated at 0.013%–0.3% [1]. Normally, the measured angle between the SMA and the aorta is 38–65° maintained by mesenteric fat padding. The pathological mechanism of intestinal obstruction is due to an exaggerated acute angularity of the SMA, leading to compression of the third part of the duodenum between the SMA and aorta, caused by excessive fat loss. There are multiple predisposing factors that can increase the angularity, leading to duodenal compression, of which the most common is significant weight loss [1]. However, substantial weight loss and low BMI are not required for development of SMA syndrome. Gastroenterologists should be cognizant of other underlying medical disorders, previous surgeries, and psychological disorders that can heighten a patient's risk. Specifically, unexpected cases have been reported due to anorexia nervosa [2], spinal cord injury and kyphoscoliosis, and bariatric surgery [1]. However, there are limited cases reported of SMA syndrome subsequent to chemotherapy.

2. Case Presentation

We present a 22-year-old female with no prior comorbidities who clinically manifested with lethargy, menometrorrhagia, and pancytopenia, and a subsequent diagnosis of aplastic anemia. She was scheduled for a stem-cell transplant, from a fully matched, unrelated donor. At time of initial medical oncology evaluation intake, she weighed 49.5 kg and was 160.7 cm tall (BMI = 19.2). Subsequently, she underwent a conditioning regimen of cyclophosphamide-fludarabine-antithymocyte globulin (Cy/Flu/ATG) prior to her allogenic bone-marrow transplant. She received all 5 days of scheduled fludarabine as well as 2 days of scheduled cyclophosphamide. On day 9 posttransplant, her weight continued to precipitously drop to 48.2 kg, to 47.9 kg, 46.6 kg, and 43.2 kg (on days 12, 14, and 50, respectively). She was drinking suboptimal amount of fluid (30–40 oz per day), and she reported no appetite and had minimal desire for food items she once enjoyed. She was refractory to antiemetics, as well as dronabinol for appetite stimulation. On consultation to gastroenterology, she complained of persistent nausea and vomiting episodes with any oral intake. Additionally, the only nutrition she was taking in regularly was 2 protein shakes with a total of 550 calories per shake. Finally, due to the intractable and intolerable nausea and vomiting, she presented to the emergency department (at a weight of 42.1 kg). Physical examination revealed peri-umbilical tenderness but was otherwise normal. Further history revealed a similar constellation of symptoms approximately 1 month prior, with a normal esophagogastroduodenoscopy, and resolution of symptoms with supportive care. During this hospitalization, however, she was initiated on total parenteral nutrition, due to malnutrition and inability to maintain >50% of caloric requirements by mouth. She was extremely fatigued, requiring even assistance to use the commode. During hospitalization, she continued to have asymptomatic sinus tachycardia, of which cardiology believed to be a physiologic response due to her volume-depleted state and acute dehydration. Her tachycardia improved with resolution of pain with vomiting and increasing physical strength. On readmission imaging, CT scan showed a massively distended stomach, first, and second portions of the duodenum, after collapse of the third portion of the duodenum as it traverses the SMA (Figure 1). CT-angiography was obtained revealing acute angulation of the SMA-aortic takeoff at approximately 20 degrees (Figures 2 and 3). A diagnosis of SMA syndrome was made. It was deduced that the chemotherapy-induced nausea, vomiting, and mucositis had led to appreciable weight loss and absence of the mesenteric fat pad, resulting with SMA syndrome. The patient underwent nasogastric decompression. By the day of surgical treatment, she dropped to 39.5 kg. Her nadir was 38.8 kg (BMI = 15) 4 days post-op. She underwent a laparoscopic duodenojejunostomy resulting in a successful bypass. Additionally, with surgical treatment and discontinuation of the chemotherapy, her weight gradually progressed to 47 kg. The patient was then followed for resolution of the preoperative symptoms. She demonstrated appropriate emptying of the duodenum and her subsequent follow up was uneventful.

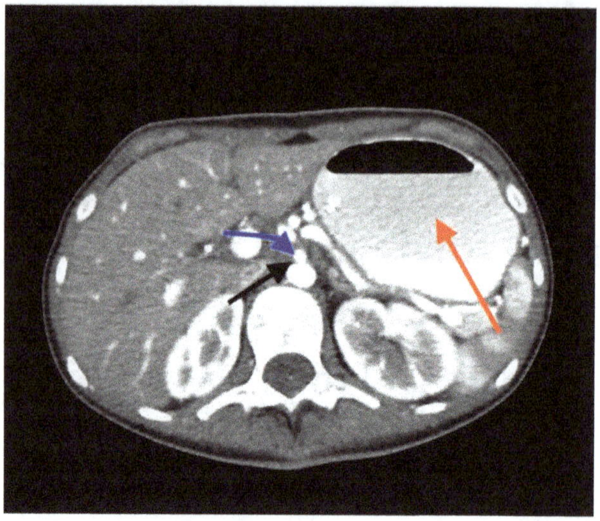

Figure 1: Axial CT abdomen showing compression of the third portion of the duodenum (black arrow) from the superior mesenteric artery (blue), with distention of the stomach (red arrow).

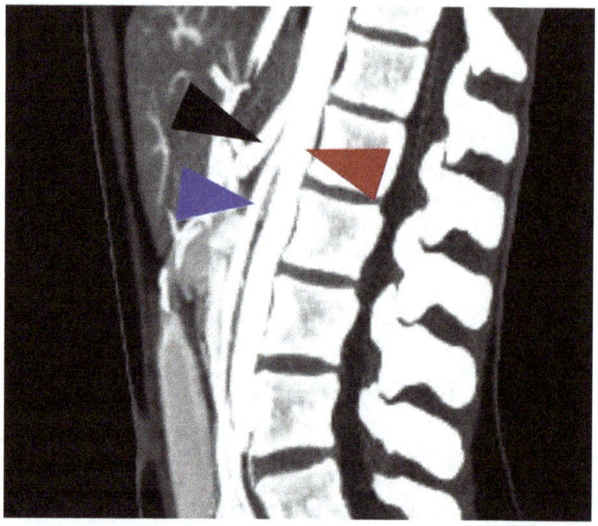

Figure 2: CT angiography revealing severe acute angularity of the SMA-aortic take off. Black arrow: celiac artery; maroon arrow: aorta; blue arrow: superior mesenteric artery.

3. Discussion

Very few cases of SMA syndrome postchemotherapy have been reported in the literature. Table 1 offers a review. Each highlights the seemingly noteworthy complications in patients receiving treatment for malignancy, who may experience weight loss and severe emesis, which likely confound the presentation of the disease. Physicians should be wary of this rare etiology of duodenal obstruction and its clinical manifestations. Usually, the diagnosis can be confused with various motility-related or anatomic causes of duodenal obstruction. Albeit rare, a high index of suspicion should be employed for young patients presenting with signs and symptoms of intestinal obstruction with a history of weight loss, to allow inclusion of SMA (Wilkie's) syndrome in the differential diagnosis. Delayed diagnosis can lead to devastating outcomes, including death from complications related to electrolyte abnormalities or perforation. Furthermore, in patients who present with persistent emesis, SMA syndrome can precipitate hypovolemia, hypokalemia, and metabolic alkalosis. In order to confirm the diagnosis in a patient with symptoms suggestive of SMA symptoms, radiological studies are required, which may include an upper gastrointestinal (GI) barium studies alongside simultaneous angiography [3] or CT abdomen for noninvasive, enhanced anatomical detail. However, even with imaging, the diagnosis may be easily overlooked [4], as radiological findings do not always correlate with clinical findings [5]. Additionally, some patients may experience intermittent symptomatic compression of the duodenum, leading to a delay in diagnosis [1]. This was illustrated with our patient, who presented with similar symptoms 1 month

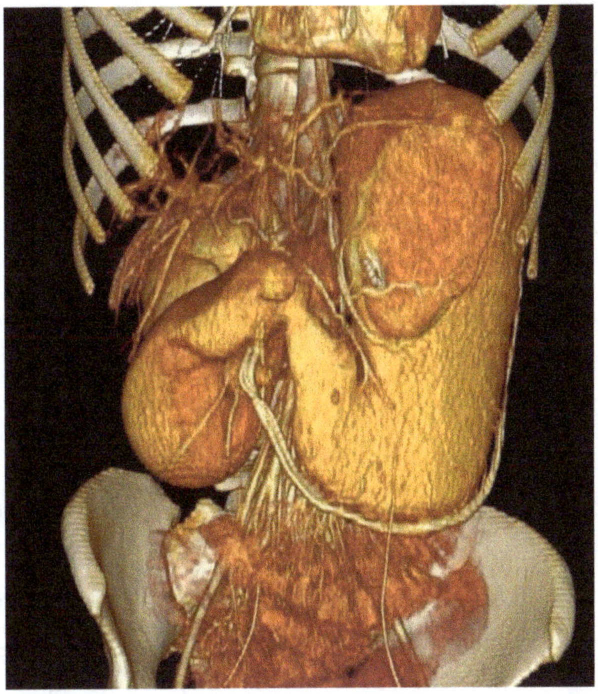

FIGURE 3: 3D reconstructed CT angiography revealing severely distended stomach and first and second portion of the duodenum.

TABLE 1: Review of reported cases of SMA syndrome following chemotherapy.

First author, year	Age (sex)	Chemotherapeutic agent	Cancer	Associated symptoms	Weight loss (kg)	Imaging	Treatment
Ushiki, 2012 [9]	61 (M)	Cisplatin	Squamous cell carcinoma, lung	Anorexia, nausea, vomiting	7	CT abdomen, upper GI series, abdominal X-ray	Tubal feeding; weight gain
Chowdhary, 2015 [10]	81 (M)	Carboplatin	Mesothelioma	Epigastric pain, nausea, vomiting	18	CT abdomen, upper GI series, esophagogram	Conservative; weight gain
Irei, 2016 [11]	~60 s (M)	Neo-adjuvant chemotherapy	Esophageal	Postprandial abdominal pain	6	CT and upper GI series	Roux-en-Y bypass of gastrostomy and jejunostomy
Lippl, 2002 [12]	31 (M)	Palliative chemotherapy	Colorectal cancer	Recurrent vomiting	7	CT abdomen, digital fluoroscopy, esophagogastroduodenoscopy	Parenteral nutrition; weight gain
Bang, 2009 [13]	57 (F)	Palliative chemotherapy	Colon cancer with peritoneal seeding	Post-prandial abdominal pain, nausea	6	CT abdomen and small bowel series	Adhesiolysis and duodenojejunostomy
Girotra, 2013 [14]	60 (F)	Chemotherapy	Breast cancer	Post-prandial pain, vomiting, nausea	36	CT abdomen, barium swallow, esophagogastroduodenoscopy	Conservative; weight gain

prior to diagnosis, with no anatomic abnormalities on esophagogastroduodenoscopy. Depending on initial management, it is recommended that once symptom free and patency of the duodenum is achieved, patients begin a dietary regimen while cautiously monitoring clinically and biochemically for refeeding syndrome. Some suggest reversal of weight as initial therapy; however, this is based off of limited evidence. In one of the largest case series of SMA syndrome, the authors concluded that surgical management is superior to medical therapy with respect to success and recurrence, and surgery should be employed when conservative management fails, with lack of consensus on timing for surgical management [3]. Medical therapy consists of supportive care such as total parenteral nutrition or small-volume meals and postural changes [6]. Ultimately, in those who do not improve with conservative management, the surgical options include mobilization of ligament of Treitz (Strong's procedure) [7], gastrojejunostomy, and laparoscopic duodenojejunostomy. Of those options, duodenojejunostomy may provide the best results [8], which is reflected in the successful outcome in our patient.

In summary, physicians should be wary of this rare etiology of duodenal obstruction and its clinical manifestations. Albeit rare, a high index of suspicion should be employed for patients presenting with signs and symptoms of intestinal obstruction in the setting of chemotherapy, to allow inclusion of SMA syndrome in the differential.

Disclosure

Corsi and Abu-Heija are co-first authors.

Authors' Contributions

NC, AAH, and MC were involved in designing, reviewing the literature, and writing up of the case. AAH, AR, and ME reviewed the manuscript and provided critical specialist input. All authors approved the final draft. Nicholas J. Corsi and Ahmad A. Abu-Heija contributed equally to this work.

Acknowledgments

The authors would like to thank the patient for her participation in the case report.

References

[1] T. Gebhart, "Superior mesenteric artery syndrome," *Gastroenterology Nursing*, vol. 38, no. 3, pp. 189–193, 2015.
[2] B. D. Pentlow and R. G. Dent, "Acute vascular compression of the duodenum in anorexia nervosa," *British Journal of Surgery*, vol. 68, no. 9, pp. 665-666, 2005.
[3] T. H. Lee, J. S. Lee, Y. Jo et al., "Superior mesenteric artery syndrome: where do we stand today?" *Journal of Gastrointestinal Surgery*, vol. 16, no. 12, pp. 2203–2211, 2012.
[4] B. Unal, A. Aktaş, G. Kemal et al., "Superior mesenteric artery syndrome: CT and ultrasonography findings," *Diagn Interv Radiol*, vol. 11, no. 2, pp. 90–95, 2005.
[5] F. Rosa-Jiménez, F. J. Rodríguez González, J. J. Puente Gutiérrez, R. Muñoz Sánchez, M. D. Adarraga Cansino, and J. L. Zambrana García, "Duodenal compression caused by superior mesenteric artery: study of 10 patients," *Revista Española de Enfermedades Digestivas*, vol. 95, no. 7, 2003.
[6] J. R. Hines, R. M. Gore, and G. H. Ballantyne, "Superior mesenteric artery syndrome," *The American Journal of Surgery*, vol. 148, no. 5, pp. 630–632, 1984.
[7] E. K. Strong, "Mechanics of arteriomesenteric duodenal obstruction and direct surgical attack upon etiology," *Annals of Surgery*, vol. 148, no. 5, pp. 725–730, 1958.
[8] G. Valiathan, M. Wani, J. Lanker, and P. K. Reddy, "A case series on superior mesenteric artery syndrome surgical management, single institution experience," *Journal of Clinical and Diagnostic Research*, vol. 11, no. 8, pp. PR01–PR03, 2017.
[9] A. Ushiki, T. Koizumi, H. Yamamoto, M. Hanaoka, K. Kubo, and M. Matsushita, "Superior mesenteric artery syndrome following initiation of cisplatin-containing chemotherapy: a case report," *Journal of Medical Case Reports*, vol. 6, no. 1, 2012.
[10] M. Chowdhary, H. P. Pansuria, B. Farooqi, and H. Goyal, "Superior mesenteric artery syndrome: a unique complication following carboplatin-based chemotherapy," *International Medical Case Reports Journal*, vol. 8, pp. 55–58, 2015.
[11] J. Straatman, M. Cuesta, J. R. Garcia et al., "Date: september 19, 2016, 08:00—10:00 FA01: featured abstracts 1: minimally invasive esophagectomy (malignant) room: topaz concourse," *Diseases of the Esophagus*, vol. 29, 2016.
[12] F. Lippl, C. Hannig, W. Weiß, H.-D. Allescher, M. Classen, and M. Kurjak, "Superior mesenteric artery syndrome: diagnosis and treatment from the gastroenterologist's view," *Journal of Gastroenterology*, vol. 37, no. 8, pp. 640–643, 2002.
[13] C. S. Bang, S. I. Lee, G. W. Park et al., "A case of superior mesenteric artery syndrome due to peritoneal seeding in a colon cancer patient," *The Korean Journal of Medicine*, vol. 76, no. 3, pp. 380–384, 2009.
[14] M. Girotra, H. R. Shah, and R. F. Rego, "An intriguing cause of intractable nausea and vomiting," *Saudi Journal of Gastroenterology*, vol. 19, no. 4, pp. 190-191, 2013.

39

Jejunal Polyps out of Place: A Case of Gastric Heterotopia of the Jejunum

Siri A. Urquhart[1] **and Nayantara Coelho-Prabhu**[2]

[1]*Division of Internal Medicine, Mayo Clinic, Rochester, MN, USA*
[2]*Division of Gastroenterology and Hepatology, Mayo Clinic, Rochester, MN, USA*

Correspondence should be addressed to Siri A. Urquhart; urquhart.siri@mayo.edu

Academic Editor: Yoshifumi Nakayama

Heterotopia is the presence of normal physiologic tissue in an atypical location. Gastric heterotopia has been described in various locations throughout the gastrointestinal tract, including the small intestine. Gastric heterotopia of the small intestine typically is asymptomatic but may present in several ways with symptoms of obstruction, bleeding, perforation, intussusception, or pain. However, gastric heterotopia is rare beyond the duodenum except for its frequent association with Meckel's diverticulum. This entity should be considered in the differential diagnosis of polypoid lesions presenting with symptoms of bleeding or obstruction especially in younger patients. We present a case of gastric heterotopia of the jejunum in a patient with a prior history of Meckel's diverticulectomy after he presented with obstructive symptoms. His symptoms improved following resection of two jejunal polyps via antegrade double-balloon assisted enteroscopy with fluoroscopy. On histopathological examination, findings were consistent with gastric heterotopia. This case highlights the importance of considering gastric heterotopia in the differential diagnosis of polypoid lesions located beyond the ligament of Treitz in younger patients presenting with obstructive symptoms.

1. Introduction

Heterotopia is the presence of mature physiologic tissue in an atypical location. Gastric heterotopia has been described in several locations throughout the gastrointestinal tract such as the esophagus, duodenum, gallbladder, Meckel's diverticulum, and other areas within the small bowel and rectum. Gastric heterotopia of the small intestine can be asymptomatic or present in various ways with symptoms of obstruction, ulceration or bleeding, perforation, intussusception, or pain [1]. Gastric heterotopia beyond the ligament of Treitz is rare but should be considered in the differential diagnosis of polypoid lesions in young patients presenting with gastrointestinal bleeding or symptoms of obstruction [2].

2. Case Presentation

A 33-year-old gentleman presented with lower abdominal pain, occasional nausea, emesis, and inability to pass stool or flatus. He did not have any fever or chills. His past medical history was notable for Meckel's diverticulectomy secondary to gastrointestinal bleeding which ultimately required ileal resection and stapled anastomosis ten years previously. The pathology following operative intervention did not demonstrate any ectopic gastric mucosa. He did not have any additional pertinent past medical, family, or social history.

His vital signs were within normal limits. Physical examination was notable for a minimally distended abdomen with tympany on percussion. Laboratory investigations were unremarkable. Coronal and axial computed tomography enterography of the abdomen and pelvis with contrast (Figure 1) demonstrated a 0.8 cm jejunal polyp in the proximal jejunum just past the ligament of Treitz. He subsequently underwent an antegrade double-balloon assisted enteroscopy with fluoroscopy which revealed a 1.5 cm semisessile polyp without bleeding at the ligament of Treitz in addition to a 0.7 cm sessile polyp in the proximal jejunum (Figure 2) which were then resected.

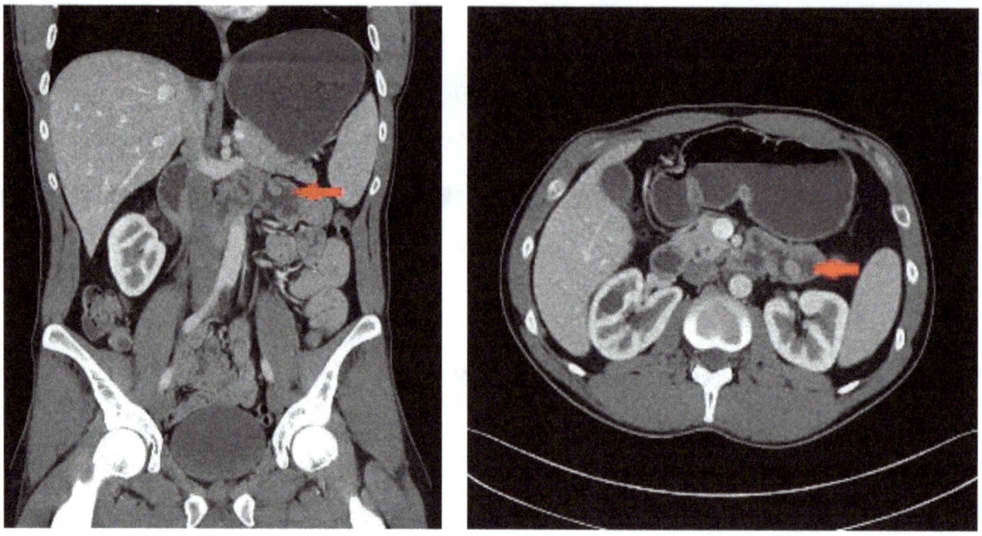

(a) (b)

FIGURE 1: Coronal (a) and axial (b) computed tomography enterography of the abdomen and pelvis with contrast demonstrating a 0.8 cm jejunal polyp in the proximal jejunum just past the ligament of Treitz.

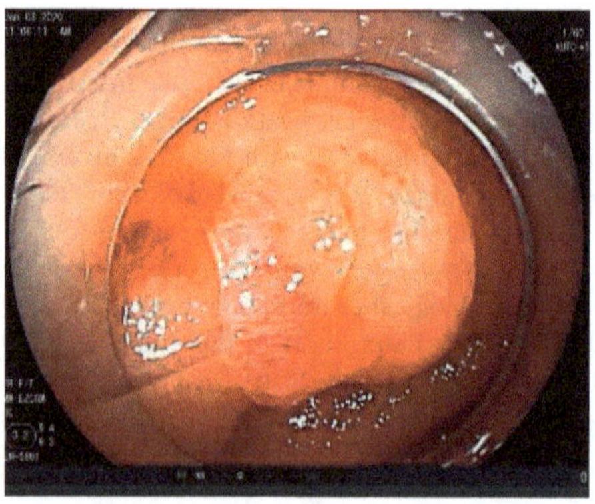

FIGURE 2: Antegrade double-balloon assisted enteroscopy with fluoroscopy demonstrating a semisessile polyp without bleeding at the ligament of Treitz.

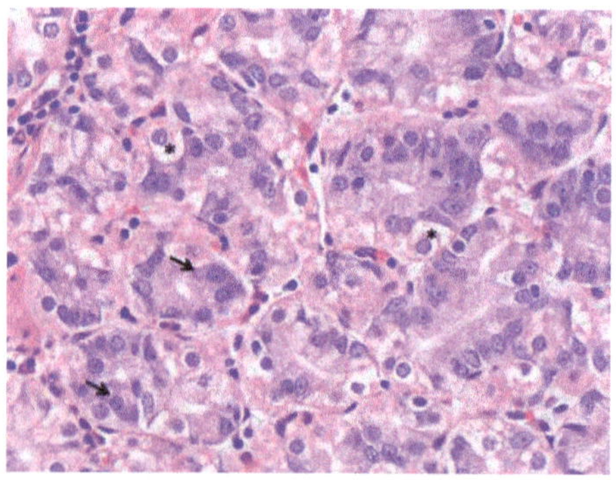

FIGURE 3: Histopathology with nodular areas of gastric fundic heterotopia without dysplasia. Oxyntic glands with chief cells (arrows) and parietal cells (asterisks) are shown at high magnification.

Histopathology demonstrated nodular areas of gastric fundic heterotopia without dysplasia. Oxyntic glands with chief cells (arrows) and parietal cells (asterisks) are shown at high magnification (Figure 3). A diagnosis of gastric heterotopia of the jejunum was made. Following endoscopic resection, the patient was advised to avoid aspirin or nonsteroidal anti-inflammatory medications and to monitor hemoglobin annually for anemia.

3. Discussion

Heterotopia is defined as the presence of normal physiologic tissue in an anatomic location where it is not normally found. Gastric heterotopia is not an uncommon lesion and can be found in several areas throughout the gastrointestinal tract. However, gastric heterotopia is rare beyond the duodenum except for its frequent association with Meckel's diverticulum [3]. Gastric heterotopia of the small intestine may be asymptomatic or present with symptoms of intestinal obstruction, ulceration or bleeding, perforation, intussusception, or pain [1]. Gross appearance is characteristically a mucosal nodularity or polypoid lesion [2, 4]. Peptic ulceration in the area of heterotopia followed by inflammation and fibrosis may result in the formation of a stricture. Polyps can cause intussusception. On microscopic examination, the surface is lined by gastric foveolar epithelium with gastric glands, typically with fundic type mucosa [2].

It is important to differentiate gastric heterotopia from gastric metaplasia. Gastric metaplasia is an acquired lesion and is usually seen in association with chronic inflammatory conditions such as inflammatory bowel disease. Unlike heterotopia which is a macroscopic lesion seen on radiographic imaging or endoscopy, ultimately requiring confirmation by biopsy, metaplasia is a microscopic lesion [2].

The typical treatment for gastric heterotopia includes endoscopic or surgical resection to prevent complications. This case is unique in that the patient had two foci of gastric

TABLE 1: Summary of previously reported cases of gastric heterotopia of the jejunum.

Author	Age	Sex	Presenting features and diagnosis	Duration	Gross appearance	Size	Treatment
Ahn, et al. [10]	5	F	Vomiting, abdominal pain; diagnosed with intussusception of proximal jejunal loops	2 weeks	Polypoid lesions with erosions on the proximal jejunum	Variable-sized with largest nearly obstructing jejunal lumen	Endoscopic resection
Ali, et al. [7]	23	M	Melena, nausea, and vomiting	Unknown	Jejunal diverticulum with white mucosal plaques 50 cm from pylorus	Unknown	Midline laparotomy and endoscopic wedge resection
Al-Jaadan, et al. [6]	1	F	Episodic abdominal distension, vomiting, diarrhea, and failure to thrive	3 years	Dilated segment of proximal jejunum followed by 8 cm narrowed segment with thickened walls	38 cm dilated segment of proximal jejunum	Laparotomy with en-bloc small bowel resection
Bhattacharya, et al. [1]	52	F	Intermittent cramping, abdominal pain, and vomiting	Unknown	Mucosal, broad-based, polypoid mass	$4 \times 2.7 \times 0.4$ cm	Exploratory laparotomy with partial resection of jejunum
Chinnery, et al. [3]	17	F	Postprandial vomiting and weight loss	3 months	Jejunal stricture 15 cm distal to ligament of Treitz	2 cm in length	Surgical excision
Isbister, et al. [18]	16	F	Abdominal pain and vomiting	1 week	Perforation and ulcer involving the jejunum, 25 cm from duodenojejunal flexure	2.5 cm in diameter	Laparotomy with surgical resection
Jimenez, et al. [8]	4	M	Abdominal pain and melena	3 days	Large polypoid mass occupying 50% of the lumen	9×4 cm	Laparotomy with en-bloc small bowel resection
Khan, et al. [11]	36	F	Abdominal pain and vomiting	Unknown	Polypoid lesion	2 cm	Laparoscopic resection
Kimpton, et al. [12]	7	F	Episodic abdominal pain, nausea, and vomiting, and intussusception	4 years	Tumor mass filling the entire lumen of the jejunum	3 cm in diameter	Surgical resection
Lee, et al. [13]	25	M	Postprandial abdominal pain and vomiting	3 weeks	Elongated, serpiginous mucosal tumors	8×3 cm and 6×3 cm	Surgical resection
Leng, et al. [9]	9	F	Gastrointestinal bleeding with melena and mild anemia	15 months	Polypoid mass	4 cm	Laparoscopic resection
Mandrekar, et al. [14]	22	F	Intestinal obstruction	Unknown	Polypoidal mass	$8 \times 6 \times 2$ cm	Emergency laparotomy and resection
Martinez, et al. [15]	21	F	Intermittent abdominal pain, nausea, and vomiting	1 year	Large intraluminal tumor of the jejunum	15 cm	Abdominal laparotomy with resection
Nasir, et al. [5]	31	M	Postprandial abdominal pain and hematochezia	10 years	Polypoid mass at duodenojejunal junction	6×2.5 cm	Endoscopic resection
Nwanze, et al. [16]	24	F	Abdominal pain, nausea and vomiting, and intussusception	12 hours	Protruding polypoid mass of the jejunum	$3.4 \times 2.7 \times 2.4$ cm	Emergent surgical resection
Omotosho, et al. [17]	17	F	Refluxlike symptoms, abdominal pain, vomiting, and intussusception	6 months	Bilobed intraluminal jejunal polyp	Unknown	Surgical resection
Vani, et al. [2]	24	M	Abdominal pain and peritonitis	Unknown	Jejunal strictures and perforation	40 cm of jejunum with multiple strictures and serosal exudate	Emergent exploratory laparotomy and resection

tissue outside of the stomach with a prior history of Meckel's diverticulectomy and prior pathology at the time of small bowel resection without any evidence of ectopic gastric mucosa.

It is important to recognize the variety of presentations associated with gastric heterotopia. A timely diagnosis of an enlarged polyp can prevent complications such as obstruction, intussusception, bleeding, or perforation. The combination of clinical presentation, radiologic imaging, and endoscopic and pathologic evaluation is helpful in making the diagnosis [5].

In most reported cases of gastric heterotopia involving the jejunum (Table 1), patients had a median age of 21.5 years with the youngest patient being one-year-old [6]. Presenting symptoms consisted of gastrointestinal bleeding [7–9] or obstructive symptoms as a result of a polypoid mass [1, 5, 10–17] and stricture [2, 3, 6]. One case report described a 16-year-old patient who developed perforation and ulceration involving the jejunum in the setting of gastric heterotopia [18]. One case report described a 21-year-old patient with a 15 cm intraluminal polypoid mass involving the jejunum [15], while two case reports described multiple strictures associated with jejunal gastric heterotopia [2, 6]. Gastric heterotopia was not suspected clinically in any of these cases and was diagnosed on histopathological examination.

Gastric heterotopia can present in various ways including masslike lesions with symptoms of obstruction, pain, or bleeding, or may even remain asymptomatic. Gastric heterotopia beyond the ligament of Treitz is a rare entity. This case highlights the importance of considering gastric heterotopia in the differential diagnosis of polypoid lesions located beyond the ligament of Treitz in younger patients presenting with obstructive symptoms [2].

References

[1] B. Bhattacharya, S. Jakate, T. J. Saclarides, and A. Keshavarzian, "Gastric heterotopia presenting as a mass in jejunum," *Archives of Pathology & Laboratory Medicine*, vol. 127, no. 4, pp. 506-507, 2003.

[2] M. Vani, A. Nambiar, K. Geetha, and B. Kundil, "Jejunal gastric heterotopia causing multiple strictures and perforation peritonitis: a case report with review of literature," *Journal of Clinical and Diagnostic Research*, vol. 11, no. 3, pp. ED11–ED12, 2017.

[3] G. E. Chinnery, M. M. Bernon, M. A. Banderker, R. Roberts, and J. E. J. Krige, "Gastric heterotopia causing jejunal ulceration and obstruction," *South African Journal of Surgery*, vol. 51, no. 4, pp. 146-147, 2013.

[4] J. Cai and H. Yu, "Giant polypoid gastric heterotopia in the small intestine in a boy: a case report and literature review," *Medicine*, vol. 96, no. 1, Article ID e5854, 2017.

[5] A. Nasir, S. K. Amateau, S. Khan, R. W. Simpson, D. C. Snover, and K. Amin, "The many faces of intestinal tract gastric heterotopia; a series of four cases highlighting clinical and pathological heterogeneity," *Human Pathology*, vol. 74, pp. 183–187, 2018.

[6] S. Al-Jadaan and O. Oda, "A rare clinical presentation of heterotopic gastric mucosa of the jejunum: a case report and review of the literature," *Journal of Pediatric Surgery Case Reports*, vol. 2, no. 7, pp. 337–340, 2014.

[7] S. M. Ali, A. A. Ahmed, L. Saaid et al., "Heterotopic gastric mucosa presenting as lower gastrointestinal bleeding: an unusual case report," *Case Reports in Surgery*, vol. 2019, Article ID 5791984, 4 pages, 2019.

[8] J. C. Jimenez, S. Emil, B. Steinmetz, S. Romansky, and M. Weller, "Recurrent gastrointestinal tract bleeding secondary to jejunal gastric heterotopia," *Journal of Pediatric Surgery*, vol. 40, no. 10, pp. 1654–1657, 2005.

[9] S. Leng, M. Ghionzoli, C. Caporalini, and A. M. Buccoliero, "Long-term intestinal bleeding in a child: a rare case of heterotopic gastric mucosa in the jejunum," *BMJ Case Reports*, vol. 2016, 2016.

[10] K. R. Ahn, J. S. Koo, H. I. Kim et al., "Endoscopic treatment of Jejunal heterotopic gastric mucosa that caused recurrent intussusception," *Clinical Endoscopy*, vol. 50, no. 6, pp. 605–608, 2017.

[11] M. J. Khan, P. Mullerat, and A. Desai, "A polypoid gastric heterotopia of jejunum diagnosed by capsule endoscopy," *Journal of the College of Physicians and Surgeons*, vol. 19, no. 10, pp. 661-662, 2009.

[12] A. R. Kimpton and A. R. Crane, "Heterotopic gastric mucosa," *New England Journal of Medicine*, vol. 218, no. 15, pp. 627–629, 1938.

[13] S. M. Lee, W. T. Mosenthal, and R. E. Weismann, "Tumorous heterotopic gastric mucosa in the small intestine," *Archives of Surgery*, vol. 100, no. 5, pp. 619–622, 1970.

[14] S. R. Mandrekar, A. Sangeeta, N. Sanjyot, and R. G. Pinto, "Giant polypoid gastric heterotopia of jejunum," *Medical Journal of Dr. D. Y. Patil University*, vol. 9, no. 5, pp. 645–647, 2016.

[15] A. Martínez, O. Decanini-Terán, and D. Soria-Céspedes, "Polypoid and hyperplastic heterotopic gastric mucosa in the jejunum as a cause of recurrent subocclusive episodes," *Annals of Gastroenterology*, vol. 26, no. 2, p. 184, 2013.

[16] J. Nwanze, V. Collins, B. Crawford, and Y. Nakanishi, "A case of small bowel intussusception in an adult caused by heterotopic gastric mucosa in the Jejunum: a case report and review of the literature," *American Journal of Clinical Pathology*, vol. 150, no. 1, p. S43, 2018.

[17] P. A. Omotosho, H. Varnholt, M. V. Tirabassi, R. Prasad, and K. P. Moriarty, "Giant polypoid gastric heterotopia of the jejunum presenting with intermittent intussusception," *Journal of Laparoendoscopic & Advanced Surgical Techniques*, vol. 17, no. 2, pp. 249–251, 2007.

[18] W. H. Isbister and D. Weedon, "Perforated jejunal ulcer and heterotopic gastric mucosa," *British Journal of Surgery*, vol. 63, no. 12, pp. 954-955, 1976.

40

Ocrelizumab-Induced Severe Colitis

Hsing Hwa Lee,[1] **Naveen Sritharan**,[1] **Daniel Bermingham**,[2] **and Gabriela Strey**[1]

[1]*Department of Medicine, Hervey Bay Hospital, Pialba, Queensland, Australia*
[2]*Department of Pharmacy, Hervey Bay Hospital, Pialba, Queensland, Australia*

Correspondence should be addressed to Hsing Hwa Lee; leehsinghwa@gmail.com

Academic Editor: Matteo Neri

We report a case of severe ocrelizumab (anti-CD20 monoclonal antibody) induced colitis in a 43-year-old woman with multiple sclerosis leading to total colectomy after failing medical therapy. Histology of the colectomy was consistent with medication-induced colitis.

1. Introduction

Ocrelizumab is a humanized monoclonal antibody that binds to the CD20 antigen on B lymphocytes and has been approved for the treatment of primary progressive multiple sclerosis (PPMS) and relapsing multiple sclerosis (RMS) in adults [1]. Ocrelizumab-induced colitis has been reported to occur within a few weeks of initiation of therapy. In this case, severe colitis involving a significant portion of the colon and requiring total colectomy occurred after only two doses of ocrelizumab.

2. Case Report/Case Presentation

A 43-year-old Caucasian female presented with multiple episodes of loose, watery, dark stools. Her presentation was associated with gradual onset, colicky, lower abdominal pain since the previous day. She otherwise denied any fever, nausea, or vomiting, history of ill contact, or any history of travelling or taking outside food. No one within her household had similar symptoms.

The patient had been diagnosed several years earlier with multiple sclerosis (MS) and is wheel-chair-bound due to that disease. She had been prescribed alemtuzumab in a clinical trial 10 years preceding this presentation and had used teriflunomide for one year prior to being prescribed ocrelizumab by her neurologist—she had received two doses six months apart. She denied any prior history of inflammatory bowel disease or bowel cancer.

Upon examination, it was noted that she was afebrile and was haemodynamically stable. Examination of the abdomen revealed a soft abdomen with tenderness at the suprapubic and iliac regions with increased bowel sounds but no evidence of peritonism or organomegaly. Digital per rectal examination established an empty rectum.

The patient was ordered a range of initial laboratory and imaging investigations and follow-up diagnostics based on those findings (Tables 1 and 2). The abdominal X-ray (Figure 1) demonstrated a classical thumbprinting sign that was nonspecific but suspicious for clostridium difficile infection. Empirical antibiotics IV metronidazole and oral vancomycin were commenced for presumed clostridium difficile infection while awaiting for laboratory tests and histology results.

The patient's venous blood gas showed lactate of 4 mmol/L (normal range, 0.6–1.8 mmol/L) which prompted a CT abdomen. The CT demonstrated a pronounced colitis extending from the transverse colon to the sigmoid colon. When the patient did not respond to IV metronidazole and oral vancomycin, a flexible sigmoidoscopy was undertaken and showed nodular mucosa with white-yellowish adherent plaques with increasing severity from the rectosigmoid to the sigmoid (Figures 2 and 3). The histology from biopsies taken from various parts of the left colon was negative for cytomegalovirus (CMV) and clostridium difficile infection, but suggestive of biological medication effect.

Accordingly, the patient was treated as ocrelizumab-induced colitis and commenced on intravenous

Table 1: Laboratory results.

Laboratory tests	Patient's sample	Normal values
Haemoglobin	172	115–160 g/L
White blood cells	15.2	4.00–11.0 × 10^9/L
Platelets	160	140–400 × 10^9/L
C-reactive protein (CRP)	187	<5.0 mg/L
Lipase	25	<60 U/L
Albumin	40	35–80 g/L
Lactate	4.0	0.6–1.8 mmol/L
Faecal calprotectin	3200	<50 μg/g
Stool culture	Normal colonic bacterial flora	
Clostridium difficile toxins	Negative	

Table 2: Imaging and procedural results.

Imaging and procedures	Relevant findings
X-ray abdomen	Dilated large bowels with thumbprinting sign
CT abdomen	Pronounced colitis primarily involving the transverse colon, splenic flexure, and descending colon of the large bowel extending to involve the sigmoid colon
Flexible sigmoidoscopy	Decreased mucosa vascular pattern in the sigmoid colon Nodular mucosa in the rectosigmoid colon and in the sigmoid colon Congested, erythematous, inflamed, and vascular pattern decreased mucosa in the rectum. Histology showed features of biological medication effect.
Laparoscopy converted to open total colectomy	Widespread inflammatory adhesions with contact bleeding. Attempted laparoscopic resection converted to open total colectomy due to disintegrating fulminant colitis of left colon and sigmoid colon falling to pieces on retraction, contact bleeding, and massive distension of large bowel. Frank pus from rectum during insertion of rectal catheter at the end of the case.
Histology of total colectomy	Mucosa in proximal colon appears normal. The rest of the colonic mucosa is completely ulcerated without residual islands of intact mucosa. There is congestion, chronic inflammation, and submucosal fibrosis. The ulceration is mostly superficial but does extend focally to the muscularis propria. Focal areas of subserosal fibrosis are noted. The pathology features are compatible with the clinical diagnosis of medication induced colitis.

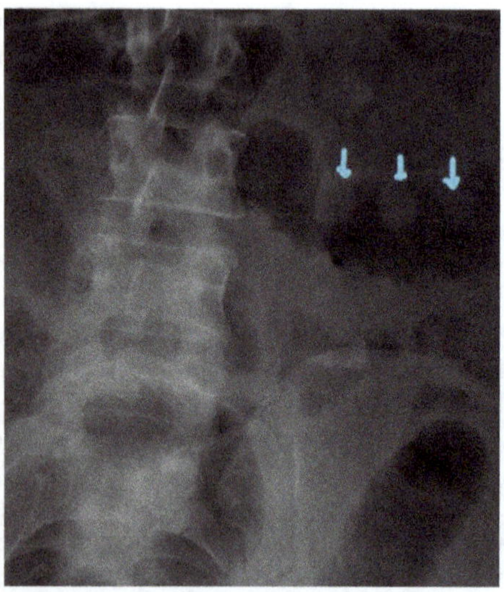

Figure 1: Abdomen X-ray showing thumbprinting sign.

hydrocortisone. Her CRP was downtrending on hydrocortisone. However, serial abdominal X-rays demonstrated ongoing gaseous distension, and she continued having watery bowel motions. The patient was referred to a tertiary hospital and colorectal surgeons for medication-resistant

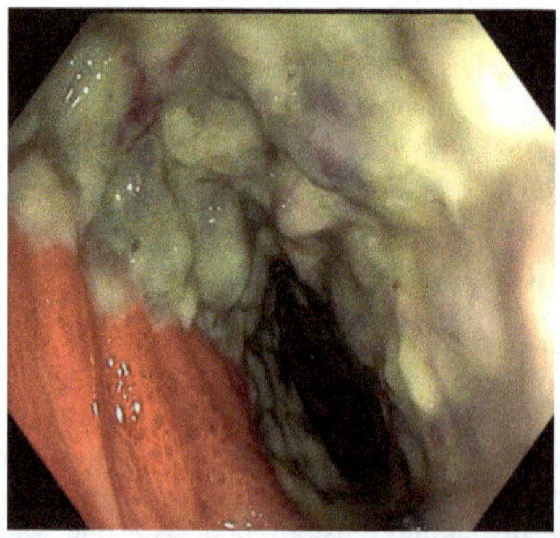

Figure 2: Distal sigmoid colon showing severe colitis.

biological medication-induced colitis. She subsequently underwent a total colectomy and ileostomy formation.

3. Discussion/Conclusion

We surmise that the most likely cause of colitis in this instance is ocrelizumab, as evidenced by both the clinical history and histopathological reports. Drug-induced colitis is a relatively new clinically recognized phenomenon with diagnosis increasing in alignment to the expansion of

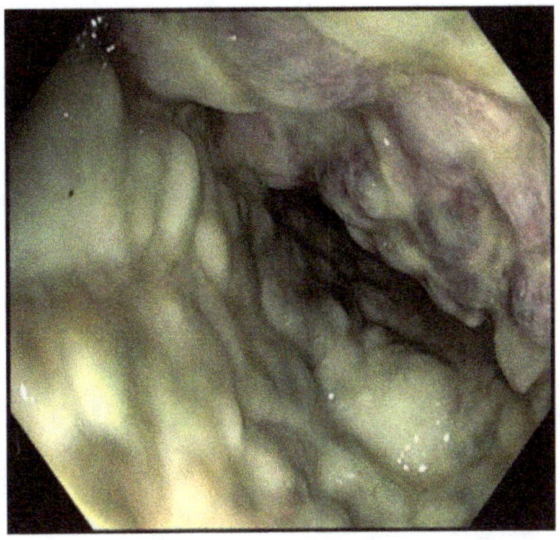

Figure 3: Midsigmoid colon showing extension of the severe colitis to the midsigmoid region.

medications and novel therapy. However, to date, we are aware of two other cases of de novo colitis associated with ocrelizumab, with one of them requiring surgical resection [2, 3].

Ocrelizumab is a humanized monoclonal antibody that binds to the CD20 antigen on B-lymphocytes and has been approved for the treatment of primary progressive multiple sclerosis (PPMS) and relapsing multiple sclerosis (RMS) in adults [1]. Ocrelizumab-induced colitis has been reported to occur within a few weeks of initiation of therapy. In this case, severe colitis involving a significant portion of the colon and requiring total colectomy occurred after only two doses of ocrelizumab. This may indicate either a cumulative effect from ocrelizumab or a delayed presentation of worsening colitis from commencement of the medication. Rituximab, which is also a humanized anti-CD20 monoclonal antibody, has been reported to be associated with colitis. However, fulminant colitis is extremely rare [4].

Ocrelizumab is likely to play a role in the development of autoimmunity resulting in severe pancolitis as described in our case. The exact mechanism of anti-CD20-induced colitis is not known, nor is the pathogenesis of ocrelizumab-induced colitis. Since ocrelizumab depletes B cells, there could be an association between colitis with the dysregulation of the gastrointestinal immune system via B-cell depletion. B cells play a vital role in the mucosal immune system by producing secretory antibodies IgA and IgM which protects the mucosal barrier [5]. B-cells also produce IL-10 which is an anti-inflammatory and has been linked to inhibit Th1-derived responses. Animal studies have shown that mice with depleted B-cells and IL-10 have severe colitis likely mediated by Th1 response profile [6]. Ocrelizumab-suppressed B-cell levels have been shown to return to pre-treatment levels at a median of 72 (27–175) weeks [7]. Therefore, the inflammatory process with T-cell dysfunction may occur and persist for up to a year. Ocrelizumab could potentially predispose patients to develop autoimmunity by causing immune dysregulation. This process might continue in the background until another immunological trigger or disruption which leads to the development of autoimmune process.

Risk factors for ocrelizumab-induced colitis remain unclear. Several cumulative risk factors may have exponentiated the presentation in this particular case. This patient had previously received teriflunomide and alemtuzumab which may have altered her immune system which concomitantly could have been affected by an already proinflammatory state of multiple sclerosis. This is consistent with literature [2, 3] describing other cases where patients received ocrelizumab after failing first-line therapy. Whether this increased risk is due to a severe refractory disease state or simply the alteration of the immune system from multiple agents remains unknown.

Treatment of ocrelizumab-induced colitis is challenging as this is extremely rare, and hence, therapeutic options are limited. Immunosuppressants such glucocorticoids were only effective in one case report but not effective in two others, including our case, and surgical intervention was needed for definitive management as a life-saving procedure [2, 3]. More studies need to be done to explore other medical therapies such as other immunosuppresants or immunomodulators which could be another option. It is unclear what the best therapeutic options are due to the novelty of this condition. However, medical management and the least invasive management will likely produce the best outcome.

In conclusion, colitis may be a potential risk with administration of ocrelizumab. Research is required to identify patients at risk and devise strategies to monitor patients who could potentially develop complications from ocrelizumab.

Authors' Contributions

Hsing Hwa Lee and Naveen Sritharan were responsible for compiling case report details, manuscript preparation, and literature search. Daniel Bermingham contributed to medication review and literature search. Gabriela Strey contributed to supervision and manuscript preparation.

Acknowledgments

The case study was performed under the guidance of the Wide Bay Hospital and Health Service with specific funding support for publication. The authors thank all medical teams and staff involved in the care of this patient and Angela Ratsch for your helpful comments on the preparation of the manuscript.

References

[1] P. Mulero, L. Midaglia, and X. Montalban, "Ocrelizumab: a new milestone in multiple sclerosis therapy," *Therapeutic Advances in Neurological Disorders*, vol. 11, 2018.

[2] D. B. Sunjaya, C. Taborda, R. Obeng, and T. Dhere, "First case of refractory colitis caused by ocrelizumab," *Inflammatory Bowel Diseases*, vol. 26, no. 6, p. e49, 2020.

[3] A. Akram, M. Valasek, and D. Patel, "P096 De novo colitis after ocrelizumab therapy," *Inflammatory Bowel Diseases*, vol. 26, no. 1, 2020.

[4] H. J. Freeman, "Colitis associated with biological agents," *World Journal of Gastroenterology*, vol. 18, no. 16, pp. 1871–1874, 2012.
[5] P. Brandtzaeg, H. S. Carlsen, and T. S. Halstensen, "The B-cell system in inflammatory bowel disease," *Immune Mechanisms in Inflammatory Bowel Disease*, vol. 579, pp. 149–167, 2006.
[6] N. J. Davidson, M. W. Leach, M. M. Fort et al., "T helper cell 1-type CD4+ T cells, but not B cells, mediate colitis in interleukin 10-deficient mice," *Journal of Experimental Medicine*, vol. 184, no. 1, pp. 241–251, 1996.
[7] A. L. Greenfield and S. L. Hauser, "B-cell therapy for multiple sclerosis: entering an era," *Annals of Neurology*, vol. 83, no. 1, pp. 13–26, 2018.

Recurrent Unprovoked Venous Thrombosis (Cerebral Sinus Thrombosis and Mesenteric Vein Thrombosis) in Young Patient with Crohn's Disease: A Case Report and Review

Abdullah Mohammed Albishi,[1] **Rafaat Chakik,**[1] **and Ali Saleh Alshamrani**[2]

[1]*Gastroenterology and Endoscopy Department, Armed Forces Hospital Southern Region, Khamis Mushayt, Saudi Arabia*
[2]*Internal Medicine Department, Armed Forces Hospital Southern Region, Khamis Mushayt, Saudi Arabia*

Correspondence should be addressed to Abdullah Mohammed Albishi; dr.abdullah6975@gmail.com

Academic Editor: Hirotada Akiho

Inflammatory bowel disease (IBD) patients have a higher risk of thrombosis. Most data about thrombosis in inflammatory bowel disease are related mainly to inpatients with disease activity, but in this article, we report one case of inflammatory bowel disease with two different sites of venous thrombosis which happened in a patient with nonactive IBD at an outpatient setting.

1. Introduction

Thrombosis in IBD is associated with a high mortality rate and directly impacts the quality of life of individuals. The literature shows that patients with ulcerative colitis and Crohn's disease have an increased risk of thrombosis, three- to fourfold higher than subjects without inflammatory bowel disease [1].

Deep venous thrombosis of the lower and upper limbs and pulmonary embolism are the most common locations of venous thromboembolism in IBD patients, but unusual sites of thrombosis, including the cerebrovascular, mesenteric, portal, or retinal veins, have also been described [2].

Here we report one case of inflammatory bowel disease with recurrent unprovoked venous thrombosis at two different rare sites which happened in a nonactive patient at an outpatient setting.

2. Case Report

A 42-year-old Saudi male patient was diagnosed as colonic inflammatory Crohn's disease 10 years ago on azathioprine. The patient presented to the emergency room (ER) complaining of headache for 2 days which started suddenly and was progressive, generalized, moderate to severe, and not relieved by analgesics. The patient had no history of seizures or decreased level of consciousness, no history of trauma or blurred vision, and no history of weakness, vomiting, fever, and neck pain. He had history of mild headache attacks, but this time it was more severe.

The patient had no history of abdominal pain, diarrhea, skin rash, joint pain, and jaundice. He was taking his medications regularly. He had no history of smoking or using of any NSAIDs and no significant family history. His Crohn's disease activity index (CDAI) was 97.

Regarding Crohn's disease, the patient was diagnosed 10 years ago as inflammatory, nonstricturing, nonfistulazing colonic Crohn's disease without perianal disease when he presented with chronic abdominal pain, chronic diarrhea, and weight loss for more than 3 years before the time of diagnosis. Colonoscopy at the time of diagnosis showed few aphthous colonic ulcers with normal terminal ileum. Colonic biopsy showed chronic colitis. CT enterography was done and showed normal small bowel. The patient was started on steroid therapy for a short period with azathioprine 150 mg orally daily as a maintenance therapy.

Since the time of diagnosis, the patient was following the gastroenterology clinic regularly. He was doing well with no abdominal pain or more diarrhea. He gained weight more than 10 kg within a 4-month period. His routine laboratory investigations were extracted and reviewed which confirm remission of disease clinically and biochemically. The patient was planned for colonoscopy to assess the mucosal and histological remission.

2.1. Examination Results. The patient was conscious and oriented to time, place, and person. He was not pale or jaundiced , with normal fundoscopy and normal vital signs and afebrile.

The chest and cardiovascular system were normal.

The abdomen was soft and lax with no tenderness and no organomegaly.

His central nervous system showed normal cranial nerves and motor and sensory and coordination.

No perianal fistula or fissure was seen in the perianal area.

2.2. Laboratory Results. CBC, liver function tests, and renal profiles were normal, CRP was 24, and ECG was normal.

At the ER, CT brain was done and was reported as no acute infarction or bleeding or space-occupying lesions.

MRI and MRV brain showed no flow within the left transverse and sigmoid sinuses and also no flow within the left internal jugular vein as shown in Figure 1.

The patient was diagnosed as cerebral sinus thrombosis, and workup for thrombosis was requested, and the patient started on therapeutic enoxaparin and then on warfarin 5 mg orally daily with target INR 2-3.

ANA, dsDNA, anticardiolipin, lupus anticoagulant, B2 glycoprotein, and JAK2 mutation were all negative. Protein C, protein S, antithrombin III, and peripheral blood smear were all normal.

The patient was following the gastroenterology clinic for 3 years every 6 months and anticoagulation clinic for warfarin adjustment dose.

He was doing well during this period taking azathioprine 150 daily and warfarin 5 mg per day. He was totally asymptomatic. His investigations during the clinic follow-up showed normal CBC, liver function tests, and renal profiles, CRP was 12, and calprotectin was 39. Follow-up MRI and MRV brain which were done after 3 years from the cerebral sinus thrombosis showed no more thrombosis.

The patient was seen by a neurologist, and hematology consultation was requested regarding the possibility of stopping anticoagulant. They labeled him as unprovoked thrombosis with normal thrombosis workup, so anticoagulant was stopped as the multidisciplinary team plan.

Colonoscopy was done to assess the remission and showed mild patchy erythema at the descending and transverse colon, no ulcers or strictures, and normal terminal ileum as shown in Figure 2.

After 1 year from stopping anticoagulation, the patient presented again to the ER complaining of abdominal pain for 1 day, which was severe mainly in the epigastrium, sudden onset, associated with vomiting and loose stool, no blood in stool or fever or jaundice, and no urinary symptoms. He was only on azathiopine 150 mg. His CDAI was 149.

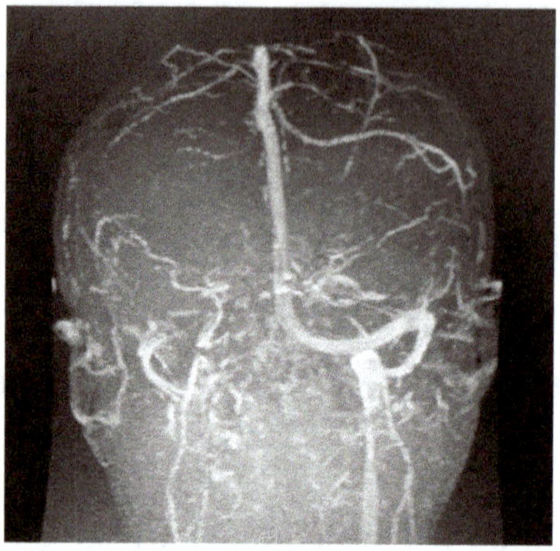

Figure 1: MRI and MRV brain showing no flow within the left transverse and sigmoid sinuses and also no flow within the left internal jugular vein.

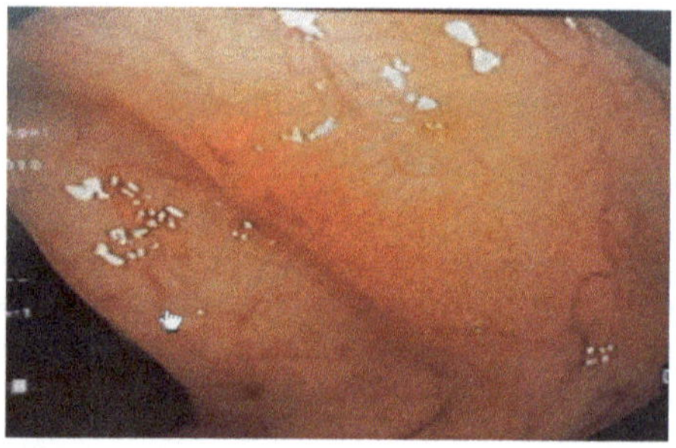

Figure 2: Colonoscopy showed mild patchy erythema at the descending and transverse colon, no ulcers or strictures, and normal terminal ileum.

2.3. Examination Results. The patient was fully conscious, oriented, and in severe pain.

Vital signs were stable apart from mild tachycardia and afebrile. O_2 saturation was 95%.

His abdomen showed moderate tenderness at the epigastrium, no rebound, and no ascites.

His perianal area showed no perianal fistula and was negative for blood or melena.

2.4. Laboratory Results. CBC, liver function tests, and renal profile were normal. Blood gases and lactate level were normal. ECG and cardiac enzymes were normal.

CT abdomen with IV contrast showed mesenteric vein thrombosis and thickening of the small bowel with skipped lesions as shown in Figure 3.

The patient was admitted under the surgery team, and he underwent diagnostic laparotomy because the pain was not relieved by analgesia. No ischemia was found. The patient was discharged on warfarin indefinitely, and he was started on adalimumab.

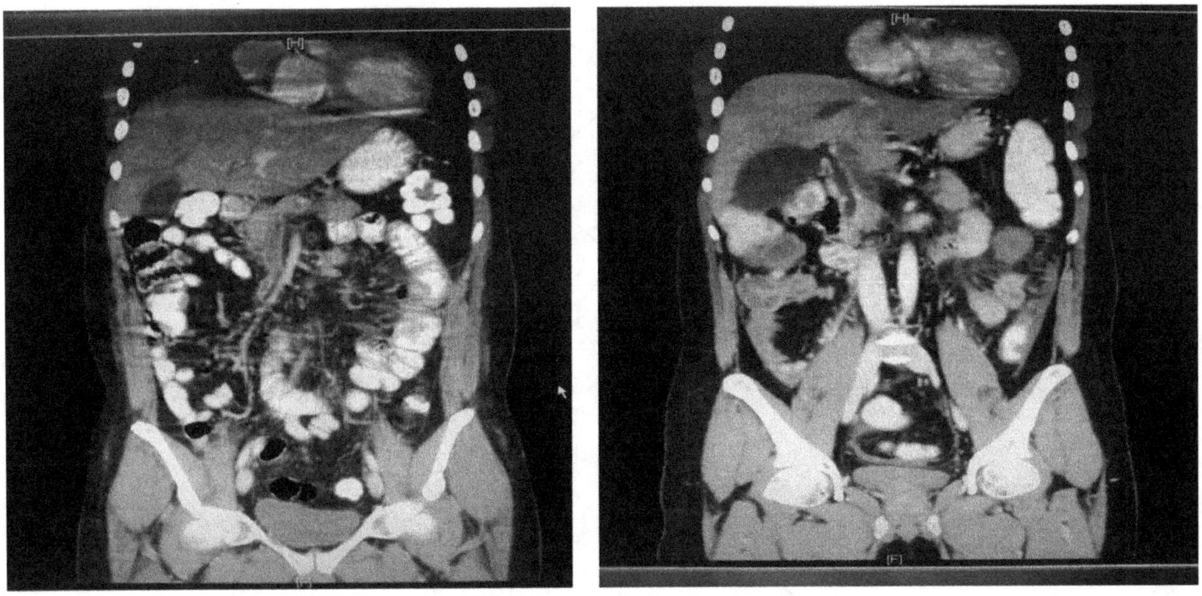

(a) (b)

FIGURE 3: CT abdomen with IV contrast showing mesenteric vein thrombosis and thickening of the small bowel with skipped lesions.

During clinic follow-up, he was doing well, taking azathioprine 150 daily and adalimumab 40 mg subcutaneously every 2 weeks and warfarin 5 mg per day. He was totally asymptomatic. Investigations during clinic follow-up showed normal CBC, liver function tests, and renal profiles, CRP was 6, and calprotectin was 27.

The patient was instructed to continue the same medications with regular follow-up in the clinic.

3. Discussion

Inflammatory bowel diseases (IBD) patients are at high risk of venous thromboembolism (VTE) as a result of the hypercoagulable state induced by chronic inflammation of the bowel [3]. Ongoing active inflammation in IBD itself appears to be a significant factor determining the VTE risk [4].

The most important risk factors for VTE in IBD are active disease, hospitalization, colonic disease, and recent surgery [5]. Around 80% of IBD patients had active disease at the time of VTE diagnosis, which was found in a study done by Dr. Craig A. Solem. Regarding the disease extension in IBD patients with VTE, 79% of Crohn's disease patients had colonic involvement, and 76% of the ulcerative colitis patients had pancolitis as seen in that study [6].

Acute and chronic episodes of intestinal inflammation lead to the elaboration of inflammatory cytokines and the development of a systemic prothrombotic state, manifested by thrombocytosis, upregulation of tissue factor and impaired fibrinolysis caused by decreased expression of tissue plasminogen activator (t-PA) and increased expression of PAI-1. The recurrent use of corticosteroids for IBD flare may exacerbate the prothrombotic state, leading to further impairment of fibrinolysis as shown in Figure 4 [7].

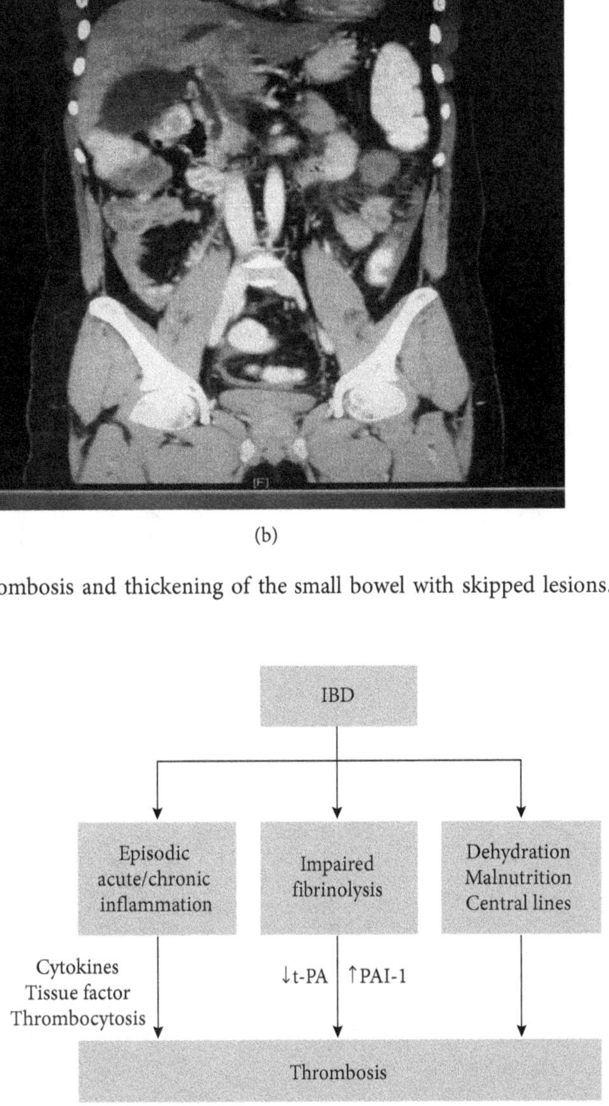

FIGURE 4: Mechanisms of thrombosis in IBD patients [7].

VTE inherited risk factors occur with a similar frequency in IBD patients and the general population [5].

The VTE overall incidence in IBD patients is estimated to be 1%–8%. IBD patients with VTE episode were generally younger and also associated with a higher risk of recurrence [8].

VTE episode in IBD patients is associated with longer hospitalization and high mortality. Half of the recurrent VTE in IBD happens in patients with active disease at recurrence [5].

Most data about VTE episode in IBD refer to hospitalized active patients. The Canadian Consensus recommends thromboprophylaxis with heparin for hospitalized active IBD flare patients without active non-severe bleeding. For outpatients, thromboprophylaxis is recommended

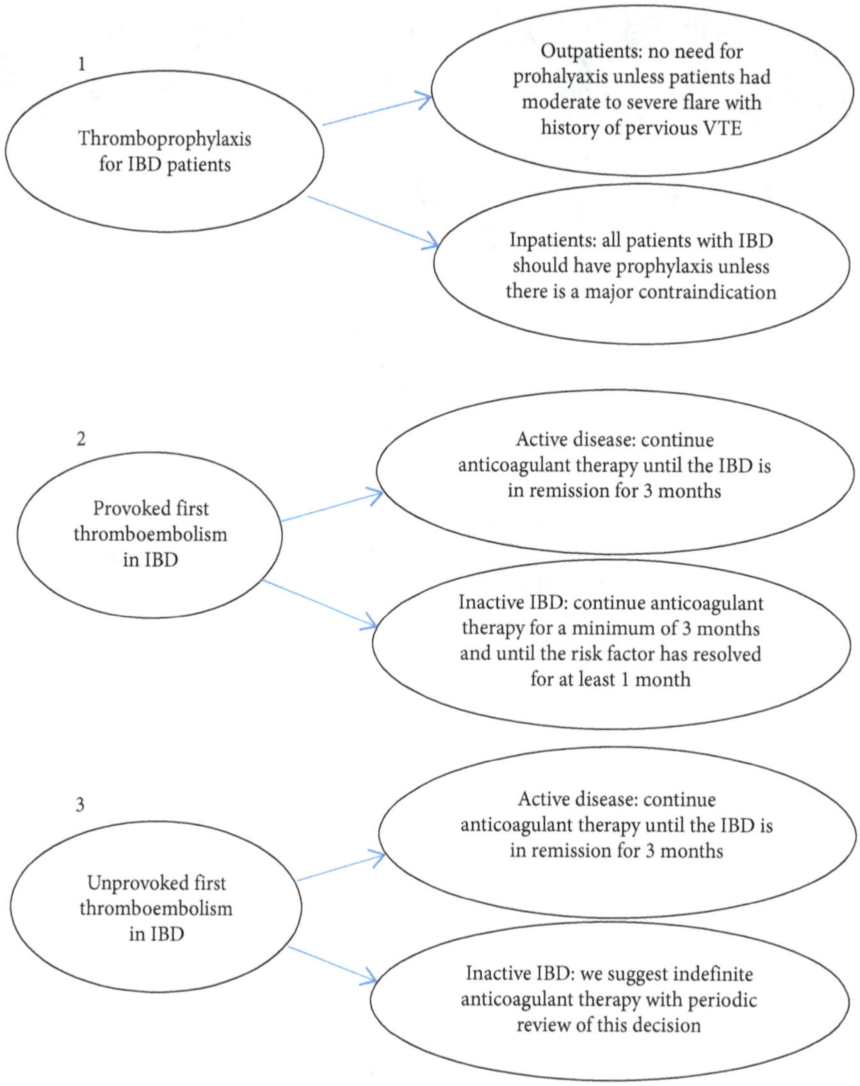

FIGURE 5: Summary of recommendations of the Canadian Association of Gastroenterology [14].

during moderate to severe IBD flares with an unprovoked previous VTE event [2].

There is no evidence for thromboprophylaxis in active IBD patients as outpatients, but the ECCO guidelines recommend that prophylaxis in IBD patients should be considered following discharge from hospital and after recent surgery and in outpatients with active disease [5].

Cerebral sinus thrombosis is rare in IBD patients. Cerebral venous thrombosis is more common in UC than in Crohn's disease [9]. The most common sign is headache, which gradually increases over a period of days or can be sudden severe headache which can mimic subarachnoid hemorrhage [10]. In IBD patients complicated by cerebral venous thrombosis, favorable outcomes are possible with early diagnosis and appropriate treatment; otherwise, the mortality rate can be as high as 50% if not treated [11].

Mesenteric vein thrombosis in IBD patients is difficult to be diagnosed which may delay the diagnosis and initiation of treatment as IBD patients frequently present with nonspecific abdominal discomfort [12].

The current practice in treatment of IBD patients with venous thromboembolism is the same as for non-IBD patients. In the acute setting, anticoagulation with low-molecular-weight heparin or unfractionated heparin is recommended, with transition to oral anticoagulation [13].

For patients with IBD at clinical remission who present with provoked venous thromboembolism other than IBD, the duration of anticoagulant therapy is a minimum of 3 months, with continuing therapy until 1 month once the risk factor has been resolved. For IBD patients at clinical remission with unprovoked venous thromboembolism, indefinite anticoagulant therapy is recommended [14]. Recommendations from the Canadian Association of Gastroenterology are summarized in Figure 5 [14].

4. Conclusion

Thrombosis either provoked or unprovoked is more reported for patients with IBD.VTE in IBD patients can occur anywhere in the body. High index of suspicion is needed for early diagnosis and appropriate treatment; otherwise, the mortality rate will be high. Management IBD patients at clinical remission with unprovoked thrombosis needs more clarifications.

References

[1] A. R. Andrade, L. L. Barros, M. F. C. Azevedo et al., "Risk of thrombosis and mortality in inflammatory bowel disease," *Clinical and Translational Gastroenterology*, vol. 9, no. 4, Article ID e142, 2018.

[2] G. Novacek, A. Weltermann, A. Sobala et al., "Inflammatory bowel disease is a risk factor for recurrent venous thromboembolism," *Gastroenterology*, vol. 139, no. 3, pp. 779.e1–787.e1, 2010.

[3] Z. Arora, X. Wu, U. Navaneethan, and B. Shen, "Non-surgical porto-mesenteric vein thrombosis is associated with worse long-term outcomes in inflammatory bowel diseases," *Gastroenterology Report*, vol. 4, no. 3, pp. 210–215, 2016.

[4] E. A. Scoville, G. G. Konijeti, D. D. Nguyen, J. Sauk, V. Yajnik, and A. N. Ananthakrishnan, "Venous thromboembolism in patients with inflammatory bowel diseases," *Inflammatory Bowel Diseases*, vol. 20, no. 4, pp. 631–636, 2014.

[5] M. Harbord, V. Annese, S. R. Vavricka et al., "The first European evidence-based consensus on extra-intestinal manifestations in inflammatory bowel disease," *Journal of Crohn's and Colitis*, vol. 10, no. 3, pp. 239–254, 2016.

[6] P. Zezos, G. Kouklakis, and F. Saibil, "Inflammatory bowel disease and thromboembolism," *World Journal of Gastroenterology*, vol. 20, no. 38, pp. 13863–13878, 2014.

[7] S. R. Lentz, "Thrombosis in the setting of obesity or inflammatory bowel disease," *Hematology*, vol. 2016, no. 1, pp. 180–187, 2016.

[8] M. Giannotta, G. Tapete, G. Emmi, E. Silvestri, and M. Milla, "Thrombosis in inflammatory bowel diseases: what's the link?" *Thrombosis Journal*, vol. 13, no. 1, pp. 1–9, 2015.

[9] F. Meloni, American Journal Experts, 2016.

[10] R. J. Nudelman, D. G. Rosen, E. Rouah, and G. Verstovsek, "Cerebral sinus thrombosis: a fatal neurological complication of ulcerative colitis," *Pathology Research International*, vol. 2010, Article ID 132754, 6 pages, 2010.

[11] Y.-H. Cho, M. K. Chae, J. M. Cha et al., "Cerebral venous thrombosis in a patient with Crohn's disease," *Intestinal Research*, vol. 14, no. 1, pp. 96–101, 2016.

[12] O. A. Hatoum, K. S. Spinelli, M. Abu-Hajir et al., "Mesenteric venous thrombosis in inflammatory bowel disease," *Journal of Clinical Gastroenterology*, vol. 39, no. 1, pp. 27–31, 2005.

[13] I. Y. Goh, S. Saric, P. Leschke, M. McFarlane, and P. K. Jha, "Thromboembolism in active ulcerative colitis," *BMJ Case Reports*, vol. 2017, Article ID bcr-2016-218608, 2017.

[14] G. C. Nguyen, C. N. Bernstein, A. Bitton et al., "Consensus statements on the risk, prevention, and treatment of venous thromboembolism in inflammatory bowel disease: Canadian association of gastroenterology," *Gastroenterology*, vol. 146, no. 3, pp. 835–848, 2014.

42

Antegrade Therapy for Management of Choledocholithiasis through Endoscopic Ultrasound-Guided Hepaticogastrostomy in a Patient with Surgically Altered Gastrointestinal Anatomy

Robert Dorrell,[1] Katelyn Madigan,[1] Swati Pawa,[2] and Rishi Pawa[2]

[1]*Department of Medicine, Wake Forest School of Medicine, Winston-Salem, USA*
[2]*Department of Medicine, Section on Gastroenterology, Wake Forest School of Medicine, Winston-Salem, USA*

Correspondence should be addressed to Rishi Pawa; rpawa@wakehealth.edu

Academic Editor: Matteo Neri

Endoscopic ultrasound-guided hepaticogastrostomy (EUS-HG) is a technique used to access the biliary tree in patients with surgically altered anatomy. Additionally, development of EUS-HG fistula permits intraductal therapy, thereby preventing patients from requiring surgery or percutaneous transhepatic biliary drainage (PTBD), thus decreasing morbidity. This clinical vignette describes an 83-year-old man with a history of gangrenous cholecystitis requiring cholecystectomy, partial gastrectomy, and Roux-en-Y gastrojejunostomy who presented to an outside hospital with abdominal pain and fever and found to have cholangitis and choledocholithiasis. He underwent two endoscopic retrograde cholangiopancreatography (ERCP) procedures at an outside hospital which were unsuccessful due to an inaccessible major papilla in the setting of the patient's surgically altered anatomy. On arrival to Wake Forest, the patient underwent EUS-HG with successful biliary drainage and resolution of cholangitis. He returned for ERCP three months later with balloon sphincteroplasty, cholangioscopy, and electrohydraulic lithotripsy (EHL) performed through the existing metal stent (hepaticogastrostomy), resulting in stone fragmentation and antegrade removal with balloon sweeps. Repeat cholangioscopy post-EHL and balloon sweeps showed complete duct clearance with no residual stones. The hepaticogastrostomy stent was subsequently removed, and the patient recovered without any complications.

1. Introduction

Endoscopic retrograde cholangiography (ERCP) is the cornerstone of accessing the biliary tree in patients requiring biliary drainage [1]. However, it is not feasible in all patients, such as those with surgically altered gastrointestinal anatomy (SAGA). Traditionally, patients with SAGA and acute biliary disease have either required invasive surgical techniques to reach the biliary tree or more often percutaneous transhepatic biliary drainage (PTBD), resulting in significant patient morbidity. Advances in the field of endoscopy have allowed for the development of novel techniques like endoscopic ultrasound-guided hepaticogastrostomy (EUS-HG), which provides patients with a safer and less-invasive option. EUS-HG involves the creation of a fistula between the stomach and the hepatic duct to access the biliary tree [2]. Through this gastrohepatic tract, ERCP can be performed for the diagnosis and management of biliary pathology [3]. This clinical vignette describes a patient with SAGA and subsequent successful treatment of choledocholithiasis and cholangitis via EUS-HG, cholangioscopy with electrohydraulic lithotripsy (EHL), and antegrade clearance of bile duct stones into the duodenum.

2. Case Description

An 83-year-old man with a history of gangrenous cholecystitis requiring cholecystectomy, partial gastrectomy, and Roux-en-Y gastrojejunostomy presented to an outside hospital with severe sepsis and recurrent unstable monomorphic ventricular tachycardia (requiring synchronized cardioversion) secondary to non-ST segment elevation myocardial infarction (NSTEMI). On examination, he was febrile (102.4°F) and hypotensive (systolic blood pressure of 85 mmHg), with generalized abdominal pain, nausea, and vomiting. Labs were notable for troponin, 1.31 ng/mL; total bilirubin, 4.0 mg/dL; aspartate aminotransferase (AST), 157 U/L; and alanine aminotransferase (ALT), 122 U/L. He was intubated and started on vasopressors. The following day, he was taken emergently to the cardiac catheterization lab during which a drug-eluting stent was placed for a coronary occlusion, and the patient was started on dual antiplatelet therapy. Following stabilization of the patient, a magnetic resonance cholangiopancreatography (MRCP) was obtained due to concerns for cholangitis, which demonstrated two large obstructing stones in the common bile duct (larger stone measuring 25 mm in diameter). He was formally diagnosed with severe acute cholangitis, grade 3, according to the Tokyo Guidelines [4]. He then underwent two unsuccessful ERCPs at an outside hospital (due to an inaccessible major papilla in the setting of SAGA) complicated by an additional cardiac arrest requiring life vest placement. On arrival to Wake Forest, he was noted to be febrile (102°F) and hemodynamically stable. After discussion with the patient and family regarding therapeutic options for choledocholithiasis and cholangitis including PTBD or EUS-HG, the patient elected to proceed with EUS-HG due to less morbidity and patient preference to avoid percutaneous drains. Given the patient's recent NSTEMI, cardiology was consulted and recommended holding dual antiplatelet therapy for no more than 3 days prior to the procedure to minimize the risk of stent thrombosis with immediate resolution 6 hours after procedure.

Upper GI endoscopy revealed a gastric pouch with a patent Roux-en-Y gastrojejunostomy anastomosis (Figure 1). EUS was then performed using a linear echoendoscope (GF-UCT140-AL5; Olympus Medical Systems, Tokyo, Japan) connected to an ultrasound processor (Aloka Prosound Alpha 10; Hitachi, Tokyo, Japan). With the scope positioned in the gastric pouch, a dilated segment 3 branch was identified in the left lobe of the liver (Figure 2). The biliary radicle was punctured with a 19-gauge fine needle aspiration (FNA) needle (EchoTip Ultra HD, Cook Medical, Winston-Salem, NC). Following aspiration of the bile, contrast was injected through the needle for cholangiography. Cholangiogram showed diffuse intrahepatic ductal dilation and a dilated common bile duct measuring 18 mm in diameter with two large filling defects consistent with stones (Figure 3). A 0.025 inch in diameter and 450 cm in length straight tip VisiGlide 2 guidewire (Olympus, Tokyo, Japan) was then advanced through the needle into the biliary tree and past the major papilla into the duodenum. The hepaticogastrostomy tract was subsequently dilated using a 4 mm × 4 cm Hurricane biliary dilation balloon (Boston Scientific, Marlborough, MA, USA) (Figure 4). An 8 mm × 80 mm GORE VIABIL biliary stent (W. L. Gore Associates, Flagstaff, AZ) was placed in the left hepatic duct with the distal end in the gastric pouch. The metal stent was anchored by a plastic

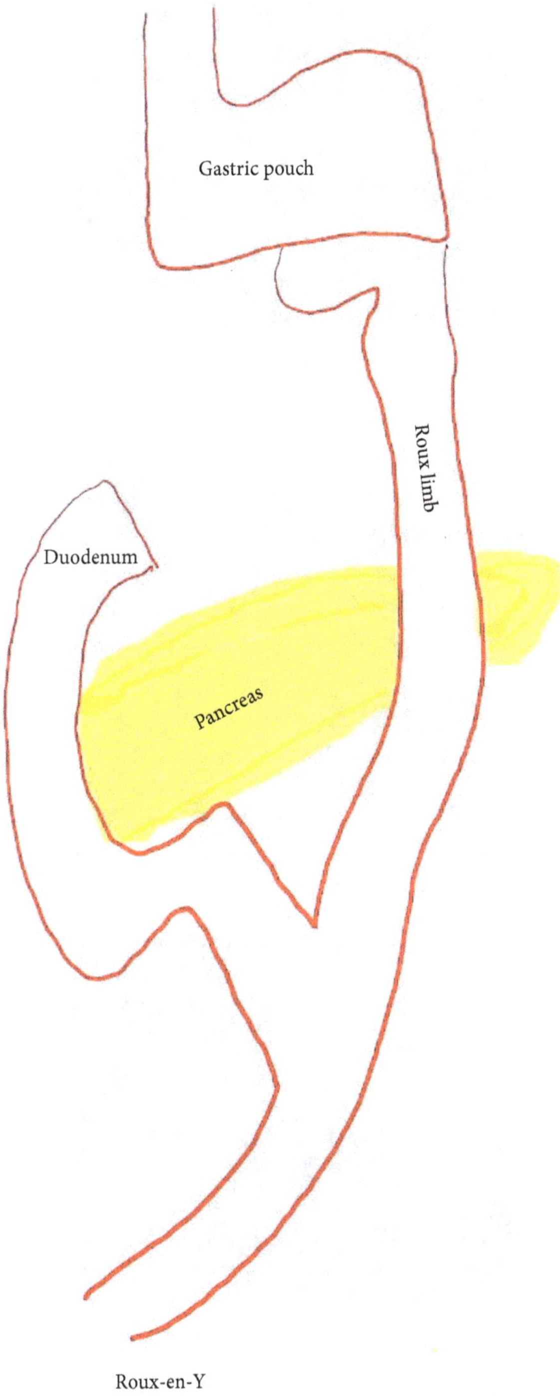

Figure 1: Schematic of surgically altered gastrointestinal anatomy: partial gastrectomy with Roux-en-Y gastrojejunostomy.

double pigtail stent (7 Fr × 18 cm) with the distal end of the plastic stent placed past the major papilla and the proximal end placed in the stomach (Figure 5). This procedure permitted decompression of the biliary tract while allowing the patient to recover from his acute infection.

The patient returned for ERCP 3 months after resolution of cholangitis and improvement of his cardiac function. Dual antiplatelet therapy was not held before procedure. Following removable of the plastic stent with a

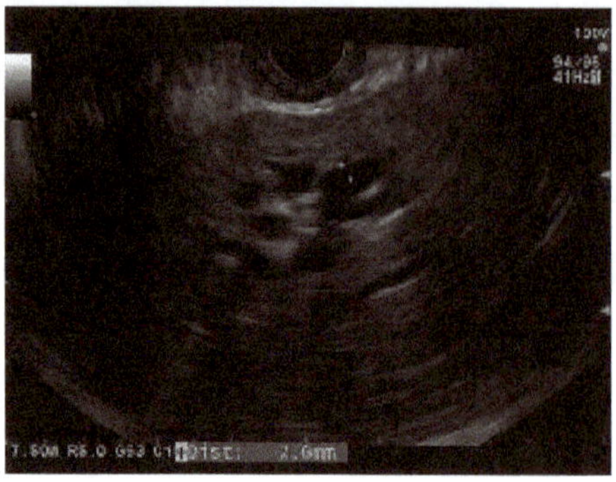

Figure 2: Endoscopic ultrasound showing a dilating segment 3 biliary radicle.

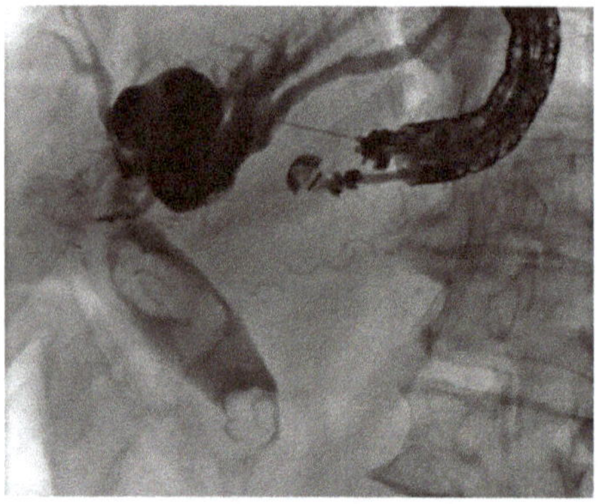

Figure 3: EUS-guided cholangiography showing a dilated biliary tree with choledocholithiasis.

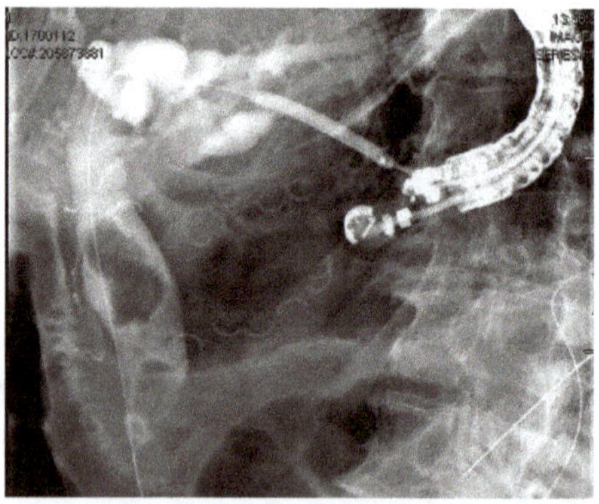

Figure 4: Balloon dilation of the HG tract.

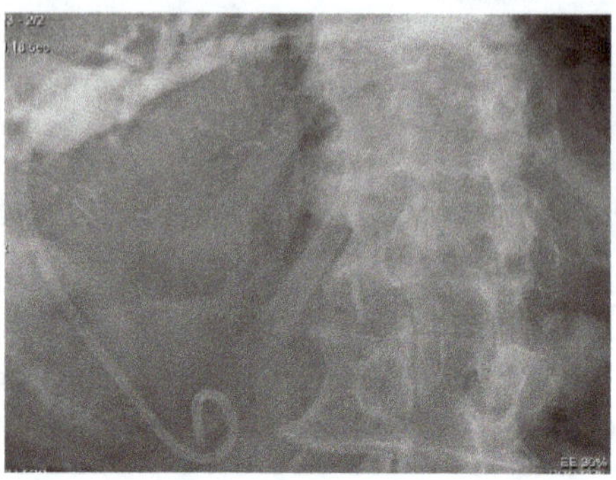

Figure 5: EUS-HG with placement of metal and double pigtail plastic stents.

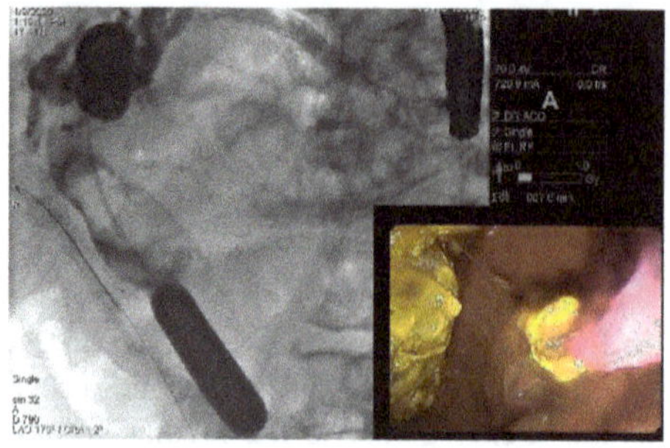

Figure 6: Antegrade balloon sphincteroplasty to facilitate stone removal.

snare from the gastric pouch, the biliary tree was accessed via the left hepaticogastrostomy using a sphincterotome preloaded with a 0.025 inch × 450 cm VisiGlide 2 guidewire. Successful balloon sphincteroplasty was performed using a CRE (controlled radial expansion) wire-guided balloon (Boston Scientific, Marlborough, MA), and the diameter was gradually increased to 15 mm (Figure 6). Cholangioscopy was then performed using a SpyScope DS (Boston Scientific, Marlborough, MA) with visualization of two large stones in the common bile duct which were fragmented using EHL (Figure 7). The biliary tree was then swept with a 15 mm stone extraction balloon (Cook Medical, Winston-Salem, NC) with antegrade advancement of stone fragments past the ampulla into the duodenum with subsequent duct clearance (Figure 8). The patient was followed up in clinic 4 weeks later, and repeat LFTs were normal.

3. Discussion

This case presents a complex patient with significant comorbidities, multiple recent cardiac arrests, and prior partial gastrectomy and Roux-en-Y gastrojejunostomy who required urgent intervention for his cholangitis. However, traditional ERCP was unsuccessful due to his SAGA, and open surgery was not preferred as he was a poor surgical candidate given his underlying condition. PTBD was offered to the patient, but he refused due to preference against external drains. Though balloon enteroscopy has a high success rate and low adverse event rate, EUS-HG was preferred given the size of stones and the likely need for cholangioscopy and EHL [5, 6]. This successful intervention was accomplished by a two-step approach. The first procedure involved creation of hepaticogastrostomy with stent placement, allowing for biliary decompression and resolution of cholangitis. The subsequent procedure involved cholangioscopy with EHL, balloon sphincteroplasty, and antegrade clearance of stone fragments from the bile duct with balloon sweeps.

Numerous retrospective and prospective studies have compared EUS-HG with other interventions. One alternative to EUS-HG is percutaneous transhepatic biliary drainage (PTBD). Sportes et al. compared EUS-HG versus PTBD as a salvage procedure for failed ERCP and showed comparable clinical success (86% vs. 83%) [7]. Sharaiha et al.

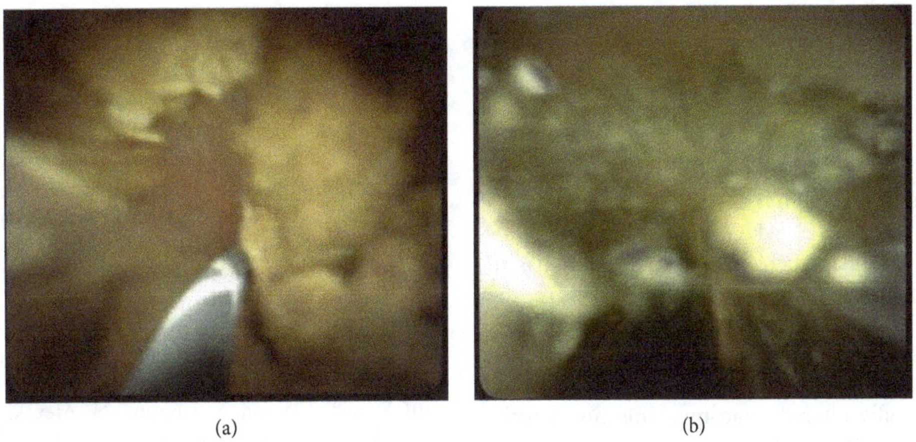

FIGURE 7: (a) Cholangioscopy showing CBD stones and (b) EHL resulting in common bile duct stone fragmentation.

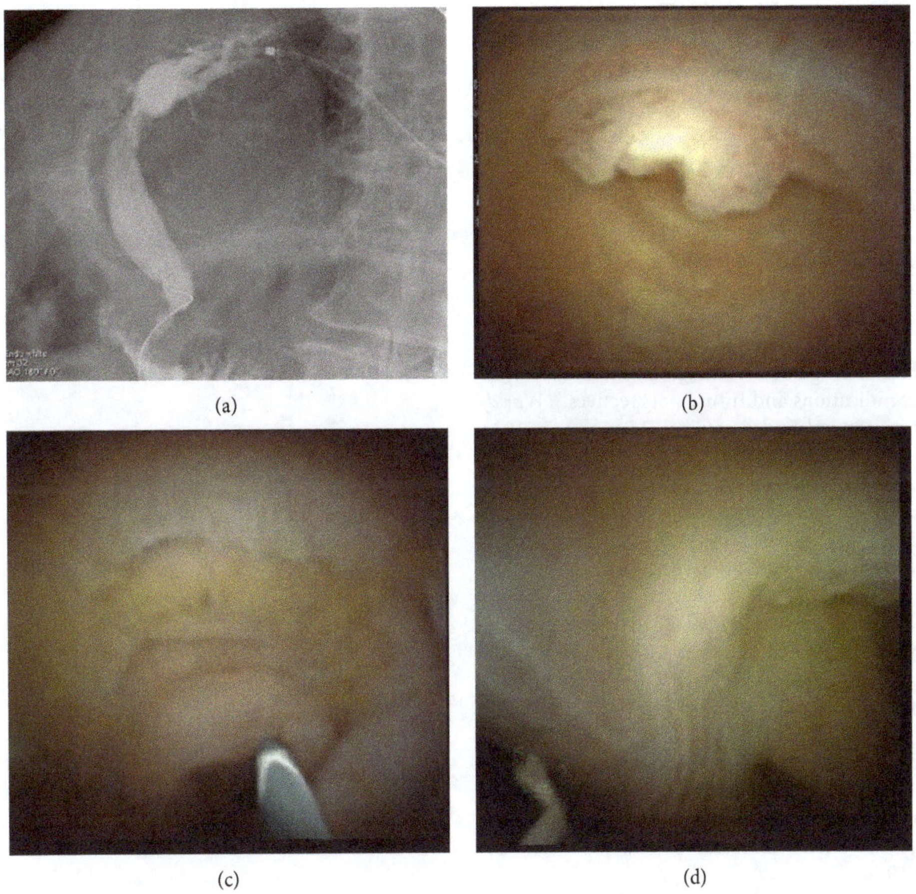

FIGURE 8: (a) Cholangiogram showing complete clearance of stones from the common bile duct. (b–d) Cholangioscopy showing normal distal common bile duct and ampulla with no residual stone disease.

performed a systematic review and meta-analysis, which found that when compared to PTBD, endoscopic ultrasound-guided biliary drainage is associated with improved clinical success, lower rate of postprocedure adverse events, and fewer reinterventions [8]. Another alternative to EUS-HG is direct surgical exploration of the bile duct. This approach intrinsically carries a higher morbidity [9]. Clayton et al. performed a meta-analysis comparing surgical bile duct clearance versus endoscopic clearance and found no significant difference in outcomes [10]. Given the lack of improved outcomes with the more invasive techniques including PTBD and surgical exploration, EUS-HG for management of choledocholithiasis is the preferred alternative.

EUS-HG is a safe treatment approach for biliary drainage in patients with SAGA. To our knowledge, this is one of the few cases reported in the literature that describes successful performance of EUS-HG, antegrade cholangioscopy, and EHL for management of choledocholithiasis in SAGA [11–13]. Of the reported cases in the literature, the clinical success rate is greater than 90%. Due to its high clinical success rate and additional therapeutic options, EUS-HG should be included in the treatment algorithm for patients with surgically altered anatomy. This novel technique has shown positive short-term outcomes; however, randomized prospective studies are needed to formulate a consensus on the long-term efficacy and safety [3].

In conclusion, EUS-HG is a safe, effective, and less-invasive therapy that should be considered in the management of biliary pathology in patients with SAGA. In this patient with multiple surgical adaptations, numerous failed ERCPs, and significant comorbidities, EUS-HG was able to facilitate biliary drainage with successful treatment of choledocholithiasis and cholangitis.

References

[1] R. Dorrell, S. Pawa, Y. Zhou, N. Lalwani, and R. Pawa, "The diagnostic dilemma of malignant biliary strictures," *Diagnostics*, vol. 10, no. 5, p. 337, 2020.

[2] P. Hindryckx, H. Degroote, D. J. Tate, and P. H. Deprez, "Endoscopic ultrasound-guided drainage of the biliary system: techniques, indications and future perspectives," *World Journal of Gastrointestinal Endoscopy*, vol. 11, no. 2, p. 103, 2019.

[3] A. Hosmer, M. Abdelfatah, R. Law, and T. Baron, "Endoscopic ultrasound-guided hepaticogastrostomy and antegrade clearance of biliary lithiasis in patients with surgically-altered anatomy," *Endoscopy International Open*, vol. 6, no. 2, p. E127, 2018.

[4] M. Hirota, T. Takada, Y. Kawarada et al., "Diagnostic criteria and severity assessment of acute cholecystitis: Tokyo guidelines," *Journal of Hepato-Biliary-Pancreatic Surgery*, vol. 14, no. 1, p. 78, 2007.

[5] Y. Tanisaka, S. Ryozawa, M. Mizuide et al., "Analysis of the factors involved in procedural failure: endoscopic retrograde cholangiopancreatography using a short-type single-balloon enteroscope for patients with surgically altered gastrointestinal anatomy," *Digestive Endoscopy*, vol. 31, no. 6, pp. 682–689, 2019.

[6] M. Shimatani, H. Hatanaka, H. Kogure et al., "Diagnostic and therapeutic endoscopic retrograde cholangiography using a short-type double-balloon endoscope in patients with altered gastrointestinal anatomy: a multicenter prospective study in Japan," *American Journal of Gastroenterology*, vol. 111, no. 12, pp. 1750–1758, 2016.

[7] A. Sportes, M. Camus, M. Greget et al., "Endoscopic ultrasound-guided hepaticogastrostomy versus percutaneous transhepatic drainage for malignant biliary obstruction after failed endoscopic retrograde cholangiopancreatography: a retrospective expertise-based study from two centers," *Therapeutic Advances in Gastroenterology*, vol. 10, no. 6, pp. 483–493, 2017.

[8] R. Z. Sharaiha, N. A. Kumta, A. P. Desai et al., "Endoscopic ultrasound-guided biliary drainage versus percutaneous transhepatic biliary drainage: predictors of successful outcome in patients who fail endoscopic retrograde cholangiopancreatography," *Surgical Endoscopy*, vol. 30, no. 12, pp. 5500–5505, 2016.

[9] W. G. Sheridan, H. O. L. Williams, and M. H. Lewis, "Morbidity and mortality of common bile duct exploration," *British Journal of Surgery*, vol. 74, no. 12, pp. 1095–1099, 1987.

[10] E. S. J. Clayton, S. Connor, N. Alexakis, and E. Leandros, "Meta-analysis of endoscopy and surgeryversus surgery alone for common bile duct stones with the gallbladderin situ," *British Journal of Surgery*, vol. 93, no. 10, pp. 1185–1191, 2006.

[11] Y. Nakai, H. Isayama, and K. Koike, "Two-step endoscopic ultrasonography-guided antegrade treatment of a difficult bile duct stone in a surgically altered anatomy patient," *Digestive Endoscopy*, vol. 30, no. 1, pp. 125–127, 2018.

[12] A. Maruta, T. Iwashita, S. Uemura et al., "Comparison of late adverse events after endoscopic sphincterotomy versus endoscopic papillary large balloon dilation for common bile duct stones: a propensity score-based cohort analysis," *Digestive Endoscopy*, vol. 30, no. 4, pp. 493–500, 2018.

[13] S. Mukai, T. Itoi, A. Sofuni et al., "EUS-guided antegrade intervention for benign biliary diseases in patients with surgically altered anatomy (with videos)," *Gastrointestinal Endoscopy*, vol. 89, no. 2, pp. 399–407, 2019.

Ischemic Colitis after Colonoscopy with Bisacodyl Bowel Preparation: A Report of Two Cases

Chris Shamatutu,[1] Daljeet Chahal,[2] Isabella T. Tai,[2] and Peter Kwan[2]

[1]*Department of Medicine, University of British Columbia, Vancouver, Canada*
[2]*Department of Medicine, Division of Gastroenterology, University of British Columbia, Vancouver, Canada*

Correspondence should be addressed to Chris Shamatutu; shamatutu@alumni.ubc.ca

Academic Editor: Hirotada Akiho

Background. Colonoscopy is widely used for the diagnosis and management of colorectal disease and requires adequate bowel preparation. Ischemic colitis is a form of intestinal ischemia that presents with abdominal pain, diarrhea, and hematochezia. Risk factors include advanced age, cardiovascular disease, and diabetes. Both colonoscopy and bisacodyl bowel preparation have been described as rare causes of ischemic colitis with less than 35 cases collectively in the literature. Our review found that of these cases, there exists significant heterogeneity within individual patient characteristics. The majority of the cases are managed conservatively without complications or sequela. Due to the risk of ischemic colitis, the FDA has withdrawn bisacodyl bowel preparations from use in the USA. Bisacodyl bowel preparations are still used in Canada. *Cases.* Here, we present two cases of ischemic colitis in previously healthy women aged 57 and 69 who underwent screening colonoscopy using bisacodyl bowel preparation. Both were treated conservatively without complications. *Conclusion.* Thus far, there has been one documented case of ischemic colitis following colonoscopy with bisacodyl bowel preparation; here, we present two additional cases with one case occurring without the presence of known risk factors for ischemic colitis. Our literature review finds that there is limited evidence surrounding bisacodyl as a causative agent of ischemic colitis. Cases often contain confounding variables such as the presence of known risk factors for ischemic colitis. Our report aims to highlight the need for a more comprehensive analysis evaluating the safety of bowel preparations as well as increasing the clinical awareness surrounding the rare risk of colonoscopy-induced ischemic colitis.

1. Introduction

Colonoscopy is a common modality for investigation and management of diseases of the colorectal tract and remains the gold standard for diagnosis and prevention of colorectal cancer [1]. Bowel preparation is required prior to colonoscopy to facilitate adequate endoscopic visualization of the mucosa. High-volume (4 L) polyethylene glycol (PEG) is a well-established, safe, and effective colon cleanser; however, up to 38% of patients do not complete this bowel preparation due to the large volume of ingested solution required and poor taste [2]. Inadequate bowel preparation occurs in up to 25% of colonoscopies [3] and results in a lower adenoma detection rate, longer colonoscopy time, and higher cost due to the need for repeat colonoscopy [4, 5].

Various preparations have been formulated in attempts to decrease the volume of solution ingested including the addition of bisacodyl, a colonic motility laxative. A combination of low-volume (2 L) PEG with 20 mg bisacodyl was first approved for use in the United States as bowel preparation in 2004. Case reports documenting episodes of ischemic colitis (IC) following the use of bisacodyl 20 mg/PEG 3350 bowel preparations resulted in the Food and Drug Administration (FDA) issuing a black box warning on these preparations in 2006. The bisacodyl 20 mg/PEG 3350 and bisacodyl 10 mg/PEG 3350 bowel preparations were eventually withdrawn from the United States market by the FDA in 2007 and 2010, respectively, due to "Reasons of Safety or Effectiveness." In Canada, the formulation Bi-Peglyte (bisacodyl 15 mg/PEG 3350) is still in use and has not been withdrawn despite these findings.

Advanced age is the strongest risk factor for IC with 90% of individuals greater than age 60 [6]. Additional identified risk factors include hypertension, cardiovascular disease, and diabetes mellitus [7, 8]. Interestingly, colonoscopy itself has been described in the literature as a cause of IC with 25 studies identified globally [9]. In these case reports, we describe two cases of IC following colonoscopy with Bi-Peglyte (15 mg Bisacodyl/PEG 3350) used as bowel preparation. We subsequently conducted a review of the literature surrounding bowel preparation and colonoscopy-induced IC.

1.1. Case Presentation 1. A 57-year-old healthy female underwent colonoscopy in the context of a positive fecal immunohistochemistry test (FIT) of 77 ng/mL. Her medical history was only significant for a remote caesarean section. Her family history was significant for her father having colonic polyps at the age of 70. The patient also endorsed occasional NSAID use. The patient had used Bi-Peglyte solution for bowel preparation.

The patient was sedated before and during the procedure with a total of 3 mg of midazolam and 100 mcg of fentanyl. CO_2 was used to insufflate the colon. The colon was quite tortuous and required repositioning of the patient on to her back and right side. Application of counter pressure was also used to reach the cecum. Bowel preparation was suboptimal, and fecal material clogged the endoscope numerous times. Extensive lavage and suction were required during withdrawal. A 1.2 cm pedunculated polyp in the descending colon was injected with methylene blue and completely removed as 2 pieces by hot snare polypectomy. Withdrawal time was 15 minutes. Overall, the patient tolerated the procedure well. Pathology of the polyp demonstrated a tubulovillous adenoma with low-grade dysplasia.

The patient subsequently presented to the emergency department (ED) 2 days after colonoscopy with severe abdominal pain but no bleeding or diarrhea. Initial bloodwork was unremarkable other than an elevated lactate of 5. A CT abdomen with IV contrast demonstrated diffuse large bowel thickening with severe involvement of the sigmoid and small volume of pelvic ascites (Figure 1). There was no hemoperitoneum, pneumoperitoneum, or bowel obstruction. The patient underwent an urgent flexible sigmoidoscopy. Starting at the rectosigmoid junction, there were patchy, dusky areas of mucosa with submucosal swelling and erythema but no frank ulcerations (Figure 2). The endoscope was only advanced to the midsigmoid, and biopsies were not taken due to the fear of inducing more complications. The proximal extent of the changes was not determined.

A diagnosis of IC was made. She ultimately deteriorated hemodynamically and required placement of central venous access for vasopressors. She was then admitted to the high acuity unit (HAU) and monitored in anticipation of possible colectomy. Interestingly, her blood cultures were positive for group A *Streptococcus* (GAS). This bacteremia was thought acquired due to an occupational hazard and likely unrelated to her IC. She stated that she had experienced symptoms of pharyngitis several weeks ago. A CT of the neck ruled out an abscess and an echocardiogram ruled out infective endocarditis. Over the next few days, the patient's abdominal pain subsided, and she recovered hemodynamically without the need for surgery. She was discharged 6 days later with oral antibiotics for her bacteremia.

1.2. Case Presentation 2. A 69-year-old healthy female underwent a surveillance colonoscopy Figure 3. Her medical history was only significant for caesarean section, hysterectomy, oophorectomy, and irritable bowel syndrome. Her family history was significant for colorectal malignancy. She endorsed daily NSAID use in the form of ibuprofen and ASA for back pain. The patient had used Bi-Peglyte solution for bowel preparation.

The patient was sedated before and during the procedure with a total of 3 mg of midazolam and 75 mcg of fentanyl. Carbon dioxide (CO_2) was used to insufflate the colon. The colonoscope was advanced without difficulty to the cecum. Bowel preparation was good. Two flat polyps of 2 mm size were removed by cold snare polypectomy in the ascending colon. Two flat, larger polyps of 1 cm size were removed from the hepatic flexure and transverse colon using methylene blue and cold snare polypectomy. Moderate diverticulosis was noted in the sigmoid colon. Pathology demonstrated normal mucosa, one tubular adenoma, and two sessile serrated lesions without dysplasia.

The patient developed abdominal pain and small volume rectal bleeding 6 days after the colonoscopy. There was no peritonitis. She underwent an urgent flexible sigmoidoscopy the next day. Starting at the distal sigmoid, a 9 cm, non-circumferential segment of erythema and friability consistent with ischemia was noted (Figure 4). There was no submucosal edema or ulceration. There was a small area of increased blood, although no active bleeding, onto which a single clip was placed. No biopsies were taken. A CT scan completed 7 days after the flexible sigmoidoscopy did not demonstrate any features consistent with ischemia. The patient did well clinically and did not require hospital admission.

2. Discussion

We have presented two cases of IC following colonoscopy with Bi-Peglyte bowel preparation in patients with no known risk factors. Our first patient's course deteriorated with hemodynamic instability requiring vasopressors, and she was concomitantly found to have GAS bacteremia and treated accordingly. Her clinical condition improved with conservative management, and she experienced resolution of symptoms after 6 days. She was discharged in stable condition on oral antibiotics. Our second patient did well with supportive management and did not require hospital admission.

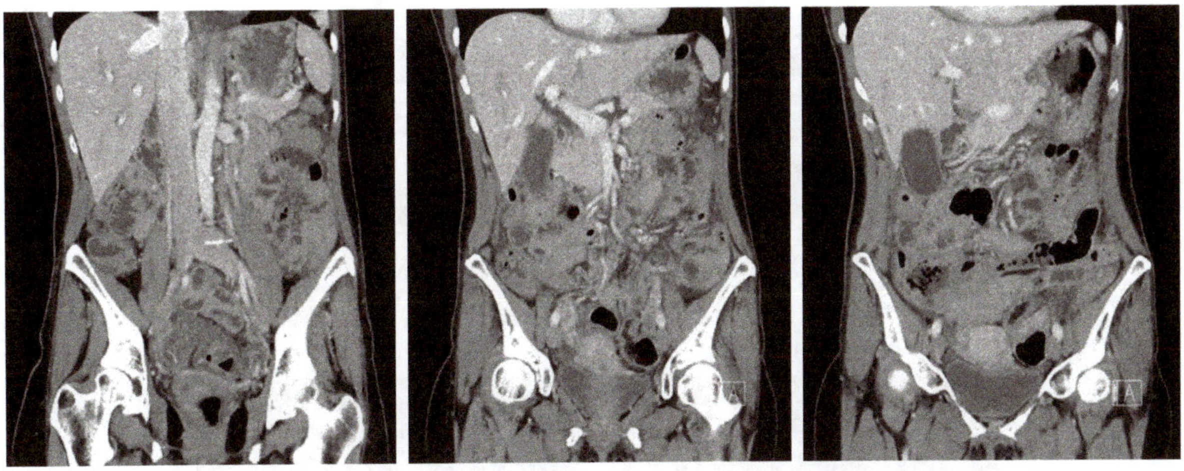

FIGURE 1: Computed tomography (CT) images demonstrated diffuse large bowel thickening consistent with ischemic colitis.

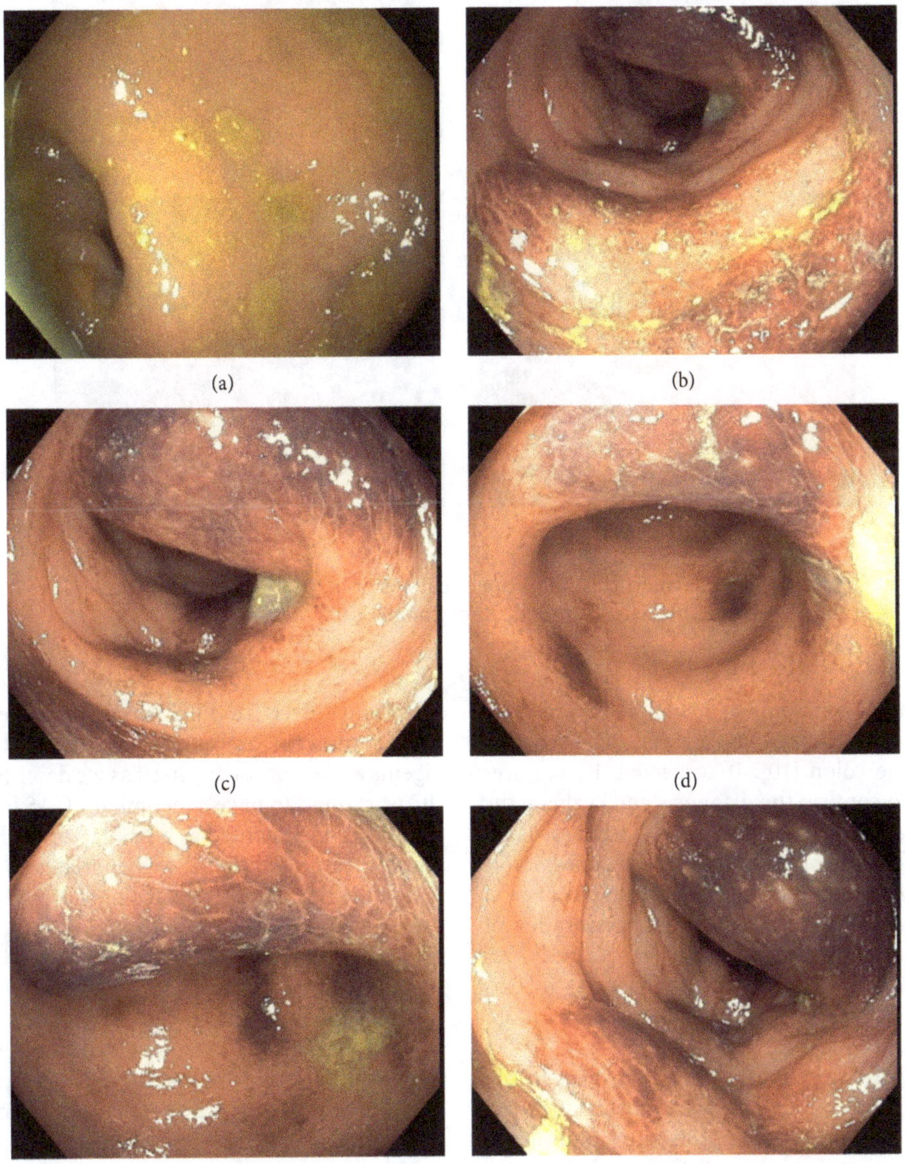

(a) (b) (c) (d) (e) (f)

FIGURE 2: Endoscopic images up to midsigmoid demonstrating patchy, dusky areas of mucosa with submucosal swelling and erythema but no frank ulcerations.

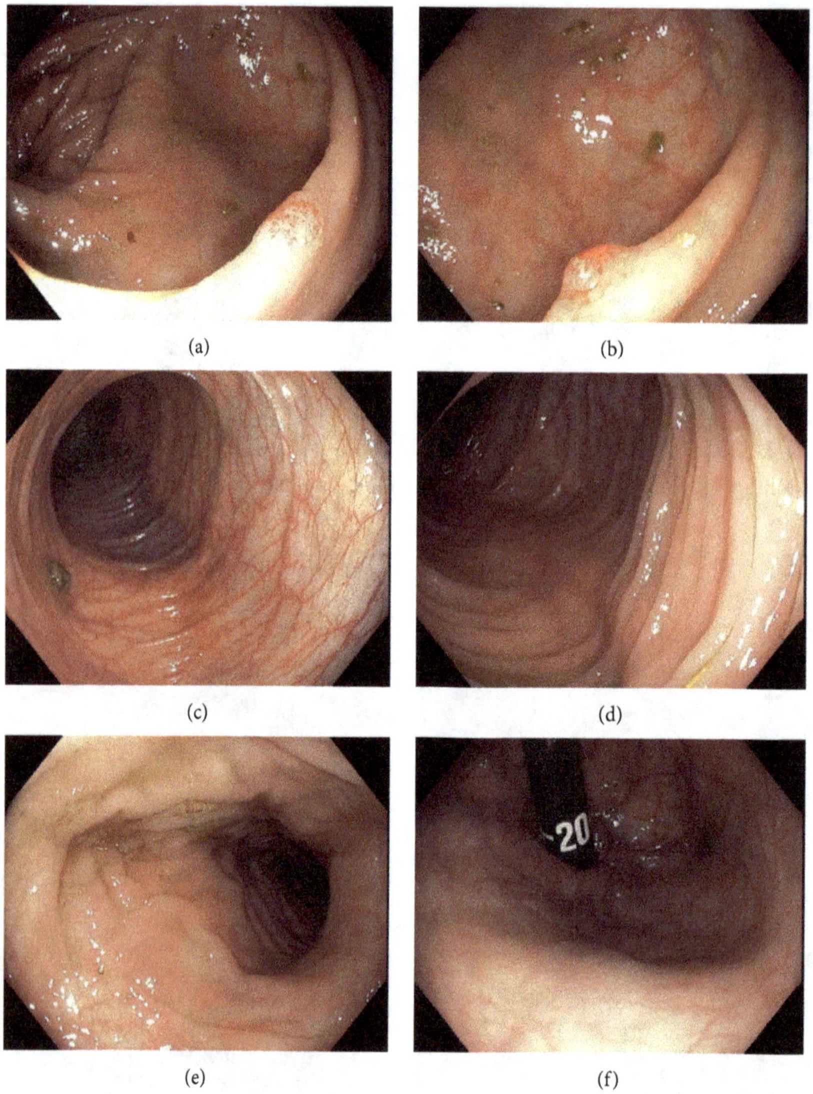

FIGURE 3: Initial endoscopic images from surveillance colonoscopy 6 days prior to the development of ischemic colitis symptoms. Images are in similar locations to their corresponding letters in Figure 4 for comparison.

IC manifests most commonly as hematochezia, colicky abdominal pain, and diarrhea as a result of transient hypoperfusion to the colon [10]. If suspected, IC requires urgent endoscopy to confirm the diagnosis and evaluate the extent of bowel wall injury ideally within 48 hours. IC is predominantly self-limiting and managed with conservative measures including intravenous fluids, analgesia, and bowel rest in 83–92% of cases [11, 12]. Necrosis and perforation of the colonic wall is a known complication of severe IC requiring emergent surgical intervention. The need for intervention is an indicator of poor prognosis with an estimated operative mortality of 40% [13].

Well-defined factors for IC include age, hypertension, coronary artery disease, dyslipidemia, diabetes mellitus, peripheral vascular disease, chronic obstructive pulmonary disease, nephropathies, and atrial fibrillation [8]. In younger individuals without traditional risk factors, IC has been associated with autoimmune diseases, coagulopathies, endurance exercise, illicit drugs, and medications such as oral contraceptives, as well as various bowel preparation agents and colonoscopy itself as we describe. Our first case of IC was found to have concomitant GAS bacteremia; this has not been documented as a risk factor in the literature prior, and we proposed that it was unrelated to the episode of IC given the timing of IC postcolonoscopy. However, it should be noted that an association with *E. coli* O157 : H7 and IC has been described [14]. History of C-section has not been documented as a risk factor.

IC secondary to laxative use was first described in 1997 by Oh et al. who documented two cases of IC following hyperosmotic laxative ingestion as bowel preparation prior to colonoscopy [15]. The mechanism of action is thought to be multifactorial and related to the laxative effect of decreased intravascular volume as well as colonic hypermobility leading to increased intraluminal pressures and subsequent hypoperfusion [16, 17]. A review of the literature

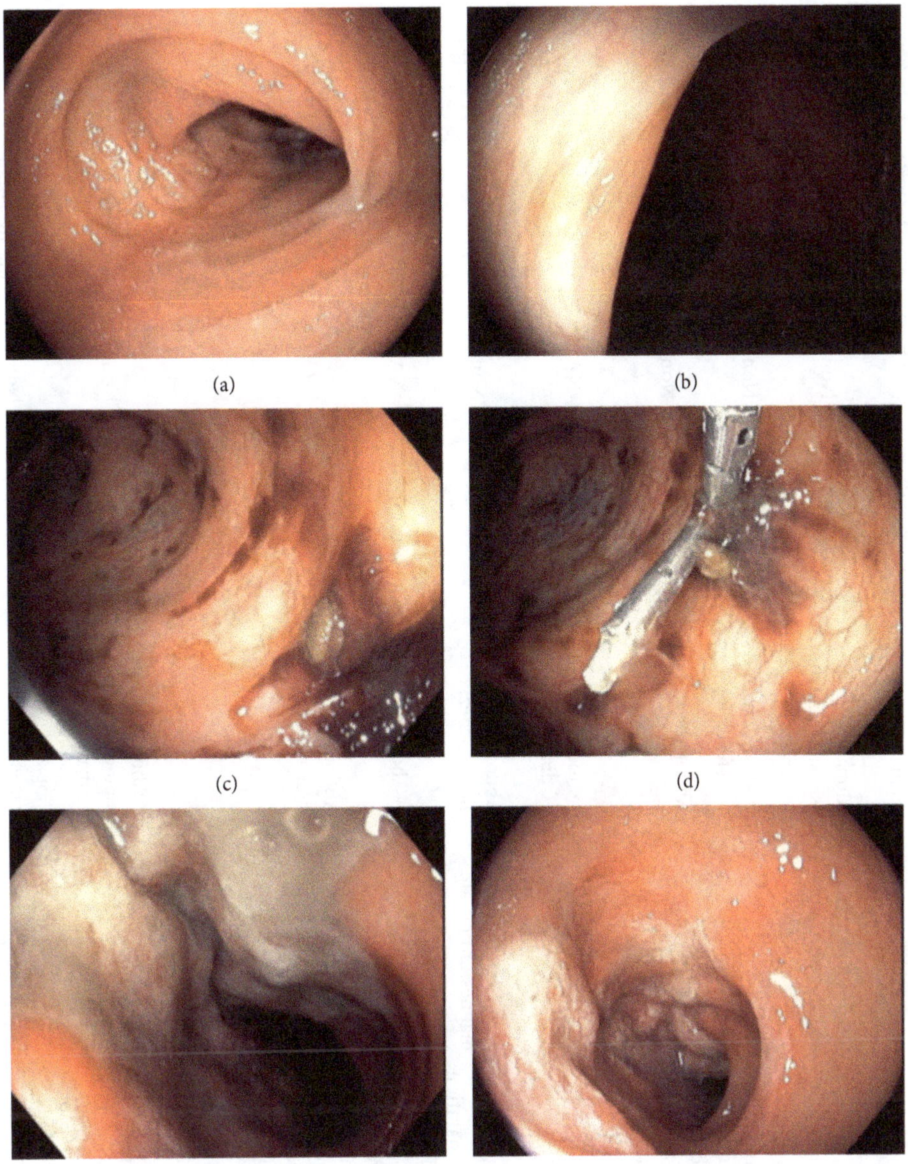

(a) (b) (c) (d) (e) (f)

FIGURE 4: Endoscopic images demonstrating the noncircumferential segment of erythema and friability without submucosal edema or ulceration (1–6). Site of increased blood where a clip was placed (4).

was conducted identifying similar cases of IC with laxative use prior to or in the absence of colonoscopy; a summary of these results is presented in Table 1. There are 12 documented cases of IC following laxative use in individuals ≤70 years of age. Common risk factors for IC were present in 6 cases. Laxative use indications in these reports included bowel preparation prior to colonoscopy ($N = 8$), bowel preparation prior to non-GI surgery ($N = 1$), and constipation ($n = 3$). Bisacodyl was the most commonly identified laxative and was implicated in 58% of cases ($n = 7$) with doses ranging from 5 mg to 20 mg and a time of onset ranging from 2 to 24 hours. Of the 7 cases of bisacodyl-associated IC, 2 were after bisacodyl tablet use for constipation and 5 were after bisacodyl/PEG 3350 for bowel preparation. Of these 5 cases, 2 are brief abstracts with limited clinical information and 3 had known risk factors for IC (hypertension, older age, and contraceptive use as well as constipation). Symptoms of abdominal pain and hematochezia were present in 66% of cases. Amongst all cases, management was conservative without complications ($n = 12$), and in most cases, patients were discharged home within 48–72 hours ($n = 11$).

Currently, the bowel preparation Bi-Peglyte and bisacodyl are still in use in Canada. Standard bowel preparation for inpatient colonoscopy at our institution involves a Bi-Peglyte equivalent, consisting of 15 mg of bisacodyl followed by 2 L of PEG 3350 in the evening prior to colonoscopy. This is followed by an additional 2 L of PEG 3350 in the morning of endoscopy as needed. Bisacodyl enemas also remain a part of our institutions constipation bowel protocol. The FDAs

Table 1: Literature review results of ischemic colitis induced by bowel cathartics. Search run, August 2019.

First author, year	Age	Sex	Risk factors	Laxative Type Dose Reason	Onset to symptoms (hours)	Symptoms	Diagnosis	Complications	Treatment	Resolution
Oh [15], 1997	69	F	Age, HTN, and DM	Magnesium citrate NA Bowel preparation	1 hour after magnesium citrate	Abdopain and hematochezia	Colonoscopy	None	Conservative	D/C 7 days
Oh [15], 1997	66	F	Age and CAD	Sodium phosphate NA Bowel preparation	0.5 hours after sodium phosphate	Abdopain, nausea, emesis, and diarrhea	Colonoscopy	None	Conservative	D/C 2 days
Lopez [18], 2005	19	M	Constipation	Bisacodyl 5 mg Constipation	Several hours after bisacodyl	Abdopain, hematochezia, and fever	Colonoscopy and CT	None	Conservative	D/C 2 days
Lopez [18], 2005	33	F	Constipation Sertraline	Bisacodyl 10 mg Constipation	6 hours after bisacodyl	Abdopain and hematochezia	Colonoscopy	None	Conservative	D/C 2 days
Vaizman [19], 2007	56	M	HTN	Bisacodyl/PEG 3350 20 mg/NA Bowel preparation	After bisacodyl/ PEG (unspecified)	Abdopain, hematochezia, and diarrhea	Colonoscopy	NA	NA	NA
Lee [20], 2008 (no English text)	39	F	None	Magnesium citrate 250 ml Bowel preparation	24 hours after magnesium citrate	Abdopain and hematochezia	Colonoscopy	None	Conservative	D/C 3 days
You [21], 2009 (no English text)	70	F	Age, COPD, and chronic constipation	SF-PEG 4 L Bowel preparation	0.5 hours after SF-PEG	Abdopain	Colonoscopy	NA	NA	NA
Baudet [16], 2010	68, 70*	M	Age	Bisacodyl/PEG 10 mg/2 L Bowel preparation	2 hours after bisacodyl	Abdopain and hematochezia	Colonoscopy	None	NA	NA
Dholakia [22], 2011 (abstract only)	37	F	None	Bisacodyl/PEG 3350 NA Bowel preparation	24 hours after bisacodyl/PEG 3350	NA	Colonoscopy	None	NA	NA
Ajani [17], 2012	54	F	Chronic constipation OCP (estradiol 0.5 mg daily)	Bisacodyl 15 mg Bowel preparation for non-GI surgery	6 hours after bisacodyl	Abdopain, hematochezia, and diarrhea	Colonoscopy and CT	None	Conservative	NA
Sherid [23], 2013	54	F	DM, HTN, dyslipidemia, and chronic constipation	Lubiprostone 24 mcg Constipation	2 hours after lubiprostone	Abdopain, nausea, clear emesis, and hematochezia	Colonoscopy	None	Stopping lubiprostone	D/C 4 days
Behzadi [24], 2015 (abstract only)	64	F	None	Bisacodyl/PEG 3350 15 mg/2 L Bowel preparation	Several hours after bisacodyl/PEG 3350	Abdopain, nausea, clear emesis, and diarrhea	Colonoscopy and biopsy	None	Conservative	D/C several days

*Recurrence in same individual 2 years later with same bowel preparation and same clinical course. Abdopain, abdominal pain; HTN, hypertension; DM, diabetes mellitus; CAD, coronary artery disease; COPD, chronic obstructive pulmonary disease; OCP, oral contraceptive pill; NA, not available; D/C, day of discharge; CT, computerized tomography. Conservative treatment in all cases consisted of IV fluids ± antibiotics.

Table 2: Literature review results of ischemic colitis following colonoscopy. Search run August 2019.

First author, year	Age	Sex	Risk factors	Bowel Preparation Type Dose	Initial endoscopy characteristics Indication for endoscopy Type of endoscopy Difficult endoscopy (Y/N) Time	Onset to symptoms (hours)	Symptoms	Diagnosis	Complications	Treatment	Resolution
Wheeldon [27], 1990	59	F	SLE	NA NA	Surveillance Colonoscopy No NA	24 hours	Abdopain, vomiting, diarrhea, and hematochezia	Colonoscopy	None	Conservative	D/C 6 days
Church [31], 1995	45	F	MCTD Methotrexate and prednisone	NA	Hematochezia Flexible sigmoidoscopy Yes: "Difficult, severe pain" NA	24 hours	Abdopain and fever	Colonoscopy	Peritonitis	Loop sigmoid colostomy	NA
Cremers [32], 1998	44	F	None	PEG 3350 4 L	Abdominal pain Colonoscopy No NA	48 hours	Abdopain and hematochezia	Colonoscopy	None	Conservative	D/C 2 days
Versaci [29], 2005	43	F	SLE	NA	Altered bowel habits Colonoscopy, polypectomy No NA	4 hours	Abdopain, hematochezia, mucous, and diarrhea	Colonoscopy	None	Conservative	D/C 12 days
Vaizman [19], 2007	78	F	HTN, age	Bisacodyl/PEG 3350 NA	Surveillance Colonoscopy NA NA	Later that day	Abdopain, hematochezia, and diarrhea	Laparotomy	Necrotic sigmoid with perforation	Left hemicolectomy	NA
Arhan [28], 2009	25	F	None	Calcium sennoside sodium phosphate enema	Constipation Colonoscopy 25 mins NA NA	1 hour	Abdopain and hematochezia	Colonoscopy	None	Conservative	D/C 5 days
Kao [30], 2009	55	M	None	NA	Screening Colonoscopy NA NA	NA	Abdopain and hematochezia	Colonoscopy	None	Conservative	NA

Table 2: Continued.

First author, year	Age	Sex	Risk factors	Bowel Preparation Type Dose	Initial endoscopy characteristics Indication for endoscopy Type of endoscopy Difficult endoscopy (Y/N) Time	Onset to symptoms (hours)	Symptoms	Diagnosis	Complications	Treatment	Resolution
Dong [33], 2009	54	F	None	NA	Abdominal pain Colonoscopy NA NA	3 hours	Abdopain and hematochezia	Sigmoidoscopy and CT	None	Conservative	NA
Singh-Ranger [34], 2011	49	F	None	Sodium picosulphate 20 mg	Abdominal pain and loose stool Colonoscopy NA NA	Later that evening	Abdopain and fever	CT	None	Conservative	NA
Cheng [35], 2012	NA	M	None	Sodium phosphate 90 mL	Screening Colonoscopy NA NA	Several hours	Abdopain, hematochezia, and diarrhea	Colonoscopy and CT	None	Conservative	D/C 7 days
Sapmaz [36], 2014	26	F	None	NA	Chronic diarrhea Colonoscopy NA NA	10 hours	Abdopain and hematochezia	Colonoscopy and CT	None	Conservative	D/C 5 days
Lee [37], 2014	47	F	None	PEG 3350 4 L	Screening Colonoscopy and polypectomy NA NA	7 hours	Abdopain and hematochezia	Colonoscopy and CT	None	Conservative	D/C 9 days
Lee [37], 2014	40	M	None	PEG 3350 4 L	Screening Colonoscopy No NA	18 hours	Abdopain and hematochezia	Colonoscopy and CT	None	Conservative	D/C 9 days
Silva [38], 2014 (abstract only)	67	F	COPD	NA	Screening Colonoscopy NA NA	6 hours	Abdopain and hematochezia	CT	None	Conservative	D/C 5 days

TABLE 2: Continued.

First author, year	Age	Sex	Risk factors	Bowel Preparation Type Dose	Initial endoscopy characteristics Indication for endoscopy Type of endoscopy Difficult endoscopy (Y/N) Time	Onset to symptoms (hours)	Symptoms	Diagnosis	Complications	Treatment	Resolution
Hai-Bo Zhou [39], 2015	30	F	None	NA	Abdopain Colonoscopy NA NA	48 hours	Abdopain and hematochezia	Colonoscopy	None	Conservative	D/C 7 days
Omar [40], 2015	70	F	Age, HTN, and dyslipidemia	PEG 3350 NA	Screening Colonoscopy No 30 mins	The next day	Abdopain and hematochezia	Colonoscopy and CT	None	Conservative	NA
Solanke [41], 2016	43	M	None	PEG 3350 4 L split	Constipation Colonoscopy NA NA	6 hours	Abdopain and hematochezia	Colonoscopy and CT	None	Conservative	D/C 2 days
Zizzo [9], 2016	43	F	None	PEG 3350 4 L	Screening Colonoscopy Yes: forced exploration, with insufflation 37 mins	12 hours	Abdopain, fever, and hematochezia	CT, laparoscopy, and laparotomy	Peritonitis Transmural infarct with necrosis	Left hemicolectomy and terminal colostomy	D/C 22 days
Current case 1, 019	57	F	None	Bisacodyl/PEG 3350 15 mg/2 L	(+) positive FITT Colonoscopy Yes: tortuous NA	48 hours	Abdopain	Flexible sigmoidoscopy and CT	Hemodynamic instability GAS bacteremia	Conservative	D/C 6 days
Current case 2, 2019	69	F	IBS	Bisacodyl/PEG 3350 15 mg/2 L	Screening Colonoscopy No NA	6 days	Abdopain and hematochezia	Flexible sigmoidoscopy	None	Conservative	D/C < 1 day (no admission)

Abdopain, abdominal pain; SLE, systemic lupus erythematosus, HTN, hypertension; MCTD, mixed connect tissue disease; NA, not available; D/C, day of discharge; CT, computerized tomography; GAS, group A *Streptococcus*.

withdrawal of Halflytely bowel preparation with 10 mg and 20 mg of bisacodyl over concerns of IC is based on a limited number of case reports. Given the growing number of recognized factors that contribute an increased risk of IC [8] causation between bisacodyl and IC is debatable. The 2010 FDA clinical review gave an estimated IC incidence rate of 1/100,000 for the 20 mg preparation [25]. The risk of IC for the 10 mg preparation is described as "markedly lower" without a numerical estimate and is based on 3 case reports. However, two of these episodes were external reports where patients consumed an unknown dosage of additional bisacodyl in addition to the 10 mg contained in the Halflytely preparation. Only one of the three cases was identified in a clinical trial, a 55-year-old woman who was found to have IC one month postcolonoscopy. Interestingly, similar to our report, she required ICU admission secondary to unstable urosepsis which was presumably bacterial in origin. *E. coli* is the most common pathogen responsible for urinary tract infections [26] and as aforementioned has been associated with IC highlighting the difficulty in assessing the validity of the causal relationships presented. Based on our review, bisacodyl at current doses in bowel preparation is unlikely to be strongly associated with IC.

IC as a rare postcolonoscopy or sigmoidoscopy complication, irrespective of bowel preparation used, was first described in 1990 by Wheeldon and Grundman who documented a case of IC in an individual with systemic lupus erythematosus 24 hours after surveillance colonoscopy [27]. Proposed mechanisms of colonoscopy-induced IC include elevated intraluminal pressures and barotrauma to the colonic wall impairing arterial oxygen delivery [28–30]. A review of the literature was conducted for cases of IC following colonoscopy in individuals ≤70 years of age, and a summary of these results is presented in Table 2. There are 24 documented cases of IC following colonic endoscopy use in individuals ≤70 years of age; 19 of these are found in English literature. Of these 19, common risk factors for IC were present in 5 cases and included autoimmune disease ($n = 3$), advanced age with hypertension ($n = 2$), and chronic obstructive pulmonary disease ($n = 1$). Screening and surveillance were the indications for colonoscopy in 53% of cases. Bowel preparation regimens prior to colonoscopy were poorly described and varied across studies. Bisacodyl was used as bowel preparation in 2 cases. A description of colonoscopy characteristics including difficulties encountered was similarly lacking across studies. The time of onset postcolonoscopy varied from 1 hour to 6 days. Management of IC was conservative in 84% of cases. There was significant heterogeneity in the time from initial presentation of IC to resolution of symptoms and subsequent discharge (2–22 days).

Colonoscopy is thought to play a role in the development of IC through its effect of elevating intraluminal pressures and barotrauma to the colonic wall, thus reducing colonic blood blow and impairing oxygen delivery [28–30, 38, 42]. Decreasing procedural time reduces the amount of time the colon experiences luminal distention and has been proposed to reduce the risk of IC. This has not been well studied, and in fact, our review found that the total procedure time is rarely reported (Table 2). In both of the cases, we presented used CO_2 as an insufflation agent. Due to its rapid absorption and vasodilatory properties, the utilization of CO_2 over room air as an insufflation agent has been proposed to decrease the risk of IC through decreased duration of distension and improved perfusion, respectively [37, 43]. While multiple randomized controlled trials and meta-analysis comparing room air to CO_2 insufflation have shown CO_2 insufflation to decrease postprocedural abdominal distension and pain, its role in decreasing episodes of ischemic colitis relative to room air insufflation has not been well studied [44, 45].In conclusion, IC after bisacodyl bowel preparation or colonoscopy is a rare complication. Currently used doses of bisacodyl in bowel preparations are unlikely to be independently associated with IC, but may contribute in at risk patients. Our first case is one of 3 cases with a complicated course. Novel to this case is the presence of GAS bacteremia with a history of pharyngitis, the significance of which is unknown to date. Case reports of this rare event thus far contain limited data on bowel preparation specifics and technical details of the colonoscopy itself. Improved documentation of such variables in future reports is needed to further characterize this event.

References

[1] K. Bibbins-Domingo et al., "Screening for colorectal cancer: US preventive services task force recommendation statement," *Jama*, vol. 315, no. 23, pp. 2564–2575, 2016.

[2] L. C. Hookey, W. T. Depew, and S. J. Vanner, "Combined low volume polyethylene glycol solution plus stimulant laxatives versus standard volume polyethylene glycol solution: a prospective, randomized study of colon cleansing before colonoscopy," *Canadian journal of gastroenterology*, vol. 20, no. 2, pp. 101–105, 2006.

[3] G. C. Harewood, V. K. Sharma, and P. de Garmo, "Impact of colonoscopy preparation quality on detection of suspected colonic neoplasia," *Gastrointest Endosc*, vol. 58, no. 1, pp. 76–79, Jul 2003.

[4] C. Hassan, J. East, F. Radaelli et al., "Bowel preparation for colonoscopy: European society of gastrointestinal endoscopy (ESGE) guideline-update 2019," *Endoscopy*, vol. 51, no. 8, pp. 775–794, 2019.

[5] D. A. Corley, C. D. Jensen, A. R. Marks et al., "Adenoma detection rate and risk of colorectal cancer and death," *New England Journal of Medicine*, vol. 370, no. 14, pp. 1298–1306, 2014.

[6] A. Theodoropoulou and I. E. Koutroubakis, "Ischemic colitis: clinical practice in diagnosis and treatment," *World Journal of Gastroenterology*, vol. 14, no. 48, pp. 7302–7308, 2008.

[7] H. I. Seo, K.-h. Choi, K. H. Han et al., "Predisposing factors of ischemic colitis: data from 14 Years of experience in a single center," *Gastroenterology Research & Practice*, vol. 2017, Article ID 1049810, 5 pages, 2017.

[8] L. J. Brandt, P. Feuerstadt, G. F. Longstreth, and S. J. Boley, "ACG clinical guideline: epidemiology, risk factors, patterns of presentation, diagnosis, and management of colon ischemia (CI)," *American Journal of Gastroenterology*, vol. 110, no. 1, pp. 18–44, 2015.

[9] M. Zizzo, C. Castro Ruiz, L. Ugoletti et al., "Transmural colonic infarction after routine colonoscopy in a young patient without risk factors," *Case Reports in Gastroenterology*, vol. 10, no. 2, pp. 479–488, 2016.

[10] J. M. Trotter, L. Hunt, and M. B. Peter, "Ischaemic colitis," *BMJ*, vol. 355, Article ID i6600, 2016.

[11] S. Yadav, M. Dave, J. E. Varayil et al., "A population-based study of incidence, risk factors, clinical spectrum, and outcomes of ischemic colitis," *Clinical Gastroenterology and Hepatology*, vol. 13, no. 4, pp. 731–738.e1-6, 2015.

[12] Y. Yngvadottir, B. R. Karlsdottir, J. P. Hreinsson et al., "The incidence and outcome of ischemic colitis in a population-based setting," *Scandinavian Journal of Gastroenterology*.vol. 52, no. 6–7, pp. 704–710, 2017.

[13] S. O'Neill and S. Yalamarthi, "Systematic review of the management of ischaemic colitis," *Colorectal Disease*, vol. 14, no. 11, pp. e751–e763, 2012.

[14] C. Su, L. J Brandt, S. H Sigal et al., "The immunohistological diagnosis of *E. coli* O157:H7 colitis: possible association with colonic ischemia," *The American Journal of Gastroenterology*, vol. 93, no. 7, pp. 1055–1059, 1998.

[15] J. K. Oh, M. Meiselman, and L. E. Lataif Jr., "Ischemic colitis caused by oral hyperosmotic saline laxatives," *Gastrointestinal Endoscopy*, vol. 45, no. 3, pp. 319–322, 1997.

[16] J.-S. Baudet, V. Castro, and I. Redondo, "Recurrent ischemic colitis induced by colonoscopy bowel lavage," *American Journal of Gastroenterology*, vol. 105, no. 3, pp. 700-701, 2010.

[17] S. Ajani, R. T. Hurt, D. A. Teeters, and L. R. Bellmore, "Ischaemic colitis associated with oral contraceptive and bisacodyl use," *BMJ Case Reports*, vol. 2012, Article ID bcr1220115451, 2012.

[18] H. A. Lopez Morra, S. N. Fine, and G. Dickstein, "Colonic ischemia with laxative use in young adults," *The American Journal of Gastroenterology*, vol. 100, no. 9, pp. 2134–2136, 2005.

[19] K. Vaizman, J. Li, K. Iswara, and S. Tenner, "Ischemic colitis induced by the combination of bisacodyl and polyethylene glycol in preparation for colonoscopy: 414," *American Journal of Gastroenterology*, vol. 102, no. 2, p. S267, 2007.

[20] C. K. Lee et al., "A case of ischemic colitis following oral osmotic laxative for bowel preparation," *Intestinal Research*, vol. 6, no. 2, pp. 135–139, 2008.

[21] J. H. You, S. T. Choi, D. H. Kim, D. W. Lee, Y. M. Kim, and H. Y. Lee, "A case of ischemic colitis by oral sulfate free-polyethylene glycol," *Intestinal Research*, vol. 7, no. 2, pp. 129–132, 2009.

[22] e. a. Dholakia A, "Colonic ischemia in a young patient: who to blame?" in *Proceedings of the Presented at the 75th Annual Scientific Meeting of the American College of Gastroenterolog*, San Antonio, TX, USA, October 2010.

[23] M. Sherid, H. Sifuentes, S. Samo, P. Deepak, and S. Sridhar, "Lubiprostone induced ischemic colitis," *World Journal of Gastroenterology*, vol. 19, no. 2, pp. 299–303, 2013.

[24] J. Behzadi, R. Kanuru, and J. R. Groce, "Biliary colic and jaundice presenting as ampullary neuroendocrine tumor," *American Journal of Gastroenterology*, vol. 110, pp. S72–S153, 2015.

[25] Z. H. Marks: HalfLytely and Bisacodyl Bowel Prep Kit.

[26] A. L. Flores-Mireles, J. N. Walker, M. Caparon, and S. J. Hultgren, "Urinary tract infections: epidemiology, mechanisms of infection and treatment options," *Nature Reviews Microbiology*, vol. 13, no. 5, pp. 269–284, 2015.

[27] N. M. Wheeldon and M. J. Grundman, "Ischaemic colitis as a complication of colonoscopy," *BMJ*, vol. 301, no. 6760, pp. 1080-1081, 1990.

[28] M. Arhan, İ. K. Önal, B. Ödemis, M. İbiş, and N. Şaşmaz, "Colonoscopy-induced ischemic colitis in a young patient with no risk factor," *The American Journal of Gastroenterology*, vol. 104, no. 1, pp. 250-251, 2009.

[29] A. Versaci, A. Macrì, G. Scuderi et al., "Ischemic colitis following colonoscopy in a systemic lupus erythematosus patient: report of a case," *Diseases of the Colon & Rectum*, vol. 48, no. 4, pp. 866–869, 2005.

[30] K. Kao, A. Jain, and A. Sheinbaum, "Ischemic colitis following routine screening colonoscopy: a case report," *Endoscopy*, vol. 41, no. Suppl 2, p. E100, 2009.

[31] J. M. Church, "Ischemic colitis complicating flexible endoscopy in a patient with connective tissue disease," *Gastrointestinal Endoscopy*, vol. 41, no. 2, pp. 181-182, 1995.

[32] M. I. Cremers, A. P. Oliveira, and J. Freitas, "Ischemic colitis as a complication of colonoscopy," *Endoscopy*, vol. 30, no. 4, p. S54, 1998.

[33] Q. Dong, Q. Wang, and Y. Li, "Ischemic colitis after colonoscopy in a female patient," *The American Journal of Gastroenterology*, vol. 104, no. 8, pp. 2123-2124, 2009.

[34] G. Singh-Ranger, A. Halls, A. Grundy, and D. Kumar, "An unusual case of severe colitis after colonoscopy," *Journal of Crohn's Colitis*, vol. 5, no. 3, pp. 267-268, 2011.

[35] Y. C. Cheng, C. C. Wu, C. C. Lee, T. Y. Lee, and K. C. Hsiao, "Rare complication following screening colonoscopy: ischemic colitis," *Digestive Endoscopy*, vol. 24, no. 5, p. 379, 2012.

[36] F. Sapmaz, I. H. Kalkan, S. Güliter, and Y. K. Bilgili, "Ischemic colitis in a young woman following colonoscopy," *Wiener Klinische Wochenschrift*, vol. 126, no. 23–24, pp. 815-816, Dec 2014.

[37] S. O. Lee et al., "Colonoscopy-induced ischemic colitis in patients without risk factors," *World Journal of Gastroenterology*, vol. 20, no. 13, pp. 3698–3702, 2014.

[38] E. da Silva, "Ischemic colitis after a routine colonoscopy: report of two cases," *American Journal of Gastroenterology*, vol. 109, p. S397, 2014.

[39] Z. Hai-Bo, "Colonoscopy induced ischemic colitis: a case report and literature review," *Journal Cytology and Histology*, vol. S329 pages, 2015.

[40] H. Omar, S. Siglin, and M. Fine, "Ischemic colitis after routine colonoscopy," *Digestive Endoscopy*, vol. 27, no. 6, p. 710, 2015.

[41] D. B. Solanke, N. M. Pipaliya, A. N. Chaubal, M. A. Ingle, and P. D. Sawant, "Post colonoscopy ischaemic colitis in a patient without risk factors for colon ischemia: a case report," *Journal of Clinical and Diagnostic Research*, vol. 10, no. 10, pp. OD10–OD11, 2016.

[42] S. J. Boley, G. P Agrawal, A. R Warren et al., "Pathophysiologic effects of bowel distention on intestinal blood flow," *American Journal of Surgery*, vol. 117, no. 2, pp. 228–234, 1969.

[43] C. Washington and J. Carmichael, "Management of ischemic colitis," *Clinics in Colon and Rectal Surgery*, vol. 25, no. 4, pp. 228–235, 2012.

[44] S. K. Lo, L. L. Fujii-Lau, B. K. Enestvedt et al., "The use of carbon dioxide in gastrointestinal endoscopy," *Gastrointestinal Endoscopy*, vol. 83, no. 5, pp. 857–865, 2016.

[45] M. S. Sajid, J. Caswell, M. I. Bhatti, P. Sains, M. K. Baig, and W. F. A. Miles, "Carbon dioxide insufflationvsconventional air insufflation for colonoscopy: a systematic review and meta-analysis of published randomized controlled trials," *Colorectal Disease*, vol. 17, no. 2, pp. 111–123, 2015.

44

Appendiceal Orifice Inflammation in Ulcerative Colitis Mimicking Mucosa-Associated Lymphoid Tissue Lymphoma in the Cecum

Masaya Iwamuro ,[1] Takahide Takahashi,[2] Takehiro Tanaka,[3] Tomohiro Toji,[3] Sakiko Hiraoka,[1] Seiji Kawano,[1] Yoshiro Kawahara,[4] and Hiroyuki Okada[1]

[1]*Department of Gastroenterology and Hepatology, Okayama University Graduate School of Medicine, Dentistry, and Pharmaceutical Sciences, Okayama 700-8558, Japan*
[2]*Division of Medical Support, Okayama University Hospital, Okayama 700-8558, Japan*
[3]*Department of Pathology, Okayama University Graduate School of Medicine, Dentistry, and Pharmaceutical Sciences, Okayama 700-8558, Japan*
[4]*Department of Practical Gastrointestinal Endoscopy, Okayama University Hospital, Okayama 700-8558, Japan*

Correspondence should be addressed to Masaya Iwamuro; pr145h2k@okayama-u.ac.jp

Academic Editor: Olga I. Giouleme

A 55-year-old Japanese woman, who had been diagnosed with ulcerative colitis at 18 years of age, underwent screening endoscopy examinations. Esophagogastroduodenoscopy revealed an extranodal marginal zone lymphoma of mucosa-associated lymphoid tissue (MALT lymphoma) of the stomach. Colonoscopy showed a slightly elevated reddish lesion with dilated microvessels but no erosions or ulcers. Although MALT lymphoma in the cecum was endoscopically suspected, flow cytometry and pathological analyses led to the diagnosis of appendiceal orifice inflammation in ulcerative colitis. This case highlights the diversity of the endoscopic appearance of appendiceal orifice inflammation in ulcerative colitis.

1. Introduction

Ulcerative colitis typically causes continuous inflammation in the colorectal mucosa extending from the rectum to the more proximal colon. However, the peri-appendiceal mucosa in the cecum is sometimes involved in a skip lesion [1–5]. This type of cecal lesion is referred to as "appendiceal orifice inflammation," "peri-appendiceal patch," or "cecal patch." The colonoscopic features of appendiceal orifice inflammation include mucosal erythema, granularity, erosion/ulceration, and friability [1].

We, herein, report a case involving a patient who had ulcerative colitis concomitant with extranodal marginal zone lymphoma of mucosa-associated lymphoid tissue (MALT lymphoma) in the stomach. Of note, although the patient's cecal lesion was initially considered to be involved with the MALT lymphoma, flow cytometry and pathological analyses led to the diagnosis of appendiceal orifice inflammation in ulcerative colitis. Typical endoscopic features of colorectal MALT lymphoma and appendiceal orifice inflammation in ulcerative colitis are discussed later in this report.

2. Case Presentation

A 55-year-old Japanese woman underwent screening esophagogastroduodenoscopy. The patient had been diagnosed with ulcerative colitis at the age of 18 years. Since palmoplantar pustulosis and arthritis of the sternoclavicular and foot joints appeared after anti-tumor necrosis factor-α antibody use, her ulcerative colitis was treated with a mesalazine and *Clostridium butyricum* preparation. She had also been taking fexofenadine, tranexamic acid, and brotizolam for sleep disturbance and prevention of drug allergy. She had a history of *Helicobacter pylori* eradication. Esophagogastroduodenoscopy revealed multiple white irregularly-shaped depressed lesions with partial redness in the gastric body (Figures 1(a) and 1(b)). Narrow-band imaging with magnification showed disappearance of the pit structure and elongated microvessels within the depressed areas (Figures 1(c) and 1(d), arrows), which are the typical features of gastric MALT lymphoma. Biopsy of the gastric lesion revealed the infiltration of small- to medium-sized lymphoid cells (Figure 2(a)), which were positive for CD20 (Figure 2(b)) and negative for CD3 (Figure 2(c)). Immunostaining for cytokeratin (CAM5.2) showed the formation of lymphoepithelial lesions (Figure 2(d)). BIRC3-MALT1 translocation was detected in the neoplastic cells. Lymphoma cells were not detected in the bone marrow on bone marrow aspiration and biopsy examinations. Computed tomography scanning with contrast media showed no lymphadenopathy. Consequently, gastric MALT lymphoma with *t*(11;18)(q21;q21) was diagnosed.

Colonoscopy revealed coarse reddish mucosa with yellowish-white pus-like deposits in the splenic flexure (Figure 3(a)), which are the representative endoscopic features of ulcerative colitis. Atrophic mucosa with multiple ulcer scars was observed in the descending to the sigmoid colon region, consistent with the characteristics of ulcerative colitis in the remission phase. In addition, a reddish flat elevated lesion was observed in the cecum (Figure 4(a)). Linked color imaging with magnification showed elongated microvessels (Figure 4(b)). The partial disappearance of the pit structure and elongated microvessels were observed on narrow-band imaging (Figure 4(c)). Indigo carmine spraying revealed that the areas with no pit structures were slightly depressed, as shown by the pooling of the indigo carmine dye (Figure 4(d)). Papular lesions resembling the lymphoid follicles were observed in the cecum and ascending colon (Figure 4(e)). Due to the similarity of the magnifying endoscopic features between the cecal lesion and the gastric MALT lymphoma, we initially considered the cecal lesion to be involved with the MALT lymphoma. However, flow cytometry analysis using an endoscopic biopsy specimen showed no light chain restriction (Figure 5). On pathological analysis of the biopsied specimens, inflammatory cell infiltration, mainly consisting of mononuclear cells, in addition to some neutrophils was observed (Figure 6). Although the CD20-positive lymphocytes were predominant, the CD3-positive cells were observed as well. Ig κ and Ig λ predominance was not observed on staining, which was consistent with the results of the flow cytometry assay. Thus, we diagnosed the cecal lesion as appendiceal orifice inflammation in ulcerative colitis, rather than being involved with the lymphoma. After discussing with the patient, we decided to manage her gastric MALT lymphoma with a watch-and-wait approach because the lesion was localized in the stomach, and she showed no symptoms, bulky adenopathy, or organ compromise.

3. Discussion

Skip inflammation of the peri-appendiceal region in patients with ulcerative colitis was first described in 1958 by Lumb and Protheroe [1, 6]. Appendiceal orifice inflammation is usually observed during colonoscopy as mucosal erythema, granularity, erosion/ulceration, and friability, all features essentially similar to those observed for continuous inflammation extending proximally from the rectum in ulcerative colitis [1]. In the present patient, a segmental skip lesion showing coarse reddish mucosa with yellowish-white pus-like deposits was observed in the splenic flexure (Figure 3(a)), while reddish flat elevated lesions were observed in the peri-appendiceal region; the skip lesion showed the typical endoscopic features of ulcerative colitis, but the latter did not.

MALT lymphoma generally develops in the stomach, and colorectal involvement in MALT lymphoma is rare. Jeon et al. investigated the endoscopic features of 51 patients with colorectal MALT lymphoma and classified the lesions as subepithelial tumors (51%), polyps (20%), epithelial masses (14%), and ileitis (16%). MALT lymphoma was most frequently observed in the rectum (39%), followed by the ileocecal area (30%) [7]. Won et al. reviewed the data for 73 patients with colorectal MALT lymphomas, 67 of whom were previously reported cases in the literature [8]. Although the endoscopic features were not categorized in detail, the MALT lymphomas were primarily observed as a single polypoid lesion (70%), while multiple polypoid lesions were also observed (30%). These tumors were located in the rectum (74%), right colon (14%), transverse colon (4%), and sigmoid colon (8%). Therefore, a single protruded lesion of a subepithelial tumor or polypoid appearance is the most commonly observed morphology of colorectal MALT lymphomas, which generally involve the rectum, followed by the right colon. However, the endoscopic features of colorectal MALT lymphomas can vary from patient to patient [9–15].

Seo et al. reported a patient with a MALT lymphoma in the transverse colon, which showed a flat elevated lesion with diffuse granularity of the mucosa and loss of vascularity. Narrow-band imaging revealed an abnormal branch-like capillary pattern in patches [16]. These macroscopic appearances were similar to those of the present patient's cecal lesion. In addition, the features of the cecal lesion of the present patient resembled those of her gastric MALT lymphoma lesions, as observed on narrow-band imaging with magnification; both lesions showed disappearance of the pit structure and elongated microvessels within the depressed areas (Figures 1(c), 1(d), and 4(c)). Based on the similarity in characteristics with those of the gastric MALT lymphoma lesion and of the previously reported patient with colonic MALT lymphoma and the dissimilarity with the typical features of ulcerative colitis, we initially considered the cecal lesion to be involved with the MALT lymphoma. However, the pathological diagnosis was appendiceal orifice inflammation, rather than a neoplastic lesion. These results underscore that appendiceal orifice inflammation in

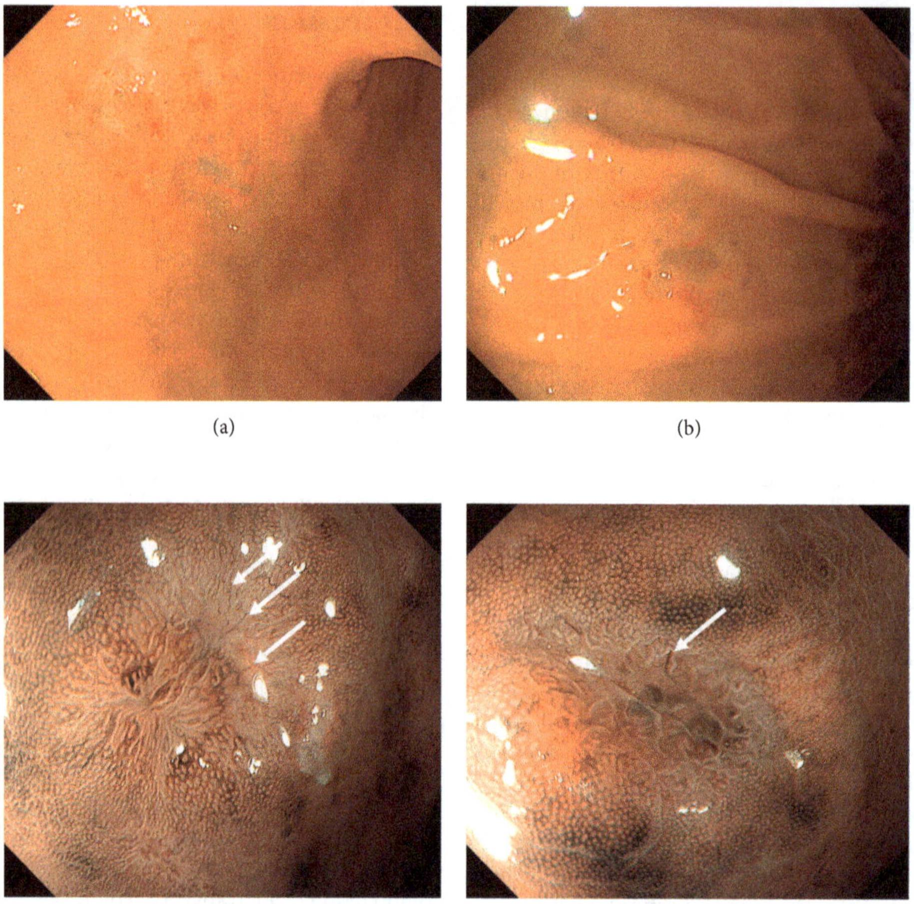

(a) (b)

(c) (d)

FIGURE 1: Esophagogastroduodenoscopy images. Multiple white irregularly shaped depressed lesions with partial redness are seen in the gastric body (a, b). Magnified narrow-band imaging images show the disappearance of the pit structure and elongated microvessels within the depressed areas (c, d, arrows). These microstructures are typical of gastric MALT lymphoma. MALT: mucosa-associated lymphoid tissue.

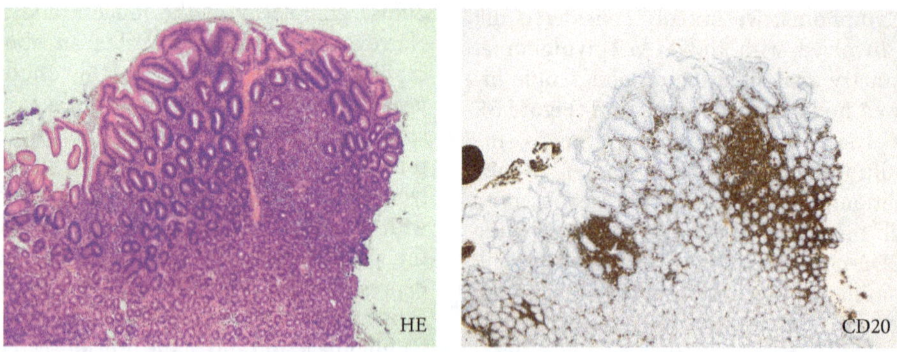

(a) (b)

FIGURE 2: Continued.

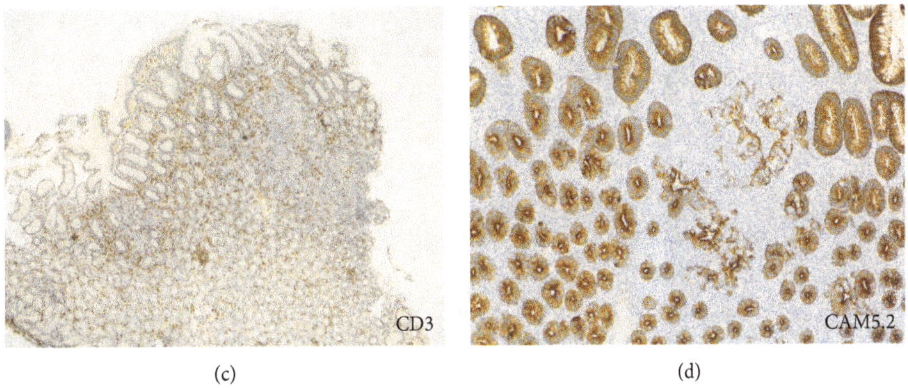

FIGURE 2: Images of the pathologic analysis of the gastric lesion. Small to medium sized lymphoid cells are observed in the biopsy specimens (a). These cells are positive for CD20 (b) and negative for CD3 (c). Immunostaining for cytokeratin (CAM5.2) shows the formation of lymphoepithelial lesions (d). Gastric MALT lymphoma was diagnosed.

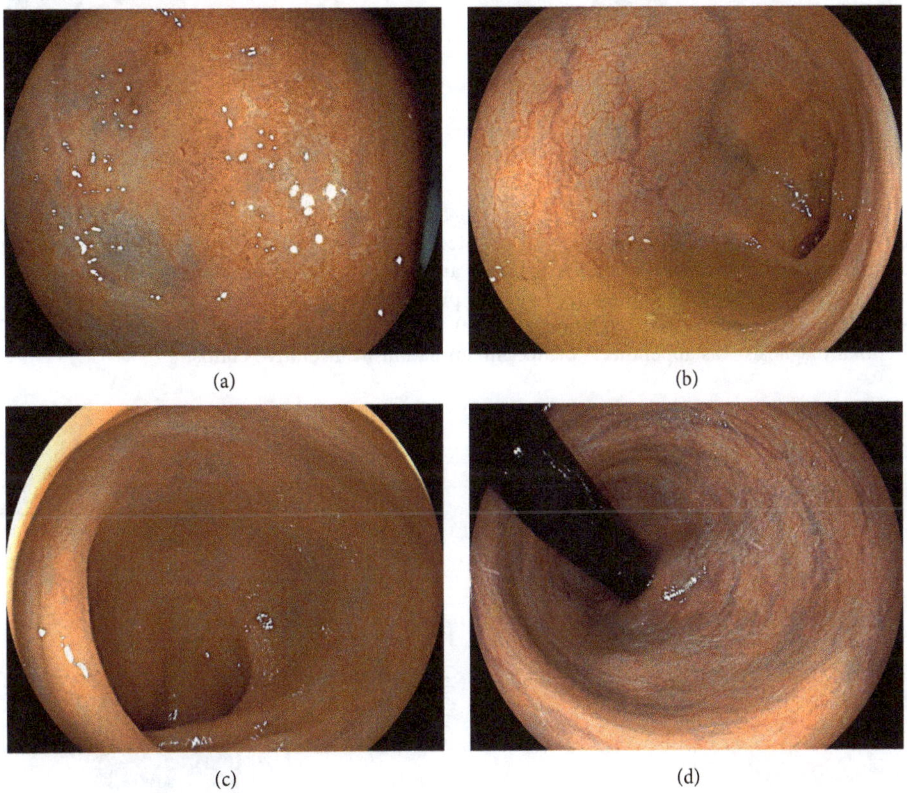

FIGURE 3: Colonoscopy images. Coarse reddish mucosa with yellowish-white pus-like deposits is observed in the splenic flexure (a). Atrophic mucosa with multiple ulcer scars is also seen in the descending to sigmoid colon region (b–d). These endoscopic findings are consistent with those for ulcerative colitis.

ulcerative colitis may present various morphologies and masquerade as a lymphoma.

For the present patient, flow cytometry analysis performed using an endoscopic biopsy specimen aided in establishing the prompt nonlymphoma diagnosis. Flow cytometric immunophenotyping is a sensitive and accurate method for the diagnosis of lymphomas that enables the detection and characterization of neoplastic lymphocytes. Since B-cell lymphomas generally develop due to the unrestricted growth of a particular clone of B cells, neoplastic cells express only one class of immunoglobulin light chain, which is either a κ or λ chain. Thus, light chain restriction is the hallmark of B-cell lymphomas. For the present patient, the flow cytometry results were obtained on the day of colonoscopy, resulting in the timely achievement of the nonlymphoma diagnosis.

In Japan, flow cytometry has not typically been used to diagnose gastrointestinal lymphoma, as an appropriate

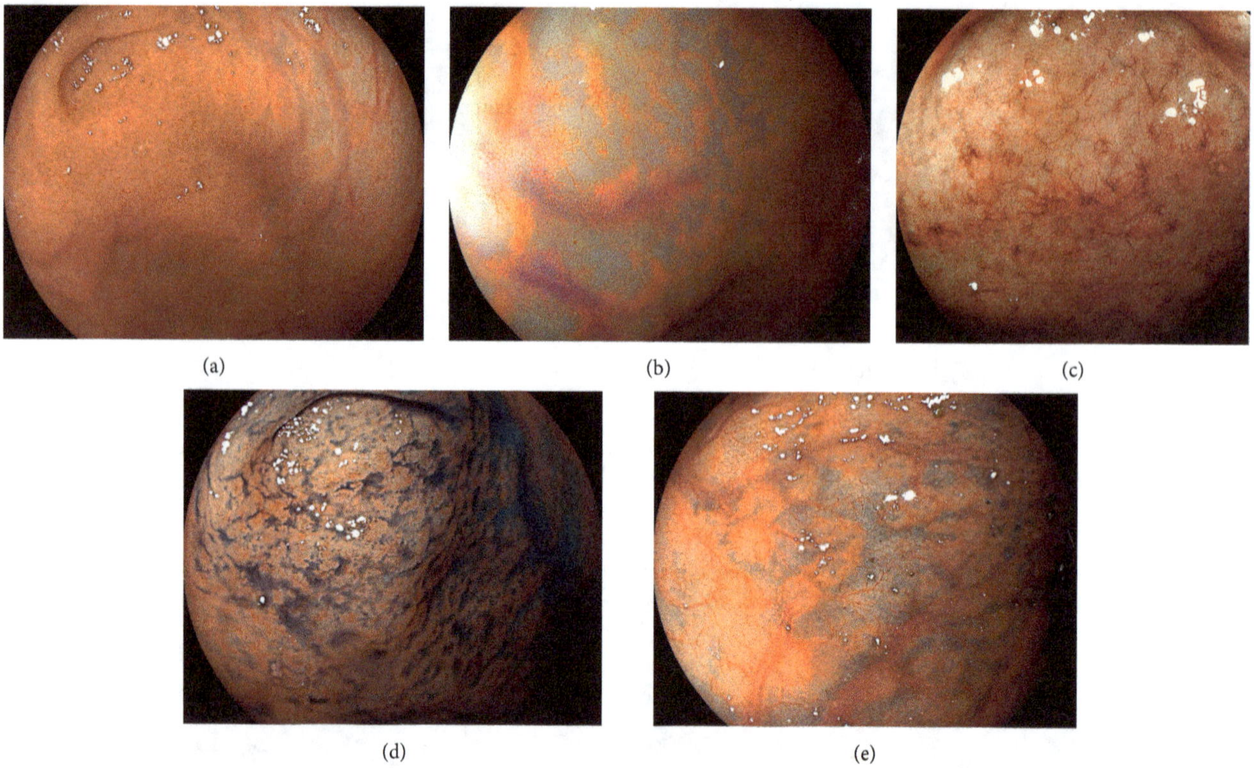

Figure 4: Colonoscopy images of the cecum. A reddish flat elevated lesion is seen (a). Magnified linked color imaging image shows elongated microvessels (b). Partial disappearance of the pit structure and elongated microvessels are observed in the narrow-band imaging image (c). Indigo carmine spraying reveals that the areas with no pit structures are slightly depressed (d). Papular lesions resembling lymphoid follicles are observed in the cecum and ascending colon (e). Although we initially considered this lesion to be involved with the MALT lymphoma, the final diagnosis was appendiceal orifice inflammation in ulcerative colitis.

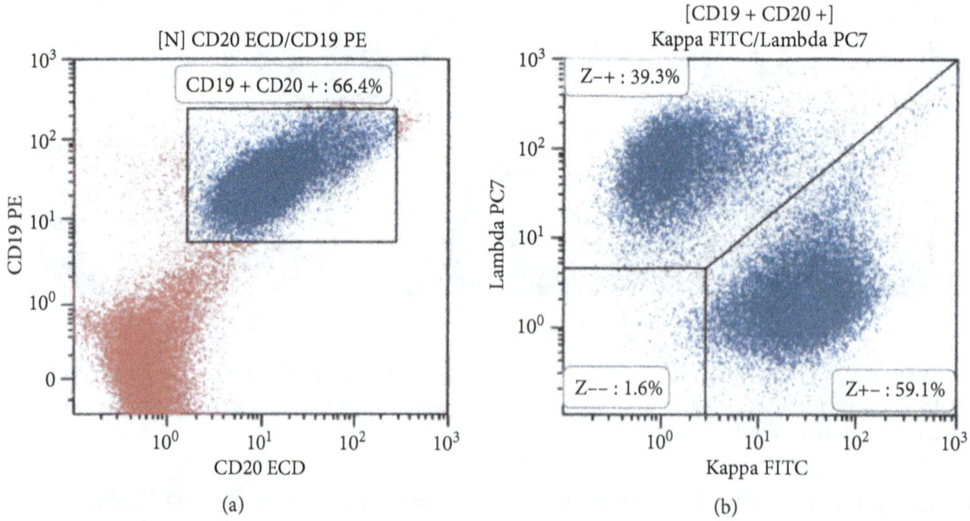

Figure 5: Flow cytometry analysis results. We used an endoscopic biopsy specimen for flow cytometry analysis; light chain restriction was not observed. $CD19^+$ and $CD20^+$ cells are gated (a), and light chain expression analysis reveals an almost equal number of Ig κ- and Ig λ-producing cells (b).

protocol has not yet been established for lymphocyte isolation from endoscopic biopsy specimens. We recently established lymphocyte isolation techniques and used them to confirm that light chain expression analysis can be performed on such specimens [17, 18]. However, even at our facility, only a limited number of endoscopists are able to

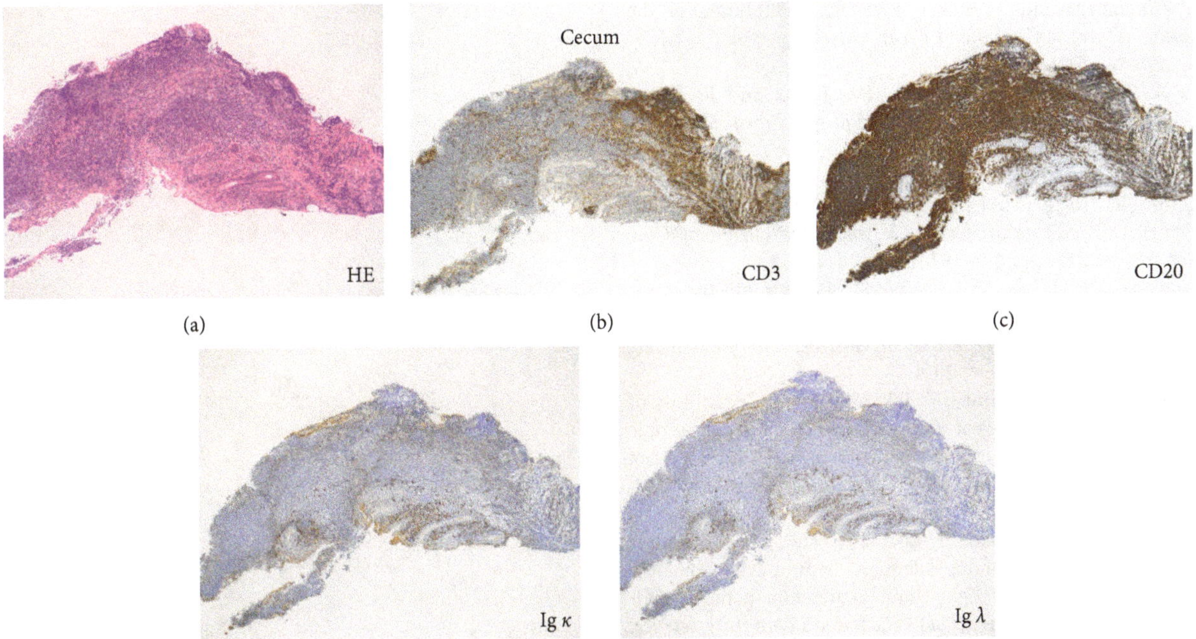

(a) (b) (c) (d) (e)

FIGURE 6: Images of the pathologic analyses of the cecal lesion. Inflammatory cell infiltration, mainly consisting of mononuclear cells, in addition to some neutrophils is observed in the biopsy specimens (a). Although CD20-positive lymphocytes are predominant (b), CD3-positive cells are observed as well (c). Predominance of neither Ig κ (d) nor Ig λ (e) is observed on staining.

perform this analysis using our newly developed methods. Therefore, flow cytometry was not performed with gastric MALT lymphoma lesion samples. Nevertheless, we anticipate that our lymphocyte isolation technique will be widely used in the future for routine clinical diagnosis of gastrointestinal lymphoma.

In conclusion, this case highlights the diversity of the endoscopic appearance of appendiceal orifice inflammation in ulcerative colitis. Although pathological analysis is essential for the differentiation of nonlymphoma lesions from lymphomas, flow cytometry analysis has the advantage of delivering results rapidly.

References

[1] S. H. Park, E. V. Loftus Jr, and S. K. Yang, "Appendiceal skip inflammation and ulcerative colitis," *Digestive Diseases and Sciences*, vol. 59, no. 9, pp. 2050–2057, 2014.

[2] P. Deng and J. Wu, "Meta-analysis of the association between appendiceal orifice inflammation and appendectomy and ulcerative colitis," *Revista Espanola de Enfermedades Digestivas*, vol. 108, no. 7, pp. 401–410, 2016.

[3] H. Anzai, K. Hata, J. Kishikawa et al., "Appendiceal orifice inflammation is associated with proximal extension of disease in patients with ulcerative colitis," *Colorectal Disease*, vol. 18, no. 8, pp. 278–282, 2016.

[4] S. H. Park, S.-K. Yang, S.-K. Park et al., "Atypical distribution of inflammation in newly diagnosed ulcerative colitis is not rare," *Canadian Journal of Gastroenterology and Hepatology*, vol. 28, no. 3, pp. 125–130, 2014.

[5] A. Parian, B. Limketkai, J. Koh et al., "Appendectomy does not decrease the risk of future colectomy in UC: results from a large cohort and meta-analysis," *Gut*, vol. 66, no. 8, pp. 1390–1397, 2017.

[6] G. Lumb and R. H. B. Protheroe, "Ulcerative colitis," *Gastroenterology*, vol. 34, no. 3, pp. 381–407, 1958.

[7] M. K. Jeon, H. So, J. Huh et al., "Endoscopic features and clinical outcomes of colorectal mucosa-associated lymphoid tissue lymphoma," *Gastrointestinal Endoscopy*, vol. 87, no. 2, pp. 529–539, 2018.

[8] J. H. Won, S. M. Kim, J. W. Kim, J. H. Park, and J. Y. Kim, "Clinical features, treatment and outcomes of colorectal mucosa-associated lymphoid tissue (MALT) lymphoma: literature reviews published in English between 1993 and 2017," *Cancer Management and Research*, vol. 11, pp. 8577–8587, 2019.

[9] N. Hasegawa, K. Kato, K. Yamada et al., "Extranodal marginal zone B-cell lymphoma of mucosa-associated lymphoid tissue (MALT) of the sigmoid colon," *Gastrointestinal Endoscopy*, vol. 52, no. 6, pp. 802–804, 2000.

[10] B. Dragosics, P. Bauer, and T. Radaszkiewicz, "Primary gastrointestinal non-Hodgkin's lymphomas. A retrospective clinicopathologic study of 150 cases," *Cancer*, vol. 55, no. 5, pp. 1060–1073, 1985.

[11] T. Matsumoto, M. Shimizu, M. Iida, K. Amano, S. Nakamura, and M. Fujishima, "Primary low-grade, B-cell, mucosa-associated lymphoid tissue lymphoma of the colorectum: clinical and colonoscopic features in six cases," *Gastrointestinal Endoscopy*, vol. 48, no. 5, pp. 501–508, 1998.

[12] T. Yoshino, K. Ichimura, T. Mannami et al., "Multiple organ mucosa-associated lymphoid tissue lymphomas often involve the intestine," *Cancer*, vol. 91, no. 2, pp. 346–353, 2001.

[13] J. Romaguera and F. B. Hagemeister, "Lymphoma of the colon," *Current Opinion in Gastroenterology*, vol. 21, no. 1, pp. 80–84, 2005.

[14] C. S. Chim, T. W. H. Shek, L. P. Chung, and R. Liang, "Unusual abdominal tumors," *Journal of Clinical Oncology*, vol. 21, no. 5, pp. 953–955, 2003.

[15] H. Abbas, M. Niazi, and J. Makker, "Mucosa-associated lymphoid tissue (MALT) lymphoma of the colon: a case report and a literature review," *American Journal of Case Reports*, vol. 18, pp. 491–497, 2017.

[16] S.-W. Seo, S. H. Lee, D. J. Lee et al., "Colonic mucosa-associated lymphoid tissue lymphoma identified by chromoendoscopy," *World Journal of Gastroenterology*, vol. 20, no. 48, pp. 18487–18494, 2014.

[17] K. Matsueda, M. Iwamuro, T. Takahashi et al., "Feasibility of flow cytometric analysis of restricted light chain in endoscopic biopsy specimens from patients with gastrointestinal tract B cell lymphoma: a pilot study," *BMC Research Notes*, vol. 12, no. 1, p. 571, 2019.

[18] M. Iwamuro, K. Matsueda, T. Takahashi et al., "An endoscopic biopsy specimen contains adequate lymphocytes for flow cytometric analysis of light chain expression in the gastrointestinal mucosa," *Annals of Clinical and Laboratory Science*, vol. 50, no. 3, pp. 348–353, 2020.

45

A Case of Gastric Intramural Hematoma Caused by Anisakis Infection

Sang Jin Lee

Department of Internal Medicine, University of Ulsan College of Medicine, Gangneung Asan Hospital, Gangneung, Republic of Korea

Correspondence should be addressed to Sang Jin Lee; sangjin@naver.com

Academic Editor: Yoshihiro Moriwaki

A sixty-year-old lady admitted complaining of epigastric pain and hematemesis. On admission, esophagogastroduodenoscopic examination revealed ruptured intramural hematoma on the antrum of stomach. Eight days later, follow-up EGD showed improving ruptured intramural hematoma and one anisakis larva. Therefore, the gastric intramural hematoma was considered to be caused by anisakis infection. She recovered after ten days of conservative treatment.

1. Introduction

Intramural hematoma of the gastrointestinal tract is a rare disease. In the upper gastrointestinal tract, most of intramural hematomas are localized either in the esophagus or in the duodenum. Gastric intramural hematoma was rarely found [1]. It can result from recurrent vomiting, endoscopic therapy, peptic ulcer disease, and trauma. It is associated with coagulopathy and anticoagulation therapy [2, 3].

Anisakis infection can occur due to ingestion of raw fish or undercooked seafood. The raw fish includes pollack, sea eel, croaker, conger, long-legged octopus, and squid. The most common symptom of anisakiasis is abdominal pain. Nausea and vomiting, hematemesis and melena, and chest discomfort are followed by abdominal pain. Endoscopic findings of anisakis infection are worms, mucosal edema, erythema, pseudotumor, mucosal fold thickening, and mucosal erosion [4].

A case of gastric intramural hematoma caused by anisakis infection is very rare. Therefore, we report this case with a review of literature.

2. Case Report

A 60-year-old female visited our emergency department complaining of epigastric pain and hematemesis. She ate sliced raw fish one day ago. She had hypertension. There was no noteworthy fact in her social and family history. She did not take any antiplatelet drug and anticoagulation drug. On her initial visit, blood pressure was 105/91 mmHg, pulse rate was 72 beats per minute, respiratory rate was 24 breaths per minute, and body temperature was 37.2°C. In abdominal physical examination, there was pain and tenderness in the epigastric area. But there was no rebound tenderness and muscle rigidity. The bowel sound was normal. In laboratory test, the white blood cell count was 14,900/mm^3, hemoglobin was 10 g/dL, and platelet count was 199,000/mm^3. The result of coagulation test was PT 1.13 (INR) and aPTT 24.4 sec. The result of blood chemistry was total protein 5.9 g/dL, albumin 3.5 g/dL, AST 27 IU/L, ALT 11 IU/L, ALP 118 IU/L, total bilirubin 0.6 mg/dL, BUN 21.2 mg/dL, creatinine 0.8 mg/dL, Na 142 mEq/L, K 3.8 mEq/L, Cl 106 mmol/L, CRP 0.08 mg/dL, and blood sugar 145 mg/dL.

Abdominal computed tomography scan showed about 8×3 cm nonenhancing mass in the stomach antrum and lower body. The Hounsfield unit of mass was 50~60 units (Figure 1(a)). It suggested submucosal hematoma in stomach.

Emergent esophagogastroduodenoscopy was performed. A pool of blood was on the greater curvature side of body in the stomach. Greater than 5 cm-sized mass was noted on the anterior wall of body and antrum. The mass was round, dark

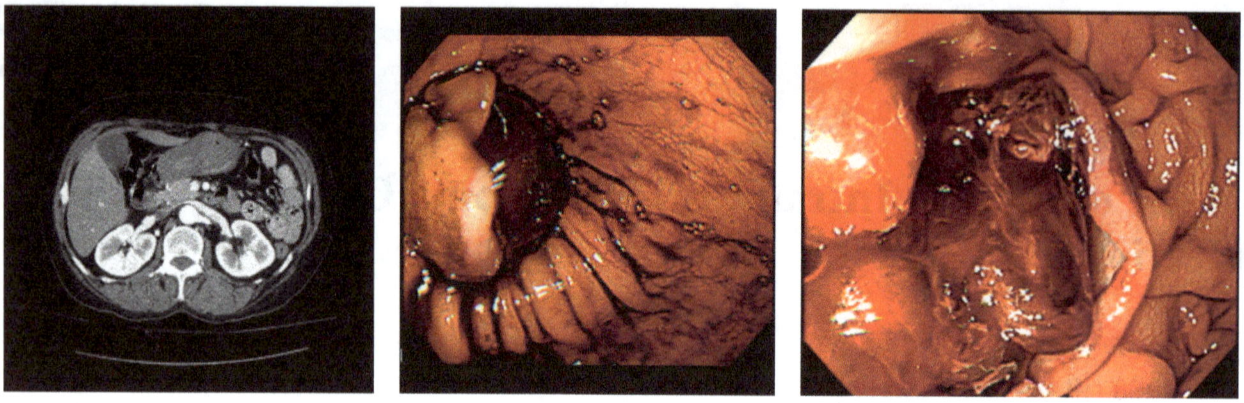

(a) (b) (c)

FIGURE 1: (a) Abdominal computed tomography scan showing about 8 × 3 cm nonenhancing mass (50~60 Hounsfield unit) in the stomach antrum and lower body, suggesting submucosal hematoma. (b) Gastroscopy showing ruptured intramural hematoma on the anterior wall of antrum and low body. (c) Gastroscopy showing ruptured mucosa and hematoma in inside the mucosa wall.

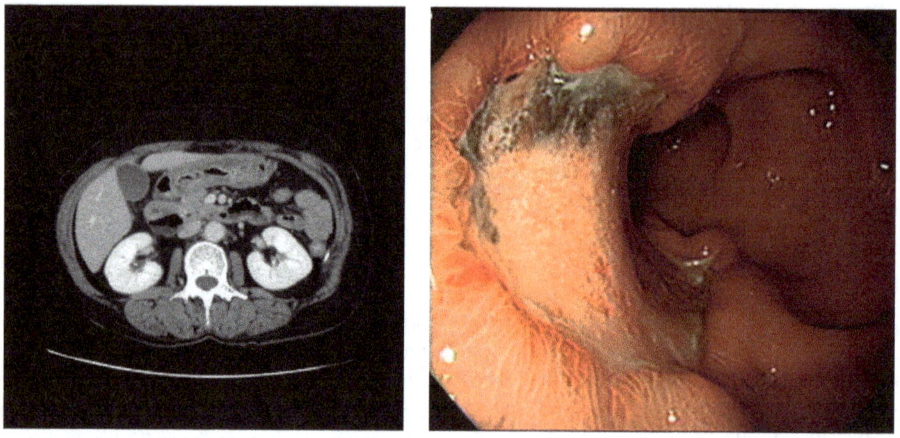

(a) (b)

FIGURE 2: (a) Significant decreased size of hematoma in the stomach antrum and lower body compared with previous computed tomography. No visible active bleeding in stomach is observed. (b) Gastroscopy showing active ulcer on the anterior wall of the antrum and low body.

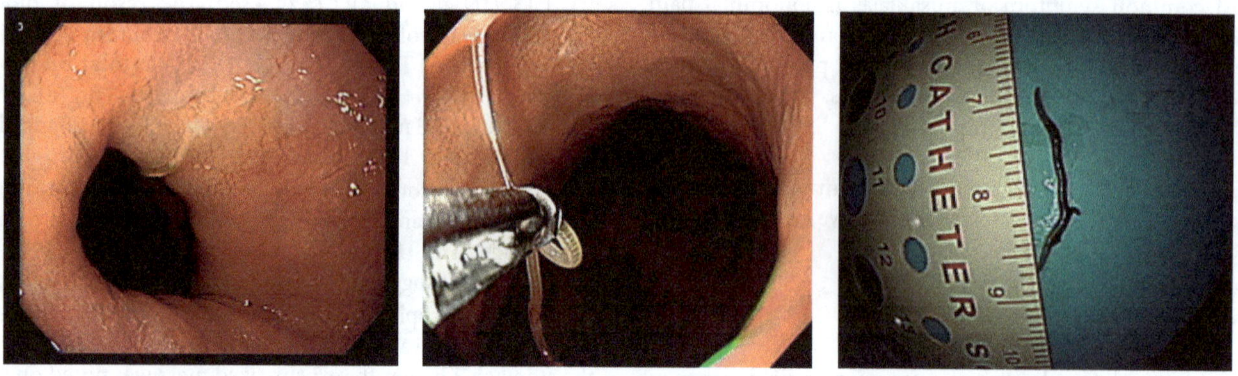

(a) (b) (c)

FIGURE 3: (a) Gastroscopy showing whitish thread-like worm on gastroesophageal junction. (b) Gastroscopic finding: the whitish thread-like worm is being removed by using a biopsy forcep. (c) Gross finding showing 2 cm whitish thread-like worm, identified as anisakis larva.

brownish. But surrounding mucosa was normal. The overlying mucosa of mass was ruptured. Dark red hematoma was noted inside the mass (Figure 1(b)). Removal of hematoma and hemostasis could not be performed owing to noncooperation of the patient.

She was diagnosed with ruptured intramural hematoma. We decided to treat conservatively because further bleeding was not occurred. We treated with intravenous proton pump inhibitor and fluids. In addition, we made her fasting for one week.

On hospital day 8, the gastric intramural hematoma has disappeared in the follow-up abdominal CT scan (Figure 2(a)). On follow-up EGD, the gastric intramural hematoma on anterior wall of low body and proximal antrum has disappeared. EGD showed active ulcer on the same site (Figure 2(b)). At that time, EGD showed a whitish worm resembling a short thread. The worm moved at the gastroesophageal junction. The worm was removed out of the body by using a biopsy forcep. The worm was a 2 cm-sized nematode. It was confirmed as anisakis (Figures 3(a)–3(c)).

Then, the meal was served. Further bleeding was not occurred. The patient was recovered and discharged without other complications.

3. Discussion

Intramural hematoma of the gastrointestinal tract is a rare disease. It can result from recurrent vomiting, endoscopic therapy, peptic ulcer disease, and trauma. It is associated with coagulopathy and anticoagulation therapy. The case of spontaneous duodenal intramural hematoma was reported in Henoch–Schönlein purpura. The case of biopsy-induced gastric intramural hematoma was reported. The case of epinephrine injection-induced intramural hematoma in liver cirrhosis was reported [5]. Rohrer et al. reported four cases of duodenal hematoma and one case of gastric hematoma in 227 bleeding peptic ulcer [3].

Anisakiasis is becoming clinical and epidemiological problem owing to the changes in diet style. Anisakis is a genus of parasitic nematodes that have lifecycles involving fish and marine mammals. Anisakiasis can be occurred due to ingestion of raw fish or undercooked seafood. The rates of anisakis infection are 68% in the stomach and 30% in the small intestine. Symptoms of anisakiasis are sudden epigastric pain, nausea, and vomiting. From two to ten hours after eating raw fish and seafood, the symptoms develop.

Intramural esophagogastric hematoma in hemophilia caused by tuberculosis infection was reported [6]. However, a report of gastric intramural hematoma caused by anisakis infection has not been published. To our knowledge, this case is the first English-written report of gastric intramural hematoma caused by anisakis infection. Anisakis larva goes through mucosa and muscle and can injure submucosal vessels. Bleeding from injured submucosal vessels can lead to intramural hematoma.

In this case, the location of anisakis and intramural hematoma was different. Intramural hematoma was at the anterior wall of body and antrum. But anisakis larva was at the gastroesophageal junction. Anisakis larva can move around inside the stomach. Therefore, the location of anisakis and intramural hematoma may be different.

Gastric intramural hematoma secondary to coagulopathy and anticoagulation therapy are treated conservatively. Conservative treatment is based on resolution of intramural hematoma due to high vascularity in the submucosa. In Vivek Dhawan et al. 's report, six reported cases of gastric hematoma secondary to hemophilia were managed with transfusion. One of them died from ongoing hemorrhage. Four cases related to anticoagulation therapy were treated conservatively. One of the four cases underwent arterial embolization [7]. If further bleeding is noted during conservative management, surgical approach is considered. In this case, the patients were recovered through conservative treatment in a week.

In summary, we reported a case of gastric intramural hematoma caused by anisakis infection. Gastric intramural hematoma may be one of the symptoms associated with anisakis infection.

References

[1] C. E. Hughes, J. Conn, and J. O. Sherman, "Intramural hematoma of the gastrointestinal tract," *The American Journal of Surgery*, vol. 133, no. 3, pp. 276–279, 1977.

[2] W. R. Jones, W. J. Hardin, J. T. Davis, and J. D. Hardy, "Intramural hematoma of the duodenum," *Annals of Surgery*, vol. 173, no. 4, pp. 534–544, 1971.

[3] B. Rohrer, J. Schreiner, P. Lehnert, H. Waldner, and W. Heldwein, "Gastrointestinal intramural hematoma, a complication of endoscopic injection methods for bleeding peptic ulcers: a case series," *Endoscopy*, vol. 26, no. 7, pp. 617–621, 1994.

[4] W. H. Lee, S. S. Yoo, H. J. Kim, T. H. Kim, and O. J. Lee, "Endoscopic and clinical characteristics of gastrointestinal parasite infections," *Clin Endosc*, vol. 35, no. 5, pp. 304–312, 2007.

[5] S. Maimone, F. Saffioti, R. Filomia et al., "Elective endoscopic variceal ligation is not a risk factor for bacterial infection in patients with liver cirrhosis," *Digestive and Liver Disease*, vol. 50, no. 4, pp. 366–369, 2018.

[6] T. Intragumtornchai, S. Israsena, V. Benjacholamard, S. Lerdlum, and S. Benjavongkulchai, "Esophageal tuberculosis presenting as intramural esophagogastric hematoma in a hemophiliac patient," *Journal of Clinical Gastroenterology*, vol. 14, no. 2, pp. 152–156, 1992.

[7] V. Dhawan, A. Mohamed, and R. N. Fedorak, "Gastric intramural hematoma: a case report and literature review," *Canadian Journal of Gastroenterology*, vol. 23, no. 1, pp. 19–22, 2009.

46

Intestinal Tuberculosis Presenting with Gastrointestinal Bleeding in Patient on Warfarin Therapy

Werimo Pascal Kuka, Joe Rakiro, Joseph Gatheru, Felix Riunga, and Allan Rajula

Aga Khan University Hospital Nairobi, 4th Floor East Tower Block, Third Avenue Parklands, P.O. Box 30270, Nairobi 00100, GPO, Kenya

Correspondence should be addressed to Werimo Pascal Kuka; wpkuka@yahoo.com

Academic Editor: Daniel C. Damin

Background. Intestinal tuberculosis (ITB) constitutes less than 5% of overall cases of extrapulmonary disease and mostly affects the ileocecal region. The presentation and radiologic findings in enteric tuberculosis can mimic Crohn's disease (CD). *Case Presentation.* We present a case report of an African woman who presented to a Kenyan hospital with lower gastrointestinal bleeding while on anticoagulation for valvular atrial fibrillation, and was diagnosed with intestinal tuberculosis after colonoscopy, biopsy, and positive staining for tuberculous bacilli. *Conclusion.* Intestinal tuberculosis causing gastrointestinal bleeding is rare but should be suspected in patients living in TB endemic regions.

1. Introduction

Tuberculosis (TB), an infection caused by *Mycobacterium tuberculosis*, is the tenth leading cause of death worldwide and the most common caused by a single infectious agent in the pre-COVID-19 pandemic era. The World Health Organization (WHO) Global Tuberculosis Report of 2020 estimated that there were 10 million cases of active tuberculosis worldwide and 1.2 million deaths in the preceding year. 90% of the infections were in thirty high TB burden countries including Kenya [1]. The country has an estimated TB prevalence of 558 per 100000 adults [2].

The primary infection site in most cases is the lungs, but virtually any other organ can be affected, which is referred to as extrapulmonary TB (EPTB). Abdominal involvement can be in solid organs, peritoneum, intestine, or lymph nodes. Intestinal tuberculosis (ITB) constitutes less than 5% of overall cases of EPTB cases, and although, it can involve the entire gastrointestinal tract (GIT), the most common sites of involvement are the ileocecal area, colon, and small bowel [3]. In contrast, the upper gastrointestinal tract, namely, the esophagus and stomach are rare sites of infection [4, 5]. Enteric TB can be a result of different modes of spread: direct infection by ingestion of bacilli from infected food or sputum, spread from an adjacent organ, and hematogenous or lymphatic spread [6].

The clinical presentation and diagnostic findings of ITB can mimic other infections, malignancies, and inflammatory bowel disease (IBD) [7]. Although infectious causes predominate in the developing nations, the prevalence of IBD is rising in these countries [8]. Crohn's disease (CD), one of the forms of IBD, shares many clinicopathologic features with GIT TB, and each can lead to misdiagnosis of the other with the risk of deleterious outcomes [9, 10]. This is compounded by the low sensitivities of tests used to ascertain the diagnosis of GIT TB [10, 11].

EPTB has been shown to have worse outcomes in treatment, compared to lung disease [5]. A source of concern in abdominal TB is the risk of complications including fistula formation, perforation, and intestinal obstruction [12]. It is essential that the diagnosis is made and appropriate treatment is initiated. Here, we describe a case of a young female who presented with gastrointestinal bleeding while on warfarin therapy for atrial fibrillation and rheumatic heart disease, whose workup including imaging, endoscopy, and histology established a diagnosis of ITB in the setting of active pulmonary disease. CD was considered a differential diagnosis during the investigation of the patient.

2. Case

A thirty-five-year-old female presented with complaints of per rectal bleeding mixed with stools. She had recurrent episodes associated with crampy lower abdominal pain over a period of five days. Upon further enquiry, she also reported a history of productive cough for three months, night sweats, and weight loss of ten kilograms over the same period. Her medical history was significant for rheumatic heart disease and atrial fibrillation. The patient had a surgical history of mitral valvuloplasty two years prior to her current presentation. Her regular medications included warfarin 5 mg daily, carvedilol 25 mg twice daily, and furosemide 40 mg daily. The examination revealed a sick-looking middle-aged female who had pallor, bipedal edema, and no palpable lymphadenopathy. The precordial examination was positive for features of mitral stenosis and aortic regurgitation. Abdominal examination did not elicit any tenderness or palpable mass. Investigations done included a complete blood count with the following results: white cell count 9.24×10^9/L, hemoglobin 5.30 g/dL, and platelets 572×10^9/L. The prothrombin time was prolonged, and the international normalized ratio (INR) was 2.78. Renal and hepatic function tests were normal. Initial management involved withholding of warfarin and transfusion of three units of packed red cells. An urgent colonoscopy performed to evaluate hematochezia revealed segmental inflammation of the ascending colon with ulcerations and polyps covered with yellowish exudate, a distended ileocecal junction, and an aberrant vascular pattern with mucosal edema extending to the hepatic flexure (Figure 1). At endoscopy, the differential diagnoses were tuberculosis or CD. In view of her respiratory complaints and accompanying systemic symptoms, a computed tomography (CT) of the chest and abdomen was performed, which demonstrated right lung consolidation, focal subsegmental consolidations in the left lung, and subcentimeter-sized lymph nodes in the small bowel mesentery (Figure 2). Given her history of chronic cough and chest imaging findings, a sputum test was requested whose staining was acid-fast bacilli (AFB) positive. Biopsies of the samples obtained during colonoscopy revealed lymphocytic infiltration, necrotizing granulomas, and positivity for AFB (Figure 3). Serologic testing for human immunodeficiency virus (HIV) was negative. A diagnosis of pulmonary and extra pulmonary tuberculosis with gastrointestinal involvement was established. The patient was initiated on the intensive phase of antituberculous therapy consisting of rifampicin (600 mg/day), isoniazid (300 mg/day), ethambutol (800 mg/day), and pyrazinamide (1 g/day). Warfarin 5 mg daily was reinstituted prior to her discharge after a five-day hospital admission. The culture in Löwenstein-Jensen medium later isolated *Mycobacterium tuberculosis* complex, which was susceptible to the first-line drugs. She is followed up at the outpatient clinic with regular INR checks to ensure a therapeutic INR range of 2.0-3.0. Her warfarin dosage was increased from the initial 35 mg/week to 52.5 mg/week by the fourth week after discharge.

3. Discussion

We present a case of ITB in a patient with concomitant pulmonary disease whose main presenting symptom was hematochezia while on warfarin therapy for atrial fibrillation and previous mitral valve surgery. The workup for an etiology of the gastrointestinal bleeding was pursued concurrently with that for her other complains identified on systemic enquiry. Although the patient is from a high TB burden country, a differential diagnosis of CD was considered during the initial investigations.

Extrapulmonary tuberculosis can be a manifestation of coexisting lung disease. The rate of coexistence of pulmonary and ITB has been reported to be in the range of 15–30% [4, 13]. The patient in our case had confirmation of active lung disease in addition to enteric TB. The likely mode of intestinal infection in such cases is ingestion of infected sputum.

The most common presentation of GIT TB is abdominal pain, which is reported by up to three quarters of patients [10, 13, 14]. Other symptoms include weight loss, fever, night sweats, and diarrhea. The patient in our case presented with hematochezia, which is a rare presentation of GIT TB, only seen in 7–20% of cases [10, 12, 13]. The cause of bleeding is postulated to be due to endarteritis caused by the bacilli [12]. A confounder in our case was the patient's use of warfarin. Mucosal inflammation due to infection is the likely major contributor to bleeding in our case. In a study to evaluate the etiology of major gastrointestinal bleeding in patients on anticoagulants, colitis was identified as the culprit lesion in 3% of patients on warfarin therapy [15]. Warfarin was resumed at discharge for our patient after a five-day admission duration. Reinitiation of anticoagulation after a clinically significant lower gastrointestinal bleeding is a challenging decision for clinicians because of the risk of recurrence of bleeding and the benefits of prevention of thromboembolism. Discontinuation of warfarin has been associated with an increased mortality in patients after admission for LGIB. The risk factors associated with mortality were age and medical comorbidities, in particular malignancies [16]. Our patient was young and had a low Charlson comorbidity index, therefore, placing her at low risk of adverse outcomes after the resumption of warfarin. The optimal timing for restarting warfarin is unknown and relies on clinical judgement of when the benefits outweigh the risks. In a review article, Kido and Scalese recommend resumption of warfarin therapy within 7–15 days after a major gastrointestinal bleed [17].

The constellations of symptoms of ITB are nonspecific, leading to either a long duration prior to diagnosis or misdiagnosis. In one report, the diagnosis of enteric TB was not considered initially in more than 60% of patients who had the eventual diagnosis [4]. The mimics include other infections, malignancies, and inflammatory bowel disease.

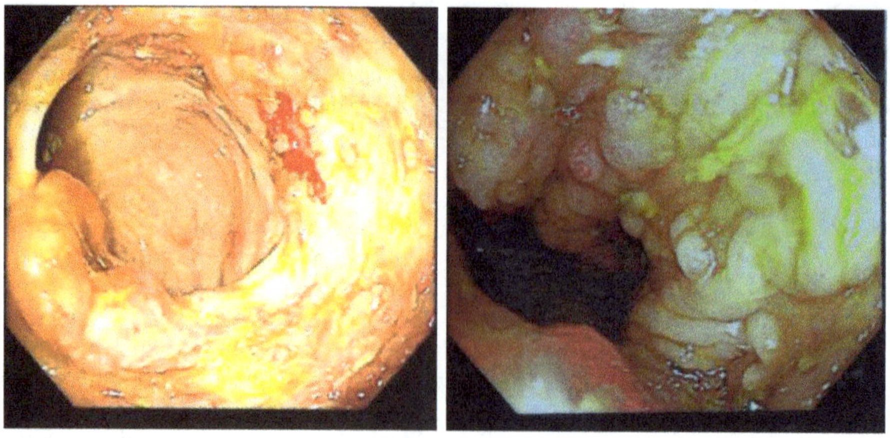

Figure 1: Colonoscopy: ulcerations and polyps in the ileocecal region and ascending colon.

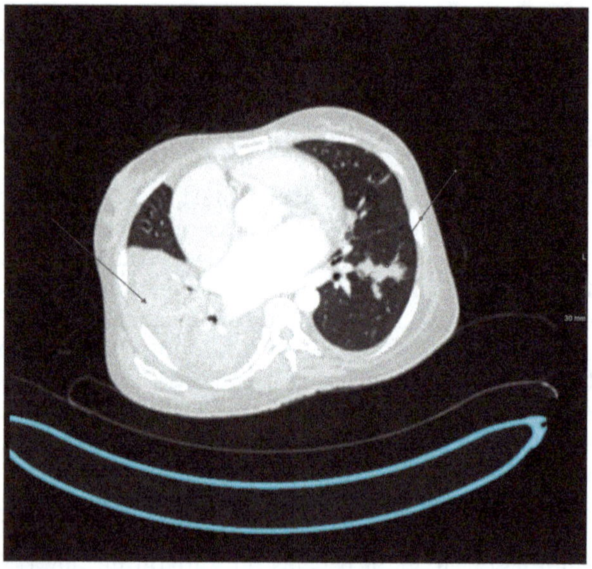

Figure 2: CT chest axial image showing bilateral lung consolidations.

CD was considered as a differential diagnosis during evaluation of our patient. Both ITB and CD have similar clinical, radiological, endoscopic, and pathological features, therefore, making it a challenging clinical problem [10]. In a report from China, in one of the high TB burden countries, up to 17% of patients with ITB were initially misdiagnosed to have CD [13]. Although TB is prevalent in the sub-Saharan African region, an increase in CD is also being reported [8]. It is crucial to identify the correct diagnosis because the use of immunosuppressive medications for CD can lead to flare up of TB with potential disastrous complications [18]. A meta-analysis showed the following features correlating with ITB more than CD: presentation with fever, night sweats, and lung disease. Other features include patulous ileocecal valve, cecal involvement, and presence of granulomas [19]. The patient in our case had all the above features favoring ITB over CD even prior to microbiological confirmation. In particular, the chest imaging findings which prompted sputum evaluation for TB was the key in our evaluation and should be performed in patients with colitis, especially in high TB endemic areas.

The colonoscopy finding of ileocecal involvement in our case was in keeping with other studies as the most common site in ITB [4, 6, 9, 20]. The reasons are postulated to be increased contact time between the mycobacteria and mucosa due to narrowing and stasis. Presence of lymphoid rich tissue in the ileocecal region, to which bacilli have a predilection for infecting, is also a possible contributory factor [21].

Biopsy of intestinal tissue for histology can be achieved by endoscopy as in our case. Other methods include percutaneously with imaging guidance, by endoscopic ultrasound, and surgically, either open or laparoscopic [6]. The demonstration of *Mycobacterium* in intestinal biopsy specimens can be by acid-fast staining, nucleic acid amplification, or culture. In addition, histologic findings of caseating granuloma are considered a hallmark in TB diagnosis [6]. The biopsy from patient in our case was positive for granulomas, AFB staining, and culture. PCR was not performed on the biopsy specimen. Although these tests are key in diagnosis, the sensitivity of any of the tests in ITB is low, with ranges of 5.3–37.5% for AFB tissue staining, 23–46% for mycobacterial culture, and 36.4–67.9% for PCR [19]. Because of the low sensitivities, a majority of patients in the high TB prevalence countries are only diagnosed retrospectively after successful empiric treatment with antituberculous medications despite initial extensive diagnostic investigations [9, 11, 13, 14].

The mainstay of treatment of ITB is medical therapy consisting of combination antituberculous therapy administered during intensive phase and maintenance phase. In drug susceptible TB, as in our case, the first-line medications during a two-month intensive phase are rifampicin, isoniazid, pyrazinamide, and ethambutol. The total duration of treatment is at least six months, though some advocate for extended durations of 9 or 12 months [4, 6]. The shorter course of treatment has been found to be just as effective as an extended period, with the added benefits of better compliance and savings on cost [22]. The role of adjuvant surgery is limited to complications such as intractable bleeding, obstruction, and fistulae [6].

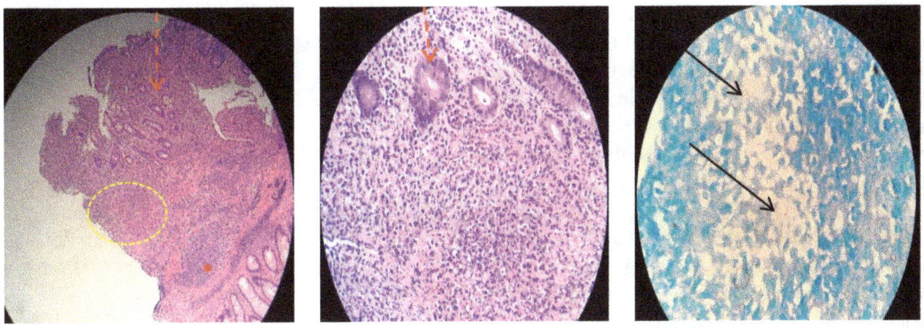

(a) (b) (c)

FIGURE 3: Colonic biopsies. (a) Lamina propria shows expansion by inflammatory cells. A lymphoid aggregate (red asterix), nonneoplastic colonic glands (red dashed arrow), and granuloma are seen (yellow dashed line) (hematoxylin and eosin, original magnification x100). (b) Goblet mucin component decreased as well as cryptitis. Edge of granuloma is seen here (original magnification x200). (c) Acid-fast bacilli (black arrows) (Ziehl–Neelsen stain).

A potential challenge in the outpatient follow-up of this case was the interaction between warfarin and rifampicin. Rifampicin is an inducer of cytochrome P450 hepatic enzymes which metabolize warfarin. Thus, there is a risk of inadequate anticoagulation in patients on both agents. It is recommended that INR be checked every two weeks in such cases and appropriate dose adjustments of warfarin be done to achieve a therapeutic INR.

4. Conclusion

ITB is a manifestation of abdominal spread of disease and should be suspected in patients presenting with gastrointestinal bleeding and constitutive symptoms in endemic areas. Although the clinical, radiologic, and endoscopic features are similar to CD, screening for pulmonary disease and microbiologic staining for specimens obtained during surgery, endoscopy, or radiologically can diagnose TB. The key treatment is a standard course of first-line antituberculous drugs.

Disclosure

An earlier version of this work was presented virtually as a poster at World Gastroenterology Organization Conference GASTRO 2021 held in Prague, December 9–11, 2021.

Authors' Contributions

WPK and JR involved in designing and writing up of the case. JG involved in review of the histology slides. FR and AR reviewed the manuscript and provided critical specialist input. All authors approved the final draft.

Acknowledgments

The authors would like to thank members of their department for their valuable input in reviewing the case.

References

[1] World Health Organization, "Global Tuberculosis Report 2020," World Health Organization, Geneva Switzerland, 2020.

[2] Ministry of Health, "National tuberculosis, leprosy and lung disease program. kenya tuberculosis prevalence survey," 2016, https://www.chskenya.org/wp-content/uploads/2018/04/Final-TB-Prevalence-Survey-Report.pdf.

[3] M. P. Golden and H. R. Vikram, "Extrapulmonary tuberculosis: an overview," *American Family Physician*, vol. 72, no. 9, pp. 1761–1768, 2005.

[4] E. H. Choi and W. J. Coyle, "Gastrointestinal tuberculosis," *Microbiology Spectrum*, vol. 4, no. 6, 2016.

[5] S. A. Ohene, M. I. Bakker, J. Ojo, A. Toonstra, D. Awudi, and P. Klatser, "Extra-pulmonary tuberculosis: a retrospective study of patients in Accra, Ghana," *PLoS One*, vol. 14, no. 1, Article ID e0209650, 2019.

[6] U. Debi, V. Ravisankar, K. K. Prasad, S. K. Sinha, and A. K. Sharma, "Abdominal tuberculosis of the gastrointestinal tract: revisited," *World Journal of Gastroenterology*, vol. 20, no. 40, pp. 14831–14840, 2014.

[7] C. Bolukbas, F. F. Bolukbas, T. Kendir et al., "Clinical presentation of abdominal tuberculosis in HIV seronegative adults," *BMC Gastroenterology*, vol. 5, no. 1, p. 21, 2005.

[8] J. W. Windsor and G. G. Kaplan, "Evolving epidemiology of IBD," *Curr Gastroenterol Reports*, vol. 21, no. 8, p. 40, 2019.

[9] R. Sharma, K. S. Madhusudhan, and V. Ahuja, "Intestinal tuberculosis versus crohn's disease: clinical and radiological recommendations," *Indian Journal of Radiology and Imaging*, vol. 26, no. 02, pp. 161–172, 2016.

[10] S. Kedia, P. Das, K. S. Madhusudhan et al., "Differentiating Crohn's disease from intestinal tuberculosis," *World Journal of Gastroenterology*, vol. 25, no. 4, pp. 418–432, 2019.

[11] S. Kumar, S. Bopanna, S. Kedia et al., "Evaluation of Xpert MTB/RIF assay performance in the diagnosis of abdominal tuberculosis," *Intestinal Research*, vol. 15, no. 2, pp. 187–194, 2017.

[12] H. K. Ha, G. Y. Ko, E. S. Yu et al., "Intestinal tuberculosis with abdominal complications: radiologic and pathologic features," *Abdominal Imaging*, vol. 24, no. 1, pp. 32–38, 1999.

[13] X. C. Shi, L. F. Zhang, Y. Q. Zhang, X. Q. Liu, and G. J. Fei, "Clinical and laboratory diagnosis of intestinal tuberculosis," *Chinese Medical Journal*, vol. 129, no. 11, pp. 1330–1333, 2016.
[14] L. Ma, Q. Zhu, Y. Li et al., "The potential role of CT enterography and gastrointestinal ultrasound in the evaluation of anti-tubercular therapy response of intestinal tuberculosis: a retrospective study," *BMC Gastroenterol*, vol. 19, no. 1, p. 106, 2019.
[15] J. M. Kolb, K. F. Flack, P. Chatterjee-Murphy et al., "Locations and mucosal lesions responsible for major gastrointestinal bleeding in patients on warfarin or dabigatran," *Digestive Diseases and Sciences publishes high-quality*, vol. 63, no. 7, pp. 1878–1889, 2018.
[16] P. Patel, N. Nigam, and N. Sengupta, "Resumption of warfarin after hospitalization for lower gastrointestinal bleeding and mortality benefits," *Journal of Clinical Gastroenterol*, vol. 52, no. 6, pp. 545–550, 2018.
[17] K. Kido and M. J. Scalese, "Management of oral anticoagulation therapy after gastrointestinal bleeding: whether to, when to, and how to restart an anticoagulation therapy," *Annals of Pharmacotherapy*, vol. 51, no. 11, pp. 1000–1007, 2017.
[18] A. P. Abadir, J. Y. Han, and F. A. Youssef, "Intestinal tuberculosis masquerading as crohn's disease? A case of disseminated tuberculosis after anti-TNF therapy for suspected crohn's disease," *Case Reports in Gastrointestinal Medicine*, vol. 2019, Article ID 6053503, 3 pages, 2019.
[19] J. Limsrivilai, A. B. Shreiner, A. Pongpaibul et al., "Meta-analytic bayesian model for differentiating intestinal tuberculosis from crohn's disease," *The American Journal of Gastroenterology*, vol. 112, no. 3, pp. 415–427, 2017.
[20] J. Kentley, J. L. Ooi, J. Potter et al., "Intestinal tuberculosis: a diagnostic challenge," *Tropical Medicine and International Health*, vol. 22, no. 8, pp. 994–999, 2017.
[21] C. Chatzicostas, I. E. Koutroubakis, M. Tzardi, M. Roussomoustakaki, P. Prassopoulos, and E. A. Kouroumalis, "Colonic tuberculosis mimicking Crohn's disease: case report," *BMC Gastroenterology*, vol. 2, no. 1, p. 10, 2002.
[22] S. H. Park, S. K. Yang, D. H. Yang et al., "Prospective randomized trial of six-month versus nine-month therapy for intestinal tuberculosis," *Antimicrobial Agents and Chemotherapy*, vol. 53, no. 10, pp. 4167–4171, 2009.

Cerebral Venous Thrombosis as an Initial Presentation of Ulcerative Colitis

Hiroshi Yamazaki,[1] **Akinori Sasaki**,[1] **Eriko Yamaguchi**,[1] **Kana Sawada**,[2] **Risa Okamoto**,[1] **Kuniyasu Saigusa**,[2] **and Yasuaki Motomura**[1]

[1]*Department of Gastroenterology, Tokyo Bay Urayasu Ichikawa Medical Center, 3-4-32 Toudaijima, Urayasu, 279-0001 Chiba, Japan*
[2]*Department of Neurosurgery, Tokyo Bay Urayasu Ichikawa Medical Center, 3-4-32 Toudaijima, Urayasu, 279-0001 Chiba, Japan*

Correspondence should be addressed to Akinori Sasaki; akinorisasaki6@gmail.com

Academic Editor: Hirotada Akiho

Cerebral venous thrombosis (CVT) is a rare complication of ulcerative colitis (UC) that is potentially fatal once it occurs. This report describes a case of CVT that led to a diagnosis of UC. A 48-year-old woman was diagnosed with CVT due to paresthesia and weakness and was hospitalized for treatment. She developed bloody diarrhea on admission and was further diagnosed with UC based on endoscopic and pathologic findings. Treatment of UC with steroids and sulfasalazine was administered immediately. Her condition improved significantly within several days following treatment. After discharge, the patient experienced no recurrence of either CVT or UC flare-up over the last five years. This report describes CVT as an initial presentation of UC. This is also the first report of a long-term follow-up following successful treatment of CVT with concomitant UC.

1. Introduction

Ulcerative colitis (UC) is a chronic disease characterized by diffuse inflammation of the rectal and colonic mucosa. In recent decades, the incidence of UC has significantly increased in several regions of the world, including Japan [1].

The clinical symptoms of UC include bloody diarrhea, abdominal pain, and tenesmus [2]. Moreover, UC may also present as a systemic disease accompanied by various extraintestinal manifestations. Thromboembolic events, such as deep venous thrombosis and pulmonary embolism, are common manifestations of UC [3]. On the other hand, cerebral venous thrombosis (CVT) is a rare but potentially fatal extraintestinal manifestation of UC [4].

A few cases of CVT due to UC have been reported in the literature, and most of these described the onset of CVT during an acute exacerbation of UC [5]. Simultaneous occurrence of CVT and UC is extremely rare in patients newly diagnosed with UC. This report describes our experience with a patient who presented with CVT, leading to a diagnosis of UC.

2. Case Presentation

A 48-year-old woman was admitted to our hospital with paresthesia and left upper extremity weakness for two days. The patient had a history of occasional bloody stools in the past few months before admission, which were assumed due to hemorrhoids. In addition, she had a recent history of nonbloody, loose stools in the past five days prior to admission. The patient was completely blind due to bilateral enucleation performed for retinoblastoma at one year of age. On physical examination, she was febrile (37.7°C) with pulse rate of 94/min and blood pressure of 132/86 mmHg. Her abdomen was flat with hyperactive bowel sounds and no abdominal tenderness. Neurological examination revealed muscle weakness of the left extremity with a manual muscle testing score of 3/5 and 4/5 in the left upper extremity and left lower extremity, respectively.

Laboratory test results showed low hemoglobin levels of 10 g/dl and a white blood cell count of 5800/mm^3. Erythrocyte sedimentation rate was 22 mm/h during the first hour. C-reactive protein level was elevated (3.26 mg/dl). Prothrombin time/international normalized ratio was 1.11 and activated partial thromboplastin time was 32.5 s. Liver and renal function tests and serum electrolyte levels were within the normal range.

A computed tomography (CT) scan of the head revealed a high-density area in the right frontoparietal lobe (Figure 1(a)). Brain magnetic resonance imaging (MRI) showed an infarction complicated by hemorrhage in the same lobe (Figure 1(c)). In addition, cerebral angiography revealed total occlusion of the right rolandic vein and inferior sagittal sinus and partial occlusion of the superior sagittal sinus (Figure 1(e)).

The patient was diagnosed with cerebral venous sinus thrombosis. Surgical hematoma evacuation was performed immediately upon hospitalization, and unfractionated heparin was administered (20,000 units/day). Prothrombotic workup such as protein C and S and antithrombin III were within the normal range. Antinuclear antibodies and anticardiolipin antibodies were negative.

She was in a stable condition following surgery. However, she experienced fever and bloody diarrhea on day seven after admission. Abdominal CT scan demonstrated thickening of the bowel wall from the rectum to the descending colon (Figure 2(a)). Rapid sigmoidoscopy revealed edematous mucosa, erythema, and loss of vascular markings, which extended continuously from the rectum (Figure 2(c)). Neither longitudinal nor discrete ulcers were seen, which were suggestive of ischemic colitis. These endoscopic findings were consistent with ulcerative colitis, Mayo endoscopic subscore (MES) of 2, and confirmed by colonic biopsies that showed crypt abscesses and goblet cell loss. Stool culture was negative. The *Clostridium difficile* toxin A/B test and indirect immunofluorescence assay antibody titer for *Entamoeba histolytica* were negative. No antibiotics responsible for drug-induced colitis were administered.

She was administered steroids (prednisolone, 60 mg/day), sulfasalazine (4 g/day), and topical mesalamine (1 g/day). Within 5 days following treatment initiation, her digestive symptoms, diarrhea, and bloody stools resolved, and her temperature returned to normal. Prednisolone was tapered without any flare-ups, and her anticoagulant medication was switched from unfractionated heparin to warfarin.

Her digestive and neurological symptoms showed significant improvement, and she was transferred to a rehabilitation hospital on day 70. By the time she was discharged from the rehabilitation hospital, clinical remission had been achieved, and her first total colonoscopy (TCS) was performed 9 months after the initial diagnosis. TCS revealed mild erythema and loss of vascular markings in mucosa of the descending and sigmoid colon and some erosions and mucosal friability in the rectum, which were consistent with MES of 1. No signs of inflammation were seen between the cecum and transverse colon, leading to a diagnosis of left-sided UC. Mesalamine suppository was added following TCS, and MES of 0 was confirmed by sigmoidoscopy 16 months later (Figure 3). Her UC has been well controlled for the last five years with mesalamine 4800 mg/d, mesalamine suppository 1 g/d, and probiotics, and her latest MES remained 0.

Warfarin was stopped after 12 months, and she experienced no recurrence of symptoms over the last five years after discontinuation of anticoagulation treatment.

3. Discussion

In the present case, the patient received treatment of both CVT and UC shortly after diagnosis, and her symptoms improved within a few days. In addition, she had an uneventful course without recurrence of CVT or UC flare-up for more than five years. To our best knowledge, this is the first report of a long-term follow-up after successful treatment of CVT with concomitant UC.

Generally, UC is a chronic idiopathic inflammatory bowel disorder (IBD) of the mucosal layer of the colon. It usually occurs in patients aged 20–30 years, with a second peak between the ages of 70 and 80 years. Patients with UC usually experience diarrhea, hematochezia, abdominal pain, tenesmus, and incontinence [2].

Furthermore, UC can be also regarded as a systemic disease with numerous extraintestinal complications. Patients with UC are at an increased risk of venous and arterial thromboembolism. Specifically, the risk of venous thromboembolism increases during UC flare-ups [6, 7]. Of these manifestations, thromboembolic events, such as deep venous thrombosis and pulmonary embolism, have been well recognized [3]. Although CVT is a rarely reported thromboembolic complication in patients with UC, it can be fatal.

It has been revealed that 0.5–6.4% of patients with UC experience CVT complications at some points in the course of their disease [8, 9]. Usually, CVT occurs in young patients with UC, with a mean age of <29 years [10]. This finding shows that patients with CVT and UC as comorbidity are significantly younger than those with CVT without UC. Cases of patients >40 years, such as the present case, are rarely reported in the literature. A previous report has shown that CVT was more common in patients with UC than in those with Crohn's disease, and female predominance has also been reported [10]. The prognosis of UC complicated with CVT was significantly worse than that of UC without CVT. One study demonstrated that the mortality rate in patients with UC with CVT could reach up to 25% [11]. The mechanism of thrombosis in UC is complex and incompletely understood [12]. However, a recent study has suggested an interaction between the coagulation cascade in the body and cytokine mediators of chronic inflammation with involvement of an inflammatory process in activating the coagulation cascade [13]. Coagulation activity in UC has been found to be related to disease activity and colonic extension of the disease [14]. Additionally, anemia, thrombocytosis, low albumin, and elevated D-dimer levels

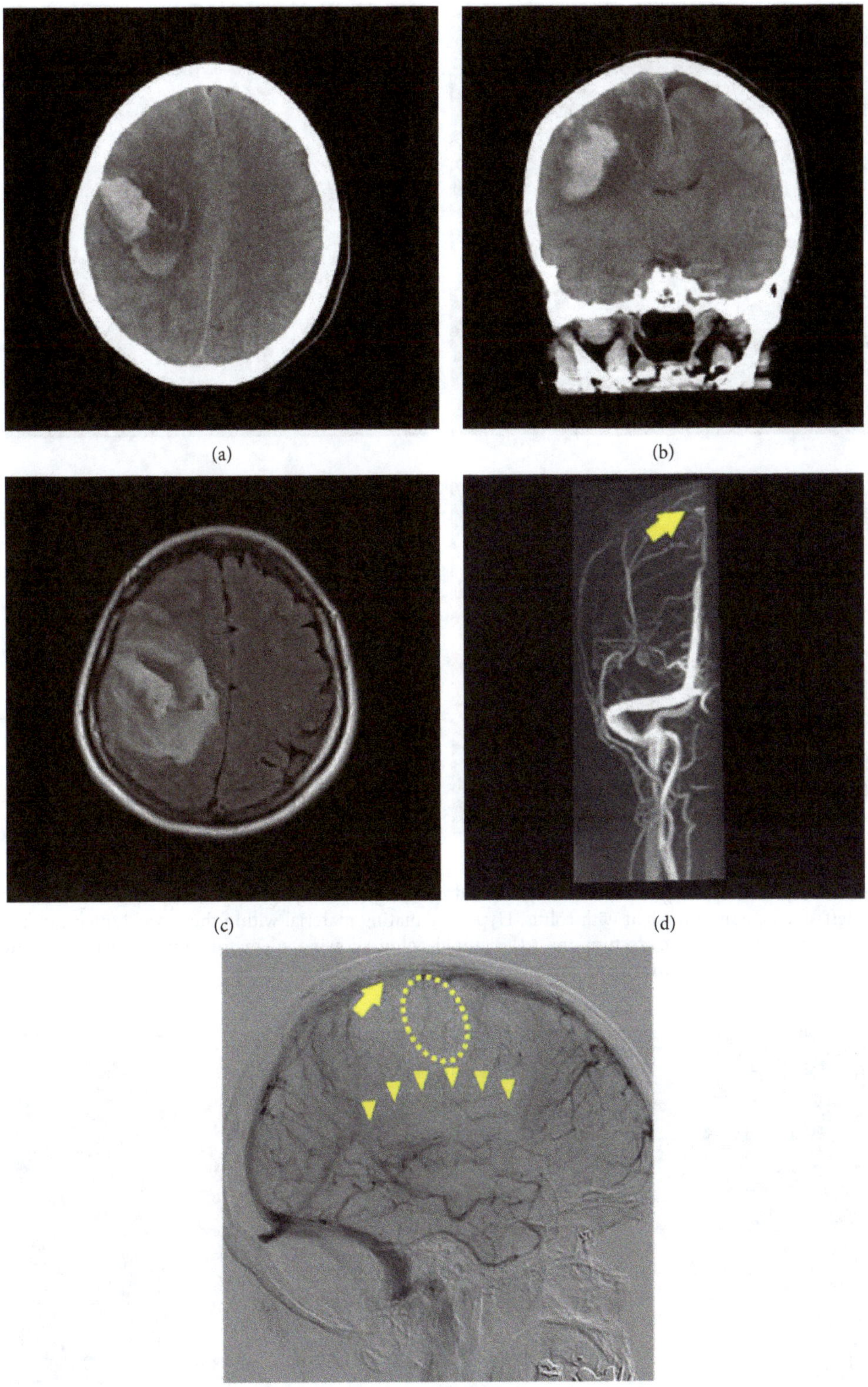

(a) (b) (c) (d) (e)

Figure 1: (a) Sagittal and (b) coronal images of nonenhanced brain computed tomography (CT) showing a high-density area in the right frontoparietal lobe, consistent with right lobar intracranial hemorrhage (ICH). (c) A head magnetic resonance image (MRI) with fluid attenuation inversion recovery (FLAIR) showing infarction surrounding subcortical hemorrhage of the frontoparietal lobe. (d) Magnetic resonance venography (MRV) revealing an absence of normal flow patterns of the superior sagittal sinus (arrow). (e) Cerebral angiogram showing total occlusion of the right rolandic vein (dotted circle) and inferior sagittal sinus (arrow heads) and partial occlusion of the superior sagittal sinus (arrow) caused by thrombosis (Figure 1(c)).

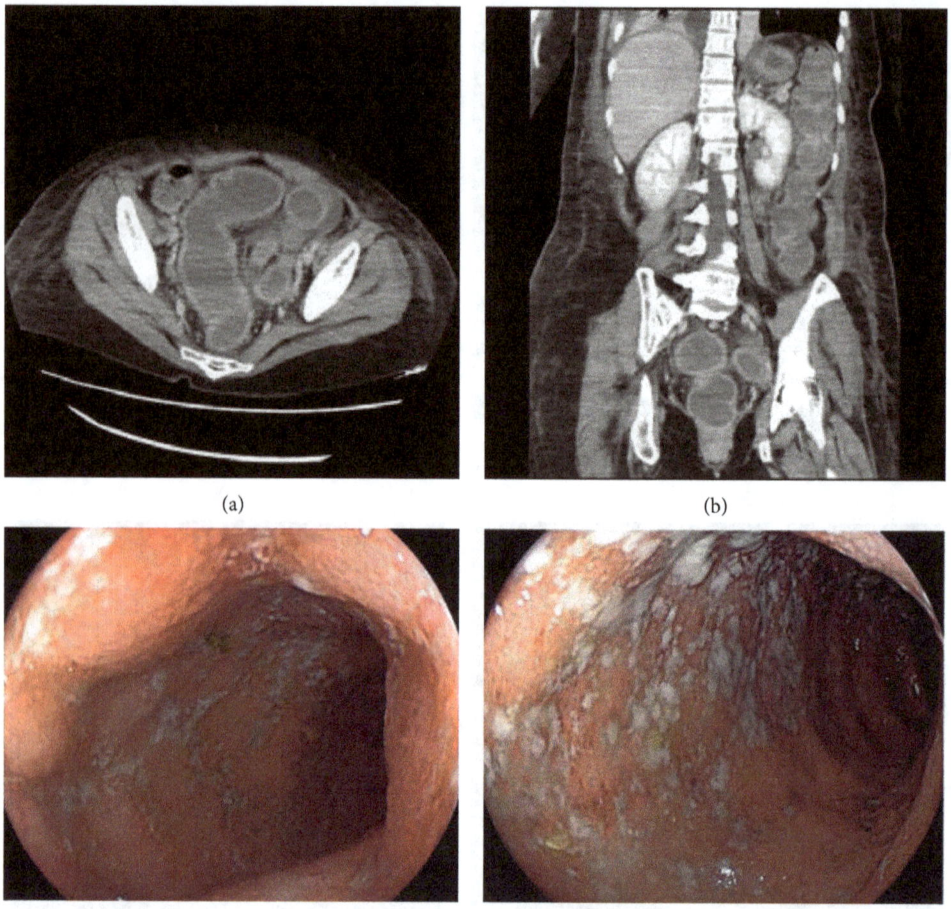

(a) (b) (c) (d)

Figure 2: (a) Axial and (b) coronal images of contrast enhanced computed tomography (CT) showing colonic mural thickening and enhancement of the left-sided colon, consistent with colitis. Hyperattenuating material within the bowel lumen can be seen, suggestive of blood clots. Endoscopic findings of the (c) rectum and (d) sigmoid colon showing edematous mucosa with marked erythema, absent vascular pattern, friability, and erosions, which are consistent with ulcerative colitis (UC).

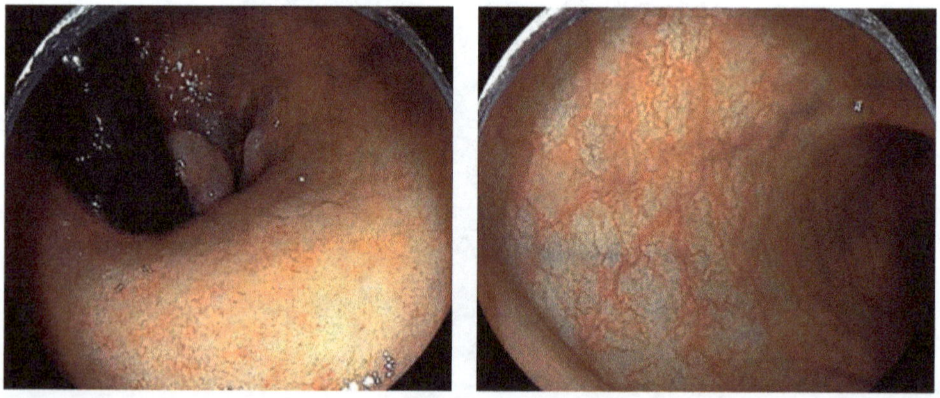

(a) (b)

Figure 3: 25 months after treatment, endoscopic findings of the (a) rectum and (b) sigmoid colon showing normal mucosa with visible vascular pattern, consistent with endoscopic remission, Mayo endoscopic subscore (MES) 0.

have been suggested as significant risk factors for CVT [10, 15]. Among these, severe iron deficiency anemia was identified as a significant risk factor for CVT in a previous study [16].

Although most case reports described CVT associated with flare-ups of established UC, this case was unique in which CVT preceded the diagnosis of UC. We suggest that in addition to chronic inflammation due to undiagnosed, hence, untreated UC, the patient experienced a flare-up in the past five days prior to admission when acute diarrhea had begun. Dehydration from diarrhea and iron deficiency were likely to have been the precipitating factors of the coagulation cascade, leading to CVT. Initially, the patient's relatively mild gastrointestinal symptom made the diagnosis of UC difficult as it seemed irrelevant to her neurological symptoms. Although physical and psychological stress due to CVT and surgery may have worsened the patient's flare-up, we hypothesize that administration of heparin ultimately provoked spontaneous bleeding from the inflamed membrane, leading to a definitive diagnosis.

The clinical manifestations of CVT comprise headache, uni or bilateral paresis, generalized or focal seizure, and encephalopathy. Headache is the most common symptom of venous sinus thrombosis, described in 89% of patients [17]. Seizure is also common in patients with CVT and reported in approximately 40% of these patients. Additionally, focal neurologic symptoms may reveal presence of venous infarction and hemorrhagic complication, which has been reported in more than one-third of patients [17].

Head CT and MRI are usually used for confirming CVT diagnosis. Moreover, CT without contrast is the initial imaging modality in patients with headaches and focal neurological symptoms [18]. Up to 30% of patients with venous sinus thrombosis would have an abnormal head CT scan without contrast. Generally, it may show hyperdensity of the cortical vein or dural venous sinus, which indicates infarct. In addition, approximately 30% of patients with CVT present with intracranial hemorrhage. Other imaging modalities such as CT venography and cerebral angiogram can assist in making a reliable diagnosis of CVT [18]. In this case, venous infarction in the superior and inferior sagittal sinuses was detected on a cerebral angiogram. However, the availability of these investigations may be influenced by institutional and regional factors and availability of specialists to perform these tests.

Currently, no guidelines are available for treatment of CVTs with concomitant UC [19]. However, several studies have shown that patients with IBD with CVT who received anticoagulation treatment showed better outcomes than those who did not [10, 20]. In addition, a previous study showed that timely diagnosis and treatment could result in a better prognosis in patients with CVT [21]. Despite concerns about hemorrhagic complications such as intestinal bleeding and intracranial hemorrhage, several studies have suggested improved survival in patients treated with anticoagulation, even in presence of intestinal bleeding and intracranial hemorrhage [10, 22]. Undifferentiated and low-molecular weight heparin is the most common drug used for prophylaxis and treatment of the acute phase of venous thromboembolism [23].

The efficacy and safety of long-term anticoagulant therapy in CVT with concomitant UC also remain unclear. The European Stroke Organization (ESO) recommends continuing anticoagulation for three months if CVT is due to a transient risk factor (e.g., pregnancy, dehydration, mechanical precipitants, and drugs) and for 6–12 months in patients with idiopathic CVT. On the other hand, these ESO guidelines recommend that anticoagulation therapy may be continued indefinitely in patients with recurrent CVT or CVT with severe thrombophilia. This severe thrombophilia is usually associated with homozygous prothrombin G20210 A mutations; homozygous factor V Leiden mutation; deficiencies in protein C, protein S, or antithrombin; combined thrombophilia defects; or antiphospholipid syndrome [24].

In presence of hypercoagulable conditions, CVT in patients with active UC should always be considered an indication for lifelong anticoagulation using warfarin [23]. However, it is unknown whether patients with CVT need to continue anticoagulant therapy after UC remission. In a previous study, CVT seldom occurred in patients with UC with stable remission [11]. In this case, warfarin was administered for 12 months and discontinued when the patient had a stable clinical course following clinical remission of UC. The patient has not experienced any recurrence of CVT without anticoagulant drugs use for more than five years.

In conclusion, in this report, we describe the case of new-onset UC after CVT. It is necessary to consider UC in patients with CVT, especially those with gastrointestinal symptoms. Early diagnosis and management of both UC and CVT may improve prognosis. Moreover, appropriate maintenance therapy for UC may prevent CVT recurrence. Further studies are warranted to further evaluate the optimal management and treatment of CVT with concomitant UC.

References

[1] Y. Murakami, Y. Nishiwaki, M. S. Oba et al., "Estimated prevalence of ulcerative colitis and Crohn's disease in Japan in 2014: an analysis of a nationwide survey," *Journal of Gastroenterology*, vol. 54, no. 12, pp. 1070–1077, 2019.

[2] M. S. Silverberg, "Toward an integrated clinical, molecular and serological classification of inflammatory bowel disease: report of a Working Party of the 2005 Montreal World Congress of Gastroenterology," *Canadian Journal of Gastroenterology*, vol. 19, 2005.

[3] C. N. Bernstein, J. F. Blanchard, D. S. Houston, and A. Wajda, "The incidence of deep venous thrombosis and pulmonary embolism among patients with inflammatory bowel disease: a population-based cohort study," *Thrombosis & Haemostasis*, vol. 85, no. 3, pp. 430–434, 2001.

[4] H. N. Gunes, B. G. Cokal, S. K. Guler et al., "Clinical associations, biological risk factors and outcomes of cerebral venous sinus thrombosis," *Journal of International Medical Research*, vol. 44, no. 6, pp. 1454–1461, 2016.

[5] S. K. Murthy and G. C. Nguyen, "Venous thromboembolism in inflammatory bowel disease: an epidemiological review," *American Journal of Gastroenterology*, vol. 106, no. 4, pp. 713–718, 2011.

[6] M. J. Grainge, J. West, and T. R. Card, "Venous thromboembolism during active disease and remission in inflammatory bowel disease: a cohort study," *The Lancet*, vol. 375, no. 9715, pp. 657–663, 2010.

[7] F. Houissa, M. Salem, S. Bouzaidi et al., "Cerebral thrombosis in inflammatory bowel disease: a report of four cases," *Journal of Crohn's and Colitis*, vol. 5, no. 3, pp. 249–252, 2011.

[8] S. Standridge and E. de los Reyes, "Inflammatory bowel disease and cerebrovascular arterial and venous thromboembolic events in 4 pediatric patients: a case series and review of the literature," *Journal of Child Neurology*, vol. 23, no. 1, pp. 59–66, 2008.

[9] A. Taous, M. A. Berri, T. Lamsiah, B. Zainoun, T. Ziadi, and A. Rouimi, "Cerebral venous thrombosis revealing an ulcerative colitis," *The Pan African medical journal*, vol. 23, Article ID 120, 2016.

[10] A. H. Katsanos, K. H. Katsanos, M. Kosmidou, S. Giannopoulos, A. P. Kyritsis, and E. V. Tsianos, "Cerebral sinus venous thrombosis in inflammatory bowel diseases," *QJM*, vol. 106, no. 5, pp. 401–413, 2013.

[11] R. W. Talbot, J. Heppell, R. R. Dozois, and R. W. Beart, "Vascular complications of inflammatory bowel disease," *Mayo Clinic Proceedings*, vol. 61, no. 2, pp. 140–145, 1986.

[12] K. Cheng and A. S. Faye, "Venous thromboembolism in inflammatory bowel disease," *World Journal of Gastroenterology*, vol. 26, no. 12, pp. 1231–1241, 2020.

[13] S. Danese, A. Papa, S. Saibeni, A. Repici, A. Malesci, and M. Vecchi, "Inflammation and coagulation in inflammatory bowel disease: the clot thickens," *American Journal of Gastroenterology*, vol. 102, no. 1, pp. 174–186, 2007.

[14] A. Stadnicki, "Involvement of coagulation and hemostasis in inflammatory bowel diseases," *Current Vascular Pharmacology*, vol. 10, no. 5, pp. 659–669, 2012.

[15] W. Shujun, Z. Huijie, B. Xia, and W. Hongjian, "Cerebral venous sinus thrombosis in patients with inflammatory bowel disease: a retrospective study," *Scientific Reports*, vol. 11, no. 1, Article ID 17004, 2021.

[16] E. Stolz, J. M. Valdueza, M. Grebe et al., "Anemia as a risk factor for cerebral venous thrombosis? An old hypothesis revisited," *Journal of Neurology*, vol. 254, no. 6, pp. 729–734, 2007.

[17] J. M. Ferro, P. Canhao, J. Stam, M.-G. Bousser, and F. Barinagarrementeria, "Prognosis of cerebral vein and dural sinus thrombosis," *Stroke*, vol. 35, no. 3, pp. 664–670, 2004.

[18] G. Saposnik, F. Barinagarrementeria, R. D. Brown et al., "Diagnosis and management of cerebral venous thrombosis," *Stroke*, vol. 42, no. 4, pp. 1158–1192, 2011.

[19] D. Joshi, T. Dickel, R. Aga, and G. Smith-Laing, "Stroke in inflammatory bowel disease: a report of two cases and review of the literature," *Thrombosis Journal*, vol. 6, no. 1, p. 2, 2008.

[20] R. J. Nudelman, D. G. Rosen, E. Rouah, and G. Verstovsek, "Cerebral sinus thrombosis: a fatal neurological complication of ulcerative colitis," *Pathology Research International*, vol. 2010, Article ID 132754, 2010.

[21] E. Cognat, I. Crassard, C. Denier, K. Vahedi, and M.-G. Bousser, "Cerebral venous thrombosis in inflammatory bowel diseases: eight cases and literature review," *International Journal of Stroke*, vol. 6, no. 6, pp. 487–492, 2011.

[22] S. S. Kupfer and D. T. Rubin, "Inflammatory bowel disease and cerebral venous sinus thrombosis," *Gastroenterology and Hepatology*, vol. 2, no. 12, pp. 914–917, 2006.

[23] I. E. Koutroubakis, "Therapy insight: vascular complications in patients with inflammatory bowel disease," *Nature Clinical Practice Gastroenterology & Hepatology*, vol. 2, no. 6, pp. 266–272, 2005.

[24] J. M. Ferro, M. G. Bousser, P. Canhão et al., "European Stroke Organization guideline for the diagnosis and treatment of cerebral venous thrombosis - endorsed by the European Academy of Neurology," *European Journal of Neurology*, vol. 24, no. 10, pp. 1203–1213, 2017.

48

Chemical Gastroenterocolitis after Dental Root Canal Therapy with Camphorated and Mentholated Chlorophenol

Mikheil Kalandarishvili, Ernst-Wolfgang Kolbe, Günther Winde, and Michael Kaspari

University Clinic of General, Abdominal and Thoracic Surgery, Hospital of Herford, Herford, Germany

Correspondence should be addressed to Mikheil Kalandarishvili; mikheil.kalandarishvili@rub.de

Academic Editor: Chia-Tung Shun

A 78-year-old man with a history of pancolitis, after the treatment of dental abscess with oral antibiotics and local application of camphorated and mentholated chlorophenol (CMCP), presented with abdominal pain of 4-day duration, as well as hair loss in the area of moustache and finger nail lifting. He was already treated with rectal application of budesonide because of pancolitis, diagnosed 6 weeks ago and interpreted as an allergic reaction to clindamycin. For further investigation, we performed gastroscopy and colonoscopy, which showed the edematous mucosa with polypus-like changes of the whole mucosa of the stomach, duodenum, first part of the jejunum, distal ileum, complete colon, and rectum. The diagnosis was complicated and was achieved in synopsis with anamnestic details, such as endodontic application of camphorated chlorophenol. The patient symptoms abated after he commenced on mesalazine therapy.

1. Case Presentation

A 78-year-old man was admitted in our surgical unit on January 2020 with lower abdominal pain of 4-day duration as well as constipation. He complained about unintended weight loss, loss of performance, loss of hair in the area of moustache, and also detachment of 3 fingernails during the last 2 months. Medical history from a third party was unremarkable. Hematologic and biochemical blood tests including serum electrolytes, liver enzymes, amylase, and renal function parameters showed no abnormalities. The C-reactive protein level was normal at 3.6 mg/L (normal range (NR): < 5 mg/L), but white blood cell count was increased to 29.7×10^9/L (NR: 4. 5–11 109/L) due to elevation of neutrophil count at 24.5×10^9/L (NR: $2–7 \times 10^9$/L) with slight elevation of the eosinophil level at 1.63×10^9/L (NR: $<0.4 \times 10^9$/L), and the protein level was slightly decreased at 55.6 G/L (NR: 66.0–87.0 G/L). Stool cultures for bacteria and viruses showed negative findings.

An abdominal CT scan was significant for previously known small left adrenal mass (remained unchanged compared to the previous examination) and small reducible incisional hernia in the area of midline laparotomy after right hemicolectomy, which was performed 5 years ago because of colon cancer. There was no sign of any changes in the gastrointestinal (GI) tract. The colon cancer was diagnosed in February 2015 with stage I, classified using the American Joint Committee on Cancer, so that there was no need for adjuvant cancer therapy. Until now, the regular cancer follow-up was unremarkable.

The patient referred himself 6 weeks ago in gastroenterology (GE) of our hospital with diarrhea of 12-day duration, which was manifested 2 days after surgical treatment of tooth abscess. At that time, his dentist incised the abscess in the area of central incisors 8 and 9, inserted camphorated and mentholated chlorophenol (CMCP) in the root canal, and prescribed the oral antibiotic clindamycin. After diarrhea manifestation in 2 days, clindamycin was rejected, and CMCP was once again locally reinserted. Diarrhea progressed despite cancelling of antibiotics, and his performance status worsened further. However, the initial colonoscopy performed in the GE unit showed the polypoid-hemorrhagic pancolitis (Figure 1). Biopsies taken from the terminal ileum, sigmoid, and rectal mucosa showed the

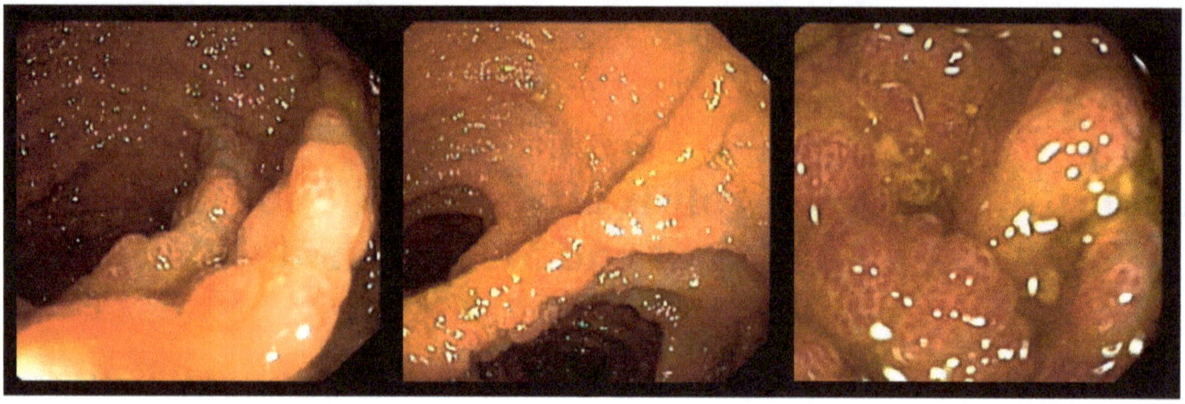

Figure 1: Colonoscopy 14 days after treatment of tooth abscess.

distorted crypt architecture as well as eosinophilic infiltration, so the allergic reaction was suggested. Primary short-term therapy with intravenous cortisone relieved his symptoms. After that, rectal application of budesonide for 8 weeks was prescribed, and the patient was discharged.

For further investigation, we performed esophagogastroduodenoscopy and colonoscopy with multiple biopsies. Endoscopic investigation showed that the whole mucosa of the stomach, duodenum, first part of the jejunum, distal ileum, complete colon, and rectum were edematous with polypus-like changes of the all aforementioned parts of the GI tract (Figures 2 and 3). Histological studies showed the ubiquitous unspecific inflammation, atrophy of the villi, and regenerative changes of all the samples collected in all the parts of the GI tract. There were no eosinophilic collections any more.

Subsequently, he was started on mesalazine to facilitate symptom relief and intestinal healing. There was an improvement in his clinical symptoms with respect to abdominal pain, and inflammation markers were declining.

Follow-up colonoscopy two months later showed no significant improvement, but there were no further changes seen, which were not grossly observed on prior colonoscopy. Over the next few months, the patient had gradual deterioration of his performance status and reported a further weight loss, hair loss, and nail loss. After this, the patient obtained parenteral nutrition. The GE of our hospital implemented the individual monitoring strategy for the patient with clinical, blood marker, and endoscopy assessment with intervals of 3 months. His further treatment was performed in gastroenterology of another university hospital at his own request.

2. Discussion

There are many types of inflammations of separate parts of the digestive tract. The followed forms of gastritis are described in literature: autoimmune, bacterial, chemical, Crohn-associated, eosinophilic, lymphocytic, radiation, and noninfectious granulomatous gastritis [1]. The common types of colitis are as follows: inflammatory bowel disease (ulcerative colitis, Crohn's disease, and indeterminate colitis) [2], microscopic (lymphocytic and collagenous colitis) [3], radiation-induced, infectious (pseudomembranous colitis caused by Clostridium difficile, enterohemorrhagic colitis caused by Shiga toxin, etc.) [4, 5], chemotherapy-induced [6], diversion [7], ischemic, checkpoint inhibitor induced, [8] and chemical colitis [9]. Even though most of the aforementioned medical conditions are single-organ diseases and have preferential areas of location, it can be, in some cases, expected that other parts of the gastrointestinal (GI) system or distant organs are also affected, for example, duodenal manifestation of Crohn's disease [10], pseudomembranous gastritis [11], and backwash ileitis in ulcerative colitis [12]. Gastroenteritis or enteritis is a general name of the condition, which is mostly infectious and characterized with diarrhea or vomiting [13].

The GI inflammation manifested in all parts of the GI system is rarely described; also, the definition "gastroenterocolitis" (GEC) is rarely used in the literature. There is no uniform classification or definition of this condition. After comprehensive search in the literature, we have identified the following types of GEC: fulminating *Staphylococci* GEC [14], PD-1 inhibitor GEC [8], nosocomial rotavirus-induced GEC [15], collagenous GEC [16], and diffuse infectious phlegmonous GEC [17].

Onycholysis is a common medical problem, which is associated with the painless separation of the nail from the nail bed. It can be a sign of many different conditions, including trauma, manicuring, psoriasis, nail fungus, phototoxic dermatitis due to drugs, hyperthyroidism, sarcoidosis, amyloidosis, connective tissue disorders, vitamin or iron deficiency, and chemotherapy [18]. The literature review showed us that clindamycin has an extremely low potential to induce a drug-induced photosensitivity [19].

Hair loss, also known as alopecia, is a very common condition. There are many types of alopecia, which is subdivided into two main categories.

2.1. *Nonscarring Alopecia*

(i) Androgenetic alopecia

(ii) Alopecia areata

(iii) Telogen effluvium

(iv) Traction alopecia

(v) Trichotillomania

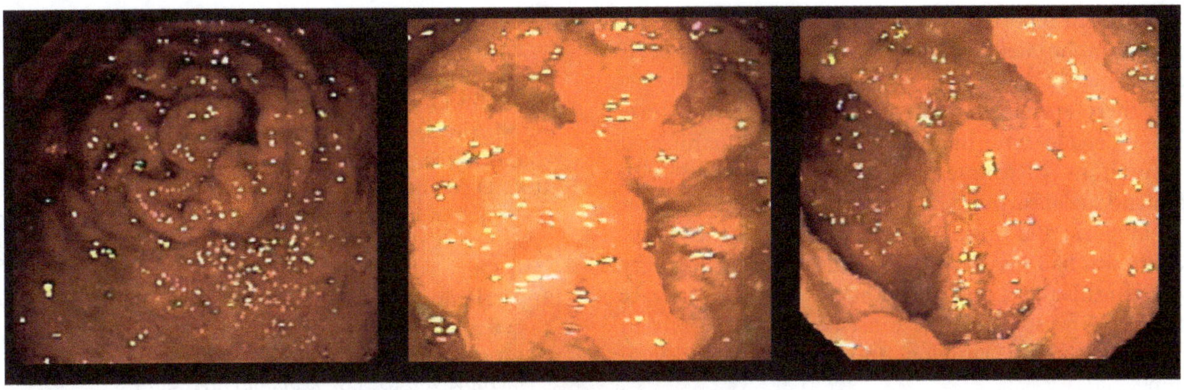

FIGURE 2: Colonoscopy 8 weeks after treatment of tooth abscess.

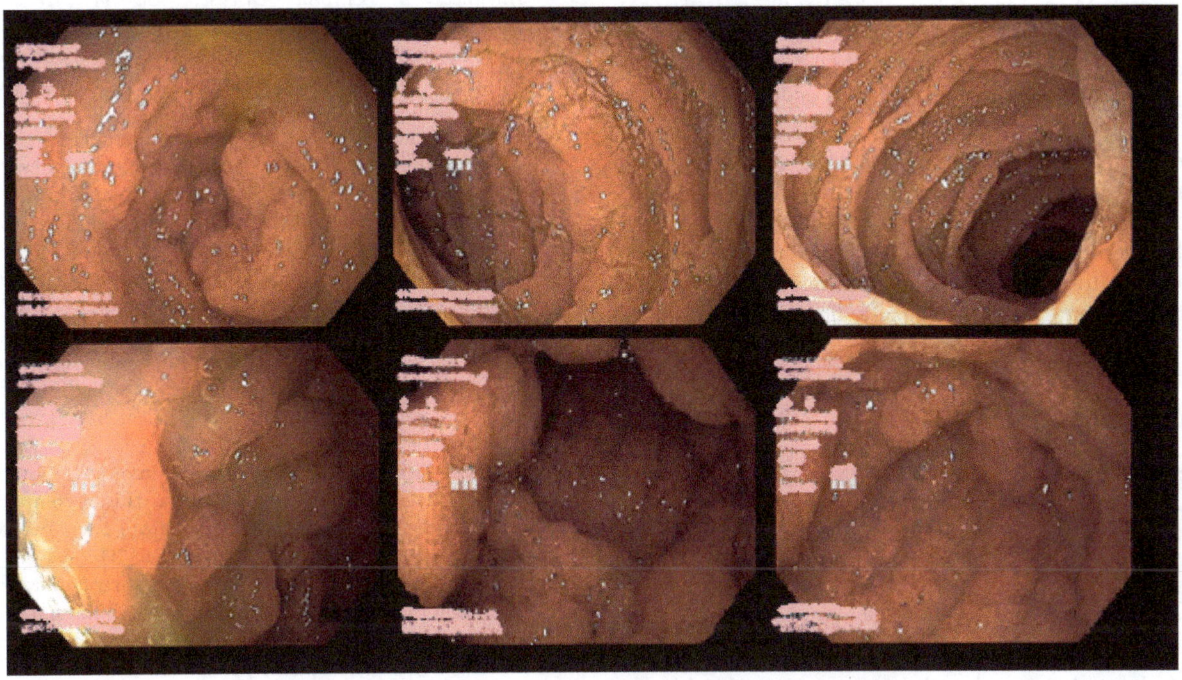

FIGURE 3: Gastroscopy 8 weeks after treatment of tooth abscess.

(vi) Anagen effluvium

2.2. Scarring Alopecia

(i) Alopecia mucinosa

(ii) Metastatic infiltrate

(iii) Favus

The pathophysiology of hair loss is predominantly well understood and depends on the alopecia type. In androgenetic alopecia, both factors, hormones and genetics, play a role in the pathogenesis. Alopecia areata is not well understood, but the most common hypothesis involves autoimmunity as a T-cell-mediated pathway. In telogen effluvium, stress and hormones are mainly described triggers. Traction alopecia is primarily caused by pulling force being applied to the hair. Trichotillomania is a mental disorder characterized with pulling out of hair. Chemotherapeutic aggression is the cause of anagen effluvium, and the infiltration of the scalp with abnormal lymphocytes causes alopecia mucinosa. Tinea capitis (favus) is dermatophytic infection responsible for alopecia [20]. There is a subtype of alopecia areata of the beard known as alopecia barbae. It is limited exclusively to the beard and characterized with losing beard hair in small circular patches [21].

Considering the etiopathogenesis of all the aforementioned diseases, the inflammation of the GI system in our case is most likely the chemical origin, and the hair and nail loss can also be explained with the chemical impact of toxins. We believe that the aforementioned changes are due to the immunotoxic effect of CMCP. We also considered the side effect or allergy to clindamycin, but it appears less feasible as the patient had a past history of 1-week antibiotics with clindamycin approximately 10 years ago. On the contrary, the selective hair loss in the area of the upper lip indicates the local effect of toxins (in our case, CMCP). Moreover, in the poison control center in Bonn, Germany, one alopecia case has already been reported after treatment with CMCP. The toxicity of camphorated chlorophenol in the animal model is also established [22].

Also, there are many similarities with the rare disease Cronkhite-Canada syndrome (CCS), which is manifested with ubiquitous gastrointestinal polyps, associated with diarrhea and malabsorption [23]. The malabsorption further leads to alopecia and onycholysis. As the first symptom of our patient was hair loss in the area of the upper lip, it is very unlikely that this was a random manifestation of a very rare disease CCS. The stool culture must be done regularly in order to exclude an antibiotic-induced colitis or viral infection.

CMCP is an antibacterial agent that is used in the treatment of dental root canal systems. The common reported side effect of chlorophenol is its toxicity, but the side effects of camphorated chlorophenol are extremely rare [24]. To the best of our knowledge and literature review, this is the first reported case of GI tract inflammation associated with the use of this medication. The use of CMCP is a widely spread dental treatment in Germany with few adverse effects reported. Because of the lack of data, it is not feasible to assess the possible risk factors for the development of the described symptom complex. Other alternative antimicrobial medicines for root canal treatment are, for example, chlorhexidine gel 2%, chlorhexidine powder 1%, povidone-iodine, and polyhexanide [24].

3. Conclusion

We experienced a case in which an oral application of CMCP caused a massive chemical inflammation of the GI tract. The chemical ignition of the GI system is rare and usually limited to one organ. The diagnosis can be challenging if the pertinent history is not obtained, and this case illustrates a delay in diagnosis. Therefore, patients with unexplained inflammation of the GI tract must be questioned about the past dental treatment. We should also bear in mind that the ingestion of CMCP can cause alopecia and nail lifting. The literature is not clear about the therapy of chemical GEC, and in our case, mesalazine was, in an initial phase, a useful treatment, but subsequently, it was not successful and encouraging. The purpose of this case report is to raise awareness about this uncommon adverse effect of CMCP.

Authors' Contributions

MKal is the main author, who wrote the paper. EWK and GW performed editing and literature search and are senior authors. MKas is the patient consultant and performed article correction.

References

[1] M. F. Dixon, R. M. Genta, J. H. Yardley, and P. Correa, "Classification and grading of gastritis," *The American Journal of Surgical Pathology*, vol. 20, no. 10, pp. 1161–1181, 1996.

[2] C. Mowat, A. Cole, A. Windsor et al., "Guidelines for the management of inflammatory bowel disease in adults," *Gut*, vol. 60, no. 5, pp. 571–607, 2011.

[3] T. Townsend, F. Campbell, P. O'Toole, and C. Probert, "Microscopic colitis: diagnosis and management," *Frontline Gastroenterology*, vol. 10, no. 4, pp. 388–393, 2019.

[4] C. D. Tanquilut, C. W. Jung, A. W. Nelson, and S. K. Lau, "Infection due to Shiga toxin-producing enterohemorrhagic *Escherichia coli* (EHEC) presenting as ischemic colitis," *IDCases*, vol. 18, Article ID e00629, 2019.

[5] C. Slimings and T. V. Riley, "Antibiotics and hospital-acquired *Clostridium difficile* infection: update of systematic review and meta-analysis," *Journal of Antimicrobial Chemotherapy*, vol. 69, no. 4, pp. 881–891, 2014.

[6] M. O'Reilly, G. Mellotte, B. Ryan, and A. O'Connor, "Gastrointestinal side effects of cancer treatments," *Therapeutic Advances in Chronic Disease*, vol. 11, Article ID 204062232097035, 2020.

[7] J. M. Geraghty and I. C. Talbot, "Diversion colitis: histological features in the colon and rectum after defunctioning colostomy," *Gut*, vol. 32, no. 9, pp. 1020–1023, 1991.

[8] R. S. Gonzalez, S. N. Salaria, C. D. Bohannon, A. R. Huber, M. M. Feely, and C. Shi, "PD-1 inhibitor gastroenterocolitis: case series and appraisal of 'immunomodulatory gastroenterocolitis," *Histopathology*, vol. 70, no. 4, pp. 558–567, Article ID 28000302, 2017.

[9] S. Sheibani and L. B. Gerson, "Chemical colitis," *Journal of Clinical Gastroenterology*, vol. 42, no. 2, pp. 115–121, 2008.

[10] M. J. Wagtmans, H. W. Verspaget, L. B. Lawers, and R. A. van Hogezand, "Clinical aspects of Crohn's disease of the upper gastrointestinal tract: a comparison with distal Crohn's disease," *American Journal of Gastroenterology*, vol. 92, pp. 1467–1471, 1997.

[11] D. L. Sanders, R. B. Pfeiffer, L. A. Hashimoto, C. Subramony, and F. Chen, "Pseudomembranous gastritis: a complication from aspergillus infection," *The American Surgeon*, vol. 69, no. 6, pp. 536–538, Article ID 12852516, 2003.

[12] N. Goldstein and M. Dulai, "Contemporary morphologic definition of backwash ileitis in ulcerative colitis and features that distinguish it from Crohn disease," *American Journal of Clinical Pathology*, vol. 126, pp. 365–376, 2006.

[13] J. By-Payne and E. Elliott, "Gastroenteritis in children," *Clinical Evidence*, vol. 12, pp. 443–454, 2004.

[14] K. Terplan, J. R. Paine, J. Sheffer, R. Egan, and H. Lansky, "Fulminating gastroenterocolitis caused by staphylococci; its apparent connection with antibiotic medication," *Gastroenterology*, vol. 24, no. 4, pp. 476–509, Article ID 13083811, 1953.

[15] A. Nitsch-Osuch, E. Kuchar, A. Kosmala, K. Zycinska, and K. Wardyn, "Nosocomial rotavirus gastroenterocolitis in a large tertiary paediatric hospital in Warsaw, 2006-2010," *Archives of Medical Science*, vol. 9, no. 3, pp. 493–498, 2013.

[16] A. Leiby, S. Khan, and D. Corao, "Clinical challenges and images in GI. Collagenous gastroduodenocolitis," *Gastroenterology*, vol. 135, no. 1, p. 17, 2008.

[17] E. D. Blei and C. Abrahams, "Diffuse phlegmonous gastroenterocolitis in a patient with an infected peritoneo-jugular venous shunt," *Gastroenterology*, vol. 84, no. 3, pp. 636–639, 1983.

[18] N. Zaias, S. X. Escovar, and M. N. Zaiac, "Finger and toenail onycholysis," *Journal of the European Academy of Dermatology and Venereology*, vol. 29, no. 5, pp. 848–853, 2015.

[19] J. Murray and A. Potts, "The phototoxic and photoallergy potential of clindamycin phosphate 1.2%/tretinoin 0.025% gel

for facial acne: results of two single-center, evaluator-blinded, randomized, vehicle-controlled phase 1 studies in healthy volunteers," *Journal of Drugs in Dermatology*, vol. 13, no. 1, pp. 16–22, 2014.

[20] Al Aboud A. M., Zito P. M. Alopecia. [Updated 2020 Sep 29]. In: StatPearls [Internet]. Treasure Island (FL): StatPearls Publishing; 2021 Jan-. Available from: https://www.ncbi.nlm.nih.gov/books/NBK538178/.

[21] E. Darwin, P. A. Hirt, R. Fertig, B. Doliner, G. Delcanto, and J. J. Jimenez, "Alopecia areata: review of epidemiology, clinical features, pathogenesis, and new treatment options," *International Journal of Trichology*, vol. 10, no. 2, pp. 51–60, 2018.

[22] A. Soekanto, S. Kasugai, S. Mataki, K. Ohya, and H. Ogura, "Toxicity of camphorated phenol and camphorated parachlorophenol in dental pulp cell culture," *Journal of Endodontics*, vol. 22, no. 6, pp. 284–289, 1996.

[23] N. Zügel, A. Tannapfel, O. Lembcke et al., "Das Cronkhite-Canada-Syndrom Epidemiologie, Symptomatik, Morphologie und Therapie anhand eines Fallberichts und der Literatur," *Chirurg*, vol. 68, pp. 710–714, 1997.

[24] T. Dammaschke, N. Jung, I. Harks, and E. Schafer, "The effect of different root canal medicaments on the elimination of *Enterococcus faecalis* ex vivo," *European Journal of Dentistry*, vol. 7, no. 4, pp. 442–448, 2013.

49

Sweet Syndrome, Not so Sweet during an Ulcerative Colitis Flare Especially When You Cannot Eat

Courtney Stead,[1] **Shahrad Hakimian**,[2] **Christina Luffman**,[3] **Zendee Elaba**,[3] **Gregory Orlowski**,[4] **and Neil Marya**[5]

[1]*Department of Medicine, University of Massachusetts Medical School, 55 Lake Avenue North, Worcester, MA 01655, USA*
[2]*Division of Digestive Diseases, University of California Health, Los Angeles, CA, USA*
[3]*Department of Pathology, University of Massachusetts Medical School, Worcester, MA, USA*
[4]*Department of Dermatology, University of Massachusetts Medical School, Worcester, MA, USA*
[5]*Division of Gastroenterology, University of Massachusetts Medical School, Worcester, MA, USA*

Correspondence should be addressed to Neil Marya; neil.marya@umassmemorial.org

Academic Editor: Matteo Neri

Sweet syndrome is a rare skin condition characterized by painful papules, nodules, or plaques with dense neutrophilic infiltrate in the upper dermis. It has been observed as idiopathic (classical), malignancy-associated, and drug-induced. The pathogenesis is not completely understood, but it is thought to involve hypersensitivity reactions to specific triggers. In some cases the etiology is unclear or may be multifactorial. We present a case of Sweet syndrome secondary to ulcerative colitis flare versus adalimumab re-induction.

1. Introduction

Sweet syndrome, or acute neutrophilic dermatosis, is a rare skin condition characterized by painful papules, nodules, or plaques with dense neutrophilic infiltrate in the upper dermis [1]. It is often accompanied by fever and peripheral neutrophilia. Less common, but reported, complications include arthralgias, myalgias, nausea, vomiting, diarrhea, headache, and conjunctivitis. This syndrome is more frequently seen in women, most prevalent in adults aged 30–70 years old, but has also been reported in children [2]. The pathogenesis of the disease remains unknown; however, it has been postulated that it may be a hypersensitivity reaction given its relation to autoimmune diseases, malignancies, and infections. Here, we report a case of Sweet syndrome in a patient with pan-ulcerative colitis recently re-induced with adalimumab.

2. Case Report

A 22-year-old male with a history of pan-ulcerative colitis (UC) recently re-induced on adalimumab presented to the hospital with odynophagia and inability to swallow secondary to significant oral ulceration and 20–25lb weight loss. He was diagnosed with UC at 20 years old and was treated with a course of prednisone along with induction with adalimumab. He remained asymptomatic on adalimumab for 8 months until he lost his insurance and self-discontinued the medication. He remained minimally symptomatic for 2 years and was lost to follow-up. However, he finally presented to clinic with one month of bloody diarrhea and weight loss and was eventually re-induced with adalimumab and a prednisone taper after being diagnosed with a UC flare. His gastrointestinal symptoms resolved quickly; however, he developed severe progression of oral mucosal ulcerations and a papular rash approximately 7–10 days after adalimumab re-induction. Due to worsening odynophagia, he presented to the hospital with severe dehydration. On admission, the patient was afebrile with laboratory investigations significant for C-reactive protein (CRP) 151.5, white blood cell count (WBC) 13.0, and neutrophils 10.18 (78.4%). Otolaryngology was consulted to perform laryngoscopy, which was significant for ulcerations along the epiglottis. Biopsy of an ulceration was collected at that time. Endoscopy was not performed. On day two of

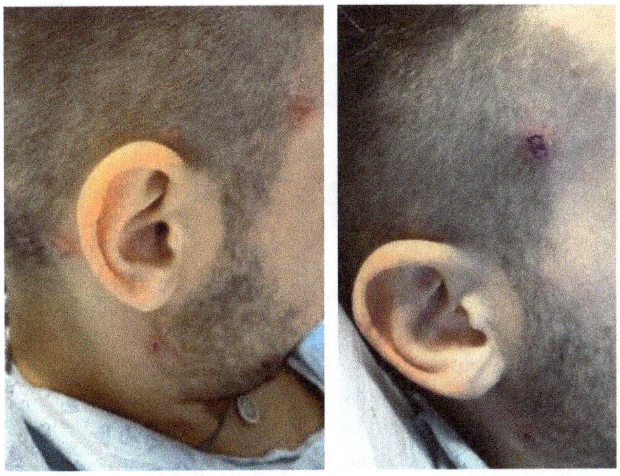

FIGURE 1: Firm, erythematous, and umbilicated papules with central erosion and crust. The lesions were observed on the face, scalp, and jaw.

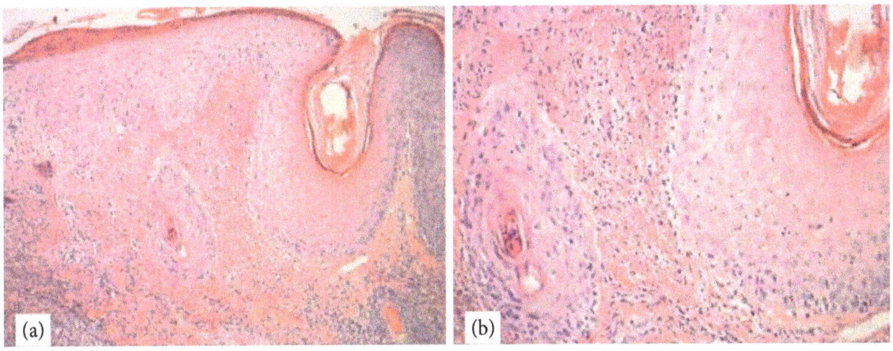

FIGURE 2: Histologic sections show subcorneal pustules and dense neutrophilic dermal infiltrate ((a)-4X and (b)-10X). Special stains including gram, AFB, and FITE were negative for definitive microorganisms.

hospitalization, he developed a fever to 38.3 C. At this time, the patient was noted to have erythematous, scaled papules, and nodules on his face, head, trunk, and buttocks that drained transparent, yellow discharge (Figure 1). Dermatology was consulted and performed a punch biopsy of the skin lesions and oral ulcers. The gingival biopsies were nonspecific; however, skin biopsy was significant for neutrophilic infiltrate in the dermis with formation of microabscesses within the epidermis and superficial dermis (Figure 2). The constellation of the patient's presenting symptoms, biopsy findings, and disease context (i.e., onset of symptoms during a UC flare two days following adalimumab induction) raised suspicion for drug-induced vs. classic Sweet Syndrome. Thus, adalimumab was discontinued, and he was switched to infliximab therapy. In addition to this management, the patient's prednisone dose was increased. At a dermatology follow-up appointment 11 days later, the patient's skin lesions were nearly resolved, and he no longer had oral ulcers.

3. Discussion

There are three clinical types of Sweet syndrome: idiopathic (classic), malignancy-associated, and drug-induced. Different diagnostic criteria have been established for each type. In the classic type, lesions may resolve after weeks to months untreated. In the malignant-associated type, symptoms may resolve following remission of the cancer. In drug-induced type, improvement may be seen after stopping the associated medication. Regardless of the subtype, systemic corticosteroids are the first-line treatment, and resolution of symptoms may begin as soon as 72 hours after initiation of therapy. In this case, the onset of skin lesions consistent with Sweet syndrome during an ulcerative colitis flare, two days post re-induction of adalimumab raises the questions of classical versus drug-induced Sweet syndrome. A 2007 review of acute neutrophilic dermatosis found that classic Sweet syndrome is often associated with upper respiratory or gastrointestinal infections, as well as inflammatory diseases such as ulcerative colitis and Crohn's Disease [1]. In 2005, a review documented that 35 cases of Sweet syndrome associated with inflammatory bowel disease had been documented worldwide [3]. Drug-induced Sweet syndrome has also been well documented as associated most commonly with granulocyte colony-stimulating factor, tretinoin, sulfamethoxazole and trimethoprim, bortezomib, and azathioprine [1]. Tumor necrosis fator (TNF) inhibitors have not been commonly documented as associated with Sweet's syndrome; however, one 2015 case report suggested its association with adalimumab re-induction in Crohn's Disease. In that case, discontinuation of adalimumab prompted full recovery of the skin lesions [4]. Oral Sweet's syndrome, presenting with mouth ulcers, has also been documented in the literature [5–8]. In one report, a patient had ulcerative colitis and was taking adalimumab. This report attributed association to be to IBD, rather than adalimumab [8].

The pathogenesis of Sweet's syndrome is not well understood. It is postulated that certain drugs or diseases may stimulate cytokines that increase neutrophil activation, leading to the syndrome's manifestations of fever, neutrophilia, and neutrophil infiltration to the dermis [9, 10]. However, in these cases, it is often pro-inflammatory drugs, or drugs that are anti, pro-inflammatory cytokines, that are associated with the syndrome. Adalimumab blocks a pro-inflammatory agent, tumor necrosis factor alpha (TNF-α), and therefore, it is unclear what the role of this drug could be in the pathogenesis of Sweet's syndrome. Alternatively, the onset of oral ulcers and skin lesions days after re-induction of adalimumab, along with a previously documented similar case, supports an association. The lack of a development of skin lesions following multiple infliximab infusions may argue against a drug-induced etiology or may suggest that the medication-induced component of this condition is medication specific. Other than one case study where Sweet's syndrome was observed after Pegfilgrastim administration but resolved following discontinuation and transition to filgrastim [11]; there is very little literature on this topic. Lastly, given the known association with inflammatory bowel disease and this patient's coinciding flare, Sweet's syndrome secondary to a UC flare cannot be excluded. Regardless of the cause, medication or IBD itself, it is important to include this syndrome as part of the differential diagnosis of rashes, skin, and oral ulceration in presence of IBD and after administration of biologic agents such as TNF inhibitor therapy including adalimumab.

References

[1] C. D. Villarreal-Villarreal, J. Ocampo-Candiani, and A. Villarreal-Martínez, "Sweet syndrome: a review and update," *Actas Dermo-Sifiliográficas*, vol. 107, no. 5, pp. 369–378, 2016.

[2] "Oxford textbook of rheumatology|R2 digital library," 2020, https://www-r2library-com.umassmed.idm.oclc.org/Resource/detail/0198509480/ch0042s3459.

[3] H. Ytting, I. Vind, D. Bang, and P. Munkholm, "Sweet's syndrome-an extraintestinal manifestation in inflammatory bowel disease," *Digestion*, vol. 72, no. 2-3, pp. 195–200, 2005.

[4] C. Banse, V. Sobocinski, G. Savoye, G. Avenel, and O. Vittecoq, "Occurrence of Sweet syndrome under anti-TNF," *Clinical Rheumatology*, vol. 34, no. 11, pp. 1993-1994, 2015.

[5] F. Femiano, F. Gombos, and C. Scully, "Sweet's syndrome: recurrent oral ulceration, pyrexia, thrombophlebitis, and cutaneous lesions," *Oral Surgery, Oral Medicine, Oral Pathology, Oral Radiology & Endodontics*, vol. 95, no. 3, pp. 324–327, 2003.

[6] J.-C. Fricain, V. Sibaud, S. Lepreux, A. Taieb, F. Boralevi, and J.-M. d'Elbée, "Sweet's syndrome revealed by oral pustulosis," *Médecine Buccale Chirurgie Buccale*, vol. 21, no. 3, pp. 177–181, 2015.

[7] N. E. Driban and M. A. Alvarez, "Oral manifestations of sweet's syndrome," *Dermatology*, vol. 169, no. 2, pp. 102-103, 1984.

[8] L. A. Nestor and A.-M. Tobin, "Oral Sweet's syndrome occurring in ulcerative colitis," *BMJ Case Reports*, vol. 2017, 2017.

[9] S. Voelter-Mahlknecht, J. Bauer, G. Metzler, G. Fierlbeck, and G. Rassner, "Bullous variant of Sweet's syndrome," *International Journal of Dermatology*, vol. 44, no. 11, pp. 946-947, 2005.

[10] J. M. L. White, G. J. Mufti, J. R. Salisbury, and A. W. P. du Vivier, "Cutaneous manifestations of granulocyte colony-stimulating factor," *Clinical and Experimental Dermatology*, vol. 31, no. 2, pp. 206-207, 2006.

[11] B. K. Draper, J. R. Robbins, and G. P. Stricklin, "Bullous Sweet's syndrome in congenital neutropenia: association with pegfilgrastim," *Journal of the American Academy of Dermatology*, vol. 52, no. 5, pp. 901–905, 2005.

50

Two Cases of Duodenal Ulcers that Developed after Transcatheter Procedures for Unruptured Visceral Artery Aneurysms

Masaya Iwamuro,[1] **Yusuke Kawai**,[2] **Mayu Uka**,[3] **Yusuke Matsui**,[3] **Takao Hiraki**,[3] **Yoshiro Kawahara**,[4] **and Hiroyuki Okada**[1]

[1]*Department of Gastroenterology and Hepatology, Okayama University Graduate School of Medicine, Dentistry, and Pharmaceutical Sciences, Okayama 700-8558, Japan*
[2]*Department of Gastroenterology, Mitoyo General Hospital, Kan'onji 769-1695, Japan*
[3]*Department of Radiology, Okayama University Graduate School of Medicine, Dentistry, and Pharmaceutical Sciences, Okayama 700-8558, Japan*
[4]*Department of Practical Gastrointestinal Endoscopy, Okayama University Hospital, Okayama 700-8558, Japan*

Correspondence should be addressed to Masaya Iwamuro; iwamuromasaya@yahoo.co.jp

Academic Editor: Haruhiko Sugimura

Herein, we report two cases of duodenal ulcers that developed after transcatheter procedures for the treatment of unruptured artery aneurysms. Both patients recovered after the administration of nothing by mouth, intravenous fluids, and proton-pump inhibitors. Notably, the duodenal ulcer was unchanged in one patient six days after endovascular treatment and improved in the other patient 13 days after angiography. These cases suggest that conservative treatment is acceptable in patients with duodenal ischemia that develops as an adverse effect of endovascular procedures. The usefulness of esophagogastroduodenoscopy in such patients has also been highlighted.

1. Introduction

Aneurysms occurring in the branches of the celiac, superior mesenteric, inferior mesenteric, or renal arteries are called abdominal visceral artery aneurysms [1–4]. Once such aneurysms rupture, mortality markedly increases, even if emergency treatment is performed. Thus, treatment of unruptured aneurysms is recommended depending on the risk factors for rupture, such as aneurysm size, morphology, and location. Currently, elective endovascular embolization is preferred for abdominal visceral artery aneurysms because it is less invasive than open surgical repair. Although endovascular treatment is safely performed in most cases, several procedure-related adverse events have been reported, including bowel ischemia and infarction, distal occlusion, arterial perforation, arterial dissection, and pancreatitis [5]. However, the detailed clinical courses of endovascular treatment-related bowel ischemia and infarction have not been sufficiently reported.

Herein, we report two patients with duodenal ulcers that developed following the transarterial approach for unruptured abdominal visceral artery aneurysms. Both patients spontaneously recovered with conservative treatment.

2. Case Presentation

2.1. Case 1. A 63-year-old woman underwent treatment for a *Helicobacter pylori* infection. Thereafter, she underwent computed tomography (CT) to investigate persistent epigastric discomfort and was diagnosed with median arcuate ligament syndrome with inferior and superior pancreaticoduodenal artery aneurysms. The patient was prescribed telmisartan, rosuvastatin, and rebamipide for hypertension, hypercholesterolemia, and epigastric symptoms, respectively, and referred to the Department of

Radiology of our hospital for further investigation and treatment. Although both endovascular treatment for visceral artery aneurysms and surgical treatment such as release or decompression of the median arcuate ligament have been proposed, endovascular embolization alone was performed as the patient did not wish to undergo surgery.

First, treatment of the superior pancreaticoduodenal artery aneurysm was planned (Figure 1(a), arrow). After coil embolization of the distal branch, the aneurysmal sac was filled with coil. However, the proximal side of the aneurysm ruptured (Figure 1(b), arrow) and the patient complained of epigastric pain. The artery was embolized using 33% n-butyl cyanoacrylate diluted with lipiodol (Figure 1(c), arrows). Although CT performed immediately after embolization showed leakage of the contrast medium into the retroperitoneum (Figure 2(a), arrows), no free air was observed in the abdomen. In addition, lipiodol retention was observed in the duodenal arteries (Figure 2(b), arrows). The patient was administered nothing orally, intravenous fluids, or proton-pump inhibitors. After the aneurysm ruptured, the patient developed epigastric pain that persisted for three days but gradually improved. Esophagogastroduodenoscopy performed three days after endovascular treatment revealed multiple ulcers in the second portion of the duodenum (Figure 3(a)). Sucralfate and sodium alginate were additionally prescribed for the duodenal ulcers. Since the duodenal ulcers did not worsen six days after endovascular treatment (Figure 3(b)), she was started on a liquid diet and discharged 10 days after endovascular treatment. Esophagogastroduodenoscopy performed 46 days after endovascular treatment revealed complete healing of duodenal ulcers (Figure 3(c)). Subsequently, the inferior pancreaticoduodenal artery aneurysm was successfully embolized using a coil.

2.2. Case 2. An 83-year-old Japanese woman underwent annual abdominal ultrasonography, which revealed a visceral artery aneurysm around the uncinate process of the pancreas. CT showed a dorsal pancreatic artery aneurysm with a diameter of 10 mm and occlusion of the celiac artery. The patient was referred to the Department of Radiology at our hospital for further investigation. The patient was prescribed ursodeoxycholic acid, ethyl icosapentate, and suvorexant for primary biliary cholangitis, hypercholesterolemia, and sleeplessness. She had a history of anterior cervical discectomy and fusion surgery for a cervical disc herniation. We attempted endovascular coiling to block blood flow into the aneurysm and prevent aneurysm rupture (Figure 4(a)).

During selective cannulation of the aneurysmal neck, retention of contrast medium was observed along the superior mesenteric artery (Figure 4(b)). CT showed separation of the inner and outer vascular layers (Figure 4(c)), confirming the diagnosis of superior mesenteric artery dissection. Stenosis of the roots of the ileocolic (Figure 4(d), arrow) and right colic arteries (Figure 4(d), arrowhead) was also observed. In contrast to the intact descending colon (Figure 4(e), asterisk), the duodenum (Figure 4(e), arrow), jejunum, and ascending colon (Figure 4(e), arrowhead) showed mural thickening and delayed reduced enhancement of the bowel wall. Although the patient complained of abdominal pain and nausea, her symptoms gradually improved. Intravascular embolization was aborted, and the patient was treated with nothing by mouth, intravenous fluids, antibiotics, heparin, and proton-pump inhibitors. As the patient had melena the day after angiography, we performed esophagogastroduodenoscopy, which revealed extensive exfoliation of the second and third portions of the duodenum (Figures 5(a) and 5(b)). The mucosa had turned black. Although there were no features of pancreatitis on computed tomography (CT), the serum amylase level was elevated to 510 U/L. Thus, nafamostat was administered and the patient was treated with total parenteral nutrition. The serum amylase levels gradually normalized, but repeat CT revealed that the superior mesenteric artery dissection and intestinal wall thickening were unchanged. No intestinal ischemia was observed on computed tomography (CT). Esophagogastroduodenoscopy performed 13 days after angiography showed an improvement in the damaged duodenal mucosa (Figures 5(c) and 5(d)). CT performed the following day revealed improvement in mural thickening of the duodenum (Figure 4(f), arrow), jejunum, and ascending colon (Figure 4(f), arrowhead). The patient was started on liquid diet. Subsequently, the patient recovered uneventfully and was discharged 31 days after angiography.

3. Discussion

The prevalence of abdominal visceral artery aneurysms has been reported to be 0.01%–0.2% of the population [3]. With regard to visceral artery aneurysms, the splenic artery is the most often involved, accounting for 60%–80% of cases, followed by the hepatic artery, mesenteric artery, celiac artery, gastric and gastroepiploic arteries, gastroduodenal artery and its pancreatic branches, jejunal and ileocolic arteries, and inferior mesenteric artery [6]. Most visceral aneurysms occur in association with arterial media degeneration due to atherosclerosis, fibromuscular dysplasia, or collagen vascular disorders [7]. Among the presented patients, Case 1 had stenosis of the celiac artery with median arcuate ligament syndrome, and Case 2 had occlusion of the celiac artery. It is known that stenosis/occlusion of the celiac axis is responsible for aneurysm formation as a consequence of increased flow in the collateral vessels [8]. Therefore, the etiology in the present two cases was suspected to be stenosis/occlusion of the celiac artery. Although a size >2 cm is considered the threshold for surgical or endovascular treatment [9, 10], rupture of visceral aneurysms <2 cm has been reported. For instance, the risk of rupture of pancreaticoduodenal artery aneurysms with celiac stenosis/occlusion is reportedly independent of aneurysmal size and is associated with a 50% mortality rate [11].

Because it is less invasive than open surgery, endovascular embolization is the first-line therapy for abdominal visceral artery aneurysms [12]. In addition to aneurysm treatment, transcatheter embolization has been used for the management of gastrointestinal bleeding refractory to

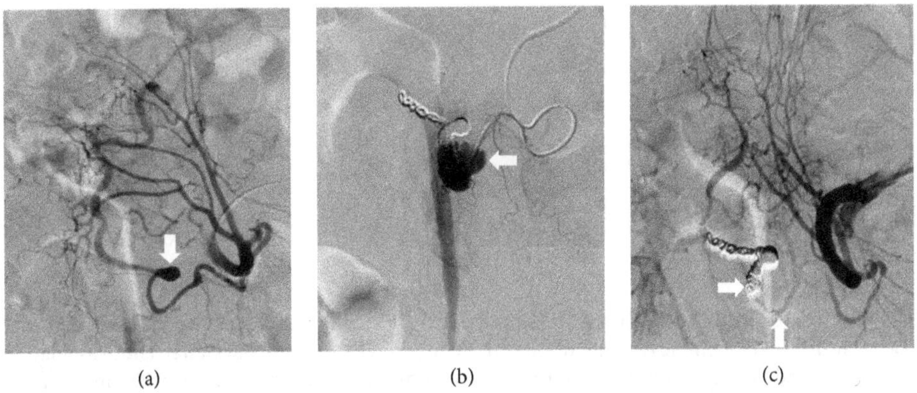

FIGURE 1: Angiography images of Case 1. A superior pancreaticoduodenal artery aneurysm is seen ((a), arrow). A rupture of the aneurysm after coil embolization of the distal branch ((b), arrow). The artery has been embolized with N-butyl cyanoacrylate ((c), arrows).

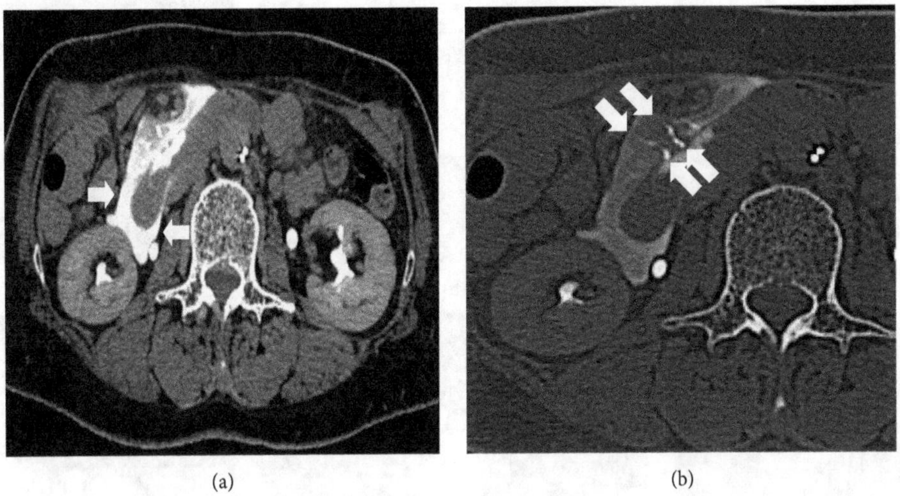

FIGURE 2: CT images of Case 1 performed immediately after embolization. CT showed leakage of the contrast medium into the retroperitoneum ((a), arrows). Lipiodol retention was observed in the duodenal arteries ((b), arrows). No free air was observed in the abdomen.

endoscopic hemostasis and transarterial chemoembolization of hepatocellular carcinoma. Adverse events related to endovascular treatment include bleeding, arterial dissection, intestinal ischemia, intestinal stenosis, coil migration [3, 13], pancreatitis [14], and access-site hematomas. Major ischemic complications of the gastrointestinal tract reportedly range from 0% to 16% [14, 15]. In Case 1, the proximal side of the aneurysm ruptured during the endovascular procedure. Although bleeding from the ruptured vessel was successfully managed with embolization using N-butyl cyanoacrylate, duodenal ulcer developed. It has been reported that the use of liquids, such as cyanoacrylates, or particulate embolic agents such as polyvinyl alcohol, is a risk factor for intestinal ischemic complications [14, 16].

In Case 2, iatrogenic dissection of the superior mesenteric artery occurred as an adverse event of an endovascular attempt to treat an aneurysm. Although the number of articles was limited, similar cases have been previously reported. Dzieciuchowicz et al. reported a case of a 42-year-old woman with pancreaticoduodenal artery aneurysms and stenosis of the celiac trunk [17]. Emergency laparotomy and thromboendarterectomy were performed, and magnetic resonance angiography performed 30 months after surgery showed patency of the superior mesenteric artery. In contrast, Tajima et al. conservatively treated a patient with superior mesenteric artery dissection that developed during angiography with peroral ticlopidine [18]. CT performed four weeks after angiography revealed patency of the lumen of the superior mesenteric artery.

We speculate that the mechanism of ischemia differed between Cases 1 and 2. In case 1, the arterial branches of the pancreaticoduodenal arcade were nonselectively clogged with N-butyl cyanoacrylate. In such patients, because vascular occlusion occurs in the peripheral parts of the artery, it is assumed that the degree of intestinal damage essentially depends on the extent of the embolic agent and the blood vessels that are affected. In contrast, in Case 2, duodenal ulceration developed due to a partial decrease in blood flow in all branches of the superior mesenteric artery, including the pancreaticoduodenal arcade and arteries supplying the small intestine and colon. In such cases, collateral circulation between the celiac and mesenteric arteries probably has

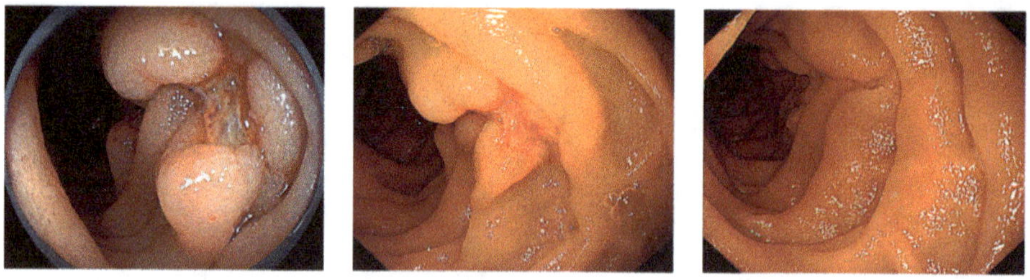

(a) (b) (c)

FIGURE 3: Esophagogastroduodenoscopy images of Case 1. Endoscopy performed three days after endovascular treatment shows multiple ulcers in the second portion of the duodenum (a). The duodenal ulcer is unchanged six days after endovascular treatment (b). Esophagogastroduodenoscopy performed 46 days after aneurysm treatment shows that duodenal ulcers are completely healed (c).

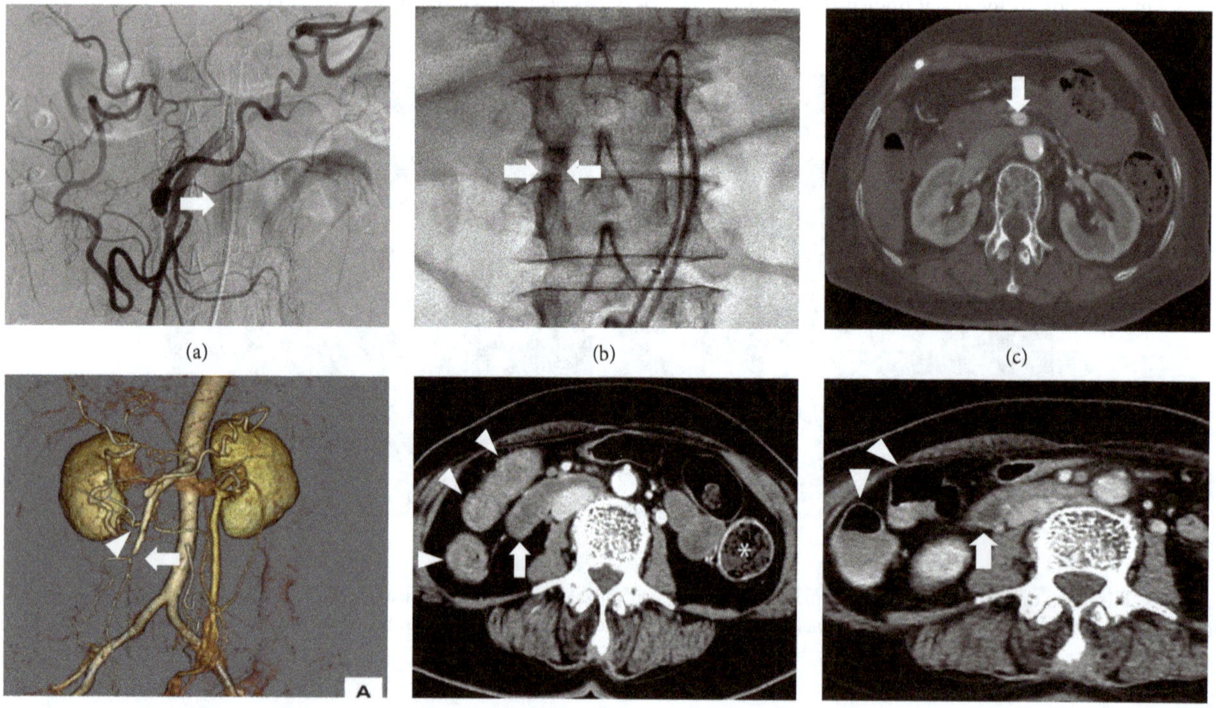

(a) (b) (c)

(d) (e) (f)

FIGURE 4: Radiology images of Case 2. A visceral artery aneurism is observed around the uncinate process of pancreas ((a), arrow). During selective cannulation to the aneurysmal neck, retention of the contrast medium is observed along the superior mesenteric artery ((b), arrows). CT shows separation of the inner and outer vascular layers ((c), arrow), confirming the diagnosis of superior mesenteric artery dissection. Stenosis of the roots of the ileocolic ((d), arrow) and right colic arteries ((d), arrowhead) is also observed. In contrast to the intact descending colon ((e), asterisk), mural thickening and delayed, reduced enhancement of the bowel wall are observed in the duodenum ((e), arrow) and ascending colon ((e), arrowhead). CT performed 14 days after angiography revealed improvement in mural thickening of the duodenum ((f), arrow), jejunum, and ascending colon ((f), arrowheads).

protective effects against ischemic insults to the intestines, while there is a potential risk of deterioration of the bowel infarction as arterial dissection progresses. These differences are merely speculation, as there was no apparent hypertrophy of the arterial arcades or emergence of arteries to compensate for the decreased blood flow in Case 2. However, these differences in the mechanisms of ischemia can theoretically influence patient management and prognosis.

Careful observation is required in patients with endovascular treatment-related bowel ischemia because cases of bowel perforation developing after arterial embolization for pancreaticoduodenal artery aneurysm [19] and hepatocellular carcinoma [20] have been previously reported. In the two patients reported herein, duodenal ulcers occurred as an adverse event of transarterial treatment of unruptured abdominal visceral artery aneurysms. However, both patients recovered spontaneously with the administration of nothing by mouth, intravenous fluids, or proton-pump inhibitors. Antibiotics and heparin were administered in Case 2. Esophagogastroduodenoscopy was useful for evaluating the degree of duodenal mucosal damage at the onset and its chronological changes during the course of treatment. We

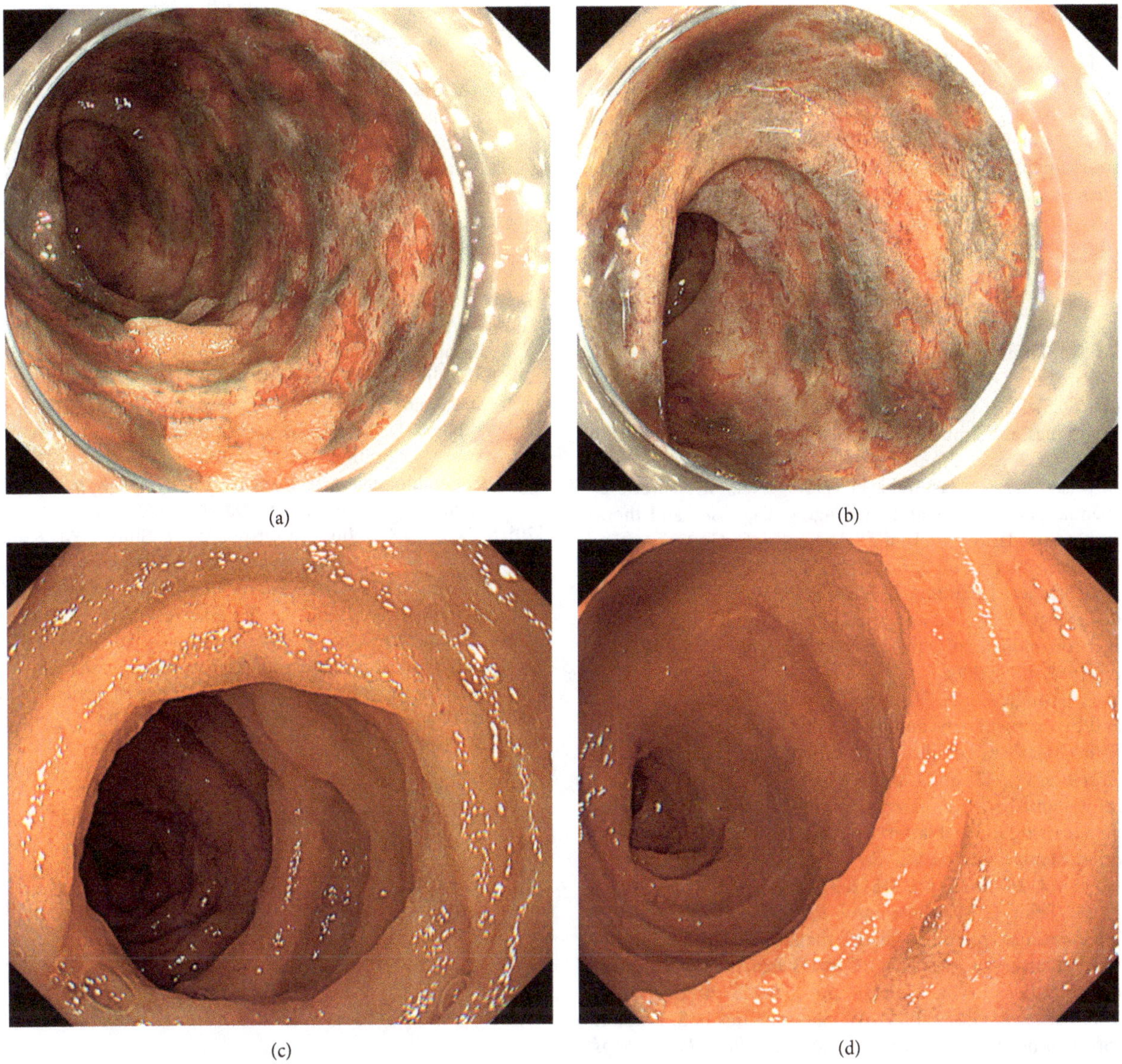

(a) (b) (c) (d)

FIGURE 5: Esophagogastroduodenoscopy images of Case 2. Esophagogastroduodenoscopy performed the day after angiography examination shows extensive exfoliation of the second and third portions of the duodenum (a, b). Thirteen days after angiography, the duodenal mucosal damage has improved (c, d).

consider that progressive deterioration or unresponsive mucosal damage during the course of treatment requires surgical management of the gastrointestinal tract, whereas conservative management is an option when improvement in mucosal damage is observed endoscopically. Thus, endoscopic examination is valuable in patients with endovascular treatment-related bowel ischemia, as it provides important information for optimal management. We recommend performing endoscopy as soon as possible, most desirably on the same day or the day after the ischemic event, to evaluate mucosal damage at onset. In Case 1, since endovascular treatment was performed on Friday, we performed endoscopy on Monday (3 days after the ischemic event), whereas we performed endoscopy the day after endovascular treatment in Case 2. Prior to performing endoscopy, it is mandatory to confirm the absence of signs of peritonitis on physical examination and CT. In addition, the use of carbon dioxide for insufflation is encouraged to decrease the risk of perforation [21].

4. Conclusions

We report two patients with duodenal ulcers that developed after transarterial embolization of unruptured abdominal visceral artery aneurysms. Both patients recovered spontaneously with conservative treatment. These cases highlight the usefulness of endoscopic observation in evaluating the degree of duodenal mucosal damage and supporting the decision-making process during conservative treatment of duodenal ulcers.

References

[1] A. D. Karaosmanoglu, A. Uysal, D. Akata, M. N. Ozmen, and M. Karcaaltincaba, "Role of imaging in visceral vascular emergencies," *Insights into Imaging*, vol. 11, no. 1, p. 112, 2020.

[2] M. A. Hosn, J. Xu, M. Sharafuddin, and J. D. Corson, "Visceral artery aneurysms: decision making and treatment options in the new era of minimally invasive and endovascular surgery," *International Journal of Angiology*, vol. 28, no. 1, pp. 11–16, 2019.

[3] B. Juntermanns, J. Bernheim, K. Karaindros, M. Walensi, and J. N. Hoffmann, "Visceral artery aneurysms," *Gefässchirurgie*, vol. 23, no. suppl 1, pp. 19–22, 2018.

[4] K. S. Madhusudhan, H. A. Venkatesh, S. Gamanagatti, P. Garg, and D. N. Srivastava, "Interventional radiology in the management of visceral artery pseudoaneurysms: a review of techniques and embolic materials," *Korean Journal of Radiology*, vol. 17, no. 3, pp. 351–363, 2016.

[5] A. Mastoraki, S. Mastoraki, E. Tziava et al., "Mesenteric ischemia: pathogenesis and challenging diagnostic and therapeutic modalities," *World Journal of Gastrointestinal Pathophysiology*, vol. 7, no. 1, pp. 125–130, 2016.

[6] J. L. Nosher, J. Chung, L. S. Brevetti, A. M. Graham, and R. L. Siegel, "Visceral and renal artery aneurysms: a pictorial essay on endovascular therapy," *RadioGraphics*, vol. 26, no. 6, pp. 1687–1704, 2006.

[7] R. A. Jesinger, A. A. Thoreson, and R. Lamba, "Abdominal and pelvic aneurysms and pseudoaneurysms: imaging review with clinical, radiologic, and treatment correlation," *RadioGraphics*, vol. 33, no. 3, pp. E71–E96, 2013.

[8] R. Kallamadi, M. A. Demoya, and S. P. Kalva, "Inferior pancreaticoduodenal artery aneurysms in association with celiac stenosis/occlusion," *Seminars in Interventional Radiology*, vol. 26, no. 3, pp. 215–223, 2009.

[9] A.-M. Belli, G. Markose, and R. Morgan, "The role of interventional radiology in the management of abdominal visceral artery aneurysms," *CardioVascular and Interventional Radiology*, vol. 35, no. 2, pp. 234–243, 2012.

[10] S. F. Pasha, P. Gloviczki, A. W. Stanson, and P. S. Kamath, "Splanchnic artery aneurysms," *Mayo Clinic Proceedings*, vol. 82, no. 4, pp. 472–479, 2007.

[11] J. A. Degheili, A. El Chediak, M. Y. R. Dergham, A. Al-Kutoubi, and A. H. Hallal, "Pancreaticoduodenal artery aneurysm associated with celiac trunk stenosis: case illustration and literature review," *Radiology Case Reports*, vol. 2017, Article ID 6989673, 7 pages, 2017.

[12] H. Bergert, I. Hinterseher, S. Kersting, J. Leonhardt, A. Bloomenthal, and H. D. Saeger, "Management and outcome of hemorrhage due to arterial pseudoaneurysms in pancreatitis," *Surgery*, vol. 137, no. 3, pp. 323–328, 2005.

[13] P. Kudaravalli, S. A. Saleem, V. S. Pendela, and M. O. Arif, "Rare complication of interventional radiology-guided arterial embolization of the gastroduodenal artery in the setting of acute gastrointestinal bleed: migrated coils in the duodenum," *Cureus*, vol. 12, no. 3, Article ID e7365, 2020.

[14] W. M. Chua, N. Venkatanarasimha, and K. Damodharan, "Acute ischemic pancreatitis: a rare complication of empirical gastroduodenal artery embolization," *Indian Journal of Radiology and Imaging*, vol. 27, no. 3, pp. 338–341, 2017.

[15] G. A. Poultsides, C. J. Kim, R. Orlando, G. Peros, M. J. Hallisey, and P. V. Vignati, "Angiographic embolization for gastroduodenal hemorrhage," *Archives of Surgery*, vol. 143, no. 5, pp. 457–461, 2008.

[16] R. Loffroy, P. Rao, S. Ota, M. De Lin, B.-K. Kwak, and J.-F. Geschwind, "Embolization of acute nonvariceal upper gastrointestinal hemorrhage resistant to endoscopic treatment: results and predictors of recurrent bleeding," *CardioVascular and Interventional Radiology*, vol. 33, no. 6, pp. 1088–1100, 2010.

[17] Ł. Dzieciuchowicz, M. Snoch-Ziółkiewicz, G. Oszkinis, and M. Frankiewicz, "Superior mesenteric artery dissection as a complication of an endovascular attempt to treat aneurysms of the pancreaticoduodenal arteries," *Interactive Cardiovascular and Thoracic Surgery*, vol. 21, no. 4, pp. 539–541, 2015.

[18] T. Tajima, H. Honda, T. Kuroiwa et al., "Spiral-shaped iatrogenic arterial dissection during superior mesenteric arteriography: a latent risk of diagnostic angiography using the power injector," *Computerized Medical Imaging and Graphics*, vol. 25, no. 5, pp. 367–371, 2001.

[19] M. Fujisawa, M. Machida, T. Kitabatake et al., "SA case of bowel perforation after arterial embolization for pancreaticoduodenal artery aneurysm," *Nihon Kyukyu Igakukai Zasshi*, vol. 20, no. 11, pp. 895–900, 2009.

[20] S. I. Kim, Y.-J. Jin, S. G. Cho, W. Y. Shin, J. M. Kim, and J.-W. Lee, "Duodenal perforation and esophageal ischemia following transarterial chemoembolization for hepatocellular carcinoma," *Medicine*, vol. 95, no. 27, Article ID e3987, 2016.

[21] J. H. Lee, P. Kedia, S. N. Stavropoulos, and D. Carr-Locke, "AGA clinical practice update on endoscopic management of perforations in gastrointestinal tract: expert review," *Clinical Gastroenterology and Hepatology*, vol. 19, no. 11, pp. 2252–2261, 2021.

Permissions

All chapters in this book were first published by Hindawi Publishing Corporation; hereby published with permission under the Creative Commons Attribution License or equivalent. Every chapter published in this book has been scrutinized by our experts. Their significance has been extensively debated. The topics covered herein carry significant findings which will fuel the growth of the discipline. They may even be implemented as practical applications or may be referred to as a beginning point for another development.

The contributors of this book come from diverse backgrounds, making this book a truly international effort. This book will bring forth new frontiers with its revolutionizing research information and detailed analysis of the nascent developments around the world.

We would like to thank all the contributing authors for lending their expertise to make the book truly unique. They have played a crucial role in the development of this book. Without their invaluable contributions this book wouldn't have been possible. They have made vital efforts to compile up to date information on the varied aspects of this subject to make this book a valuable addition to the collection of many professionals and students.

This book was conceptualized with the vision of imparting up-to-date information and advanced data in this field. To ensure the same, a matchless editorial board was set up. Every individual on the board went through rigorous rounds of assessment to prove their worth. After which they invested a large part of their time researching and compiling the most relevant data for our readers.

The editorial board has been involved in producing this book since its inception. They have spent rigorous hours researching and exploring the diverse topics which have resulted in the successful publishing of this book. They have passed on their knowledge of decades through this book. To expedite this challenging task, the publisher supported the team at every step. A small team of assistant editors was also appointed to further simplify the editing procedure and attain best results for the readers.

Apart from the editorial board, the designing team has also invested a significant amount of their time in understanding the subject and creating the most relevant covers. They scrutinized every image to scout for the most suitable representation of the subject and create an appropriate cover for the book.

The publishing team has been an ardent support to the editorial, designing and production team. Their endless efforts to recruit the best for this project, has resulted in the accomplishment of this book. They are a veteran in the field of academics and their pool of knowledge is as vast as their experience in printing. Their expertise and guidance has proved useful at every step. Their uncompromising quality standards have made this book an exceptional effort. Their encouragement from time to time has been an inspiration for everyone.

The publisher and the editorial board hope that this book will prove to be a valuable piece of knowledge for researchers, students, practitioners and scholars across the globe.

List of Contributors

Catherine Gisi and Lawrence Ku
Department of Internal Medicine, Harbor-UCLA Medical Center, Torrance, CA, USA

Anamaria Munteanu and Samuel French
Department of Pathology, Harbor-UCLA Medical Center, Torrance, CA, USA

Michael Fleischman and Viktor Eysselein
Department of Internal Medicine, Division of Gastroenterology, Harbor-UCLA Medical Center, Torrance, CA, USA

Gregor Krstevski, Urim Isahi and Vladimir Andreevski
University Clinic of Gastroenterohepatology, Medical Faculty, Ss. Cyril and Methodius University, Boulevard Mother Teresa 17, Skopje 1000, North Macedonia

Hamza Mohammed and Mahmoud Mosli
Departments of Medicine, King Abdulaziz University, Jeddah, Saudi Arabia

Rana Bokhary
Departments of Pathology, King Abdulaziz University, Jeddah, Saudi Arabia

Mohammed Nassif
Departments of Surgery, King Abdulaziz University, Jeddah, Saudi Arabia

Kevin J. Yang
University of California, Berkeley, CA, USA

C. K. Chang
Kaiser Permanente, Oakland, CA, USA

Clive Jude Miranda, Murad Hayatt Ali, Muddasir Ayaz, Yousef Soofi and Thomas Christopher Mahl
Department of Gastroenterology, University at Buffalo, 955 Main Street, Buffalo 14203, New York, USA

Muaaz Masood and Michael Coles
Department of Internal Medicine, Medical College of Georgia at Augusta University, Augusta, Georgia, USA

Humberto Sifuentes
Department of Gastroenterology and Hepatology, Medical College of Georgia at Augusta University, Augusta, Georgia, USA

Jonathan Kopel
Texas Tech University Health Sciences Center School of Medicine, Lubbock, TX, USA

Rebeccah Baucom
Department of Surgery, Texas Tech University Health Sciences Center, Lubbock, TX, USA

Samuel Campbell
Department of Surgery Division of Vascular Surgery, Texas Tech University Health Sciences Center, Lubbock, TX, USA

Gregory L. Brower
Department of Medical Education, Texas Tech University Health Sciences Center, Lubbock, TX, USA

Aye-Mya-Mya Kyaw and Than-Than Aye
Gastroenterology Department, thingangyun General Hospital, Yangon, Myanmar

Lin-Lin Htun
Pathology Department, thingangyun General Hospital, Yangon, Myanmar

Adil Salyani, Linda Barasa, Allan Rajula and Sayed K. Ali
Department of Medicine, Aga Khan University Hospital, Nairobi, Kenya

Andrawus Beany and Tova Rainis
Division of Gastroenterology, Bnai Zion Medical Center, Haifa, Israel
The Ruth and Bruce Rappaport Faculty of Medicine, Technion, Haifa, Israel

Varag Abed, Alexis Faber, Cristina Jageka, Ryan Goleniak and Raef Fadel
Henry Ford Health System, 2799 W Grand Blvd, Detroit, MI 48202, USA

Jenny Roselli, Tommaso Innocenti, Erica Nicola Lynch, Laura Parisio, Pasquale Apolito, Tommaso Mello, Maria Rosa Biagini, Mirko Tarocchi, Stefano Milani and Andrea Galli
Department of Biomedical, Experimental and Clinical Sciences, University of Florence, Florence, Italy

Giuseppe Macrì and Monica Milla
Azienda Ospedaliero-Universitaria Careggi, Florence, Italy

Masaya Iwamuro, Kenta Hamada, Hiroyuki Okada, Sakiko Hiraoka, Seiji Kawano and Shohei Oka
Department of Gastroenterology and Hepatology, Okayama University Graduate School of Medicine, Dentistry and Pharmaceutical Sciences, Okayama 700-8558, Japan

Somay Yamagata Murayama
Department of Fungal Infection, National Institute of Infectious Diseases, Tokyo 162-8340, Japan

Masahiko Nakamura
Omura Satoshi Memorial Institute, Kitasato University, Tokyo 108-8641, Japan

Takehiro Tanaka
Department of Pathology, Okayama University Graduate School of Medicine, Dentistry and Pharmaceutical Sciences, Okayama 700-8558, Japan

Akifumi Matsumura
Department of Hematology and Oncology, Okayama University Graduate School of Medicine, Dentistry and Pharmaceutical Sciences, Okayama 700-8558, Japan

Yoshiro Kawahara
Department of Practical Gastrointestinal Endoscopy, Okayama University Hospital, Okayama 700-8558, Japan

T. Lai
Community Memorial Health System, Graduate Medical Education, Ventura, CA, USA

A. Frugoli
Community Memorial Health System, Graduate Medical Education, Department of Internal Medicine, Pacific Inpatient Physicians, Ventura, CA, USA

B. Barrows
Community Memorial Hospital, Department of Pathology, Ventura, CA, USA

M. Salehpour
Community Memorial Hospital, Department of General Surgery, Ventura, CA, USA

Ilias Galanis, Georgios Floros, Christophoros Theodoropoulos, Myriam Metaxa, Panagiotis Theodoropoulos, Panagiotis Tsintavis, Dimitrios Bartziotas, Georgios Giannos, Georgios Stylianidis and Georgios Papadopoulos
Department of Surgery, Evaggelismos General Hospital, Athens, Greece

Steven Park
Department of Internal Medicine, University of Rochester Medical Center, Rochester, NY, USA

John Miller, Janice Cheong Asad Ullah, Lawrence Saubermann and Arthur Decross
Division of Gastroenterology & Hepatology, University of Rochester Medical Center, Rochester, NY, USA

Marcus Juan Esteban, Daniel Herlihy, Sherif Elhanafi and Marc J. Zuckerman
Division of Gastroenterology, Texas Tech University Health Sciences Center, El Paso, TX, USA

Amit Sureen
Department of Internal Medicine, Texas Tech University Health Sciences Center, El Paso, TX, USA

Abdullah Mohammed Albishi and Rafaat Chakik
Gastroenterology and Endoscopy Department, Armed Forces Hospital Southern Region, Khamis Mushayt, Saudi Arabia

Mohammed Bazeed
Radiology Department, Armed Forces Hospital Southern Region, Khamis Mushayt, Saudi Arabia

Michael Coles
Augusta University, Department of Internal Medicine, 1120 15th Street, Augusta, Georgia, USA

Pearl Uy, John Erikson Yap and Subbaramiah Sridhar
Augusta University, Department of Gastroenterology and Hepatology, 1120 15th Street, Augusta, Georgia, USA

Victoria Madray
Augusta University, Medical College of Georgia, 1120 15th Street, Augusta, Georgia, USA

Akwe Nyabera, Nso Nso, Saphwat Eskaros and Negar Niknam
Icahn School of Medicine at Mount Sinai (NYC Health+Hospitals/Queens) Program, New York City, NY, USA

Keya Shah
NYIT College of Osteopathic Medicine, Old Westbury, NY, USA

Yousaf Bashir Hadi and Syeda Fatima Zehra Naqvi
Department of Medicine, West Virginia University, Morgantown, WV, USA

John Lindsay IV
West Virginia University School of Medicine, Morgantown, WV, USA

Hatim Al-Jaroushi
Department of Medicine, Section of Pulmonary and Critical Care Medicine, West Virginia University, Morgantown, WV, USA

Jacky Ng
Touro University California, 1310 Club Dr, Vallejo, CA 94592, USA

David Zezoff and Hanadi Abou Dargham
Graduate Medical Education, St. Joseph's Medical Center,1800 N California St, Stockton, CA 95204, USA

Krystal Mills, Shaheen Fatima and Norberto Fas
Internal Medicine Program, Morehouse School of Medicine, 720 Westview Drive SW, Atlanta, GA 30310, USA

Hossain Salehi
Gastroenterology Ward, Baharlo Hospital, Tehran University of Medical Sciences, Tehran, Iran

Amir Mohammad Salehi
Medical Student, School of Medicine, Hamadan University of Medical Sciences, Hamadan, Iran

Youseung Kim
Virginia Tech Carilion School of Medicine, Department of Internal Medicine, Roanoke, VA, USA

Douglas Grider
Virginia Tech Carilion School of Medicine, Department of Internal Medicine, Roanoke, VA, USA
Virginia Tech Carilion School of Medicine, Department of Basic Science Education, Roanoke, VA, USA
Dominion Pathology Associates, Roanoke, VA, USA

Varun Kesar and Maithili V. Chitnavis
Virginia Tech Carilion School of Medicine, Department of Internal Medicine, Division of Gastroenterology and Hepatology, Roanoke, VA, USA

Gregorios Christodoulidis, Konstantinos Perivoliotis, Alexandros Diamantis, Dimitrios Magouliotis and Dimitrios Zacharoulis
Department of Surgery, University Hospital of Larissa, Mezourlo 41110, Larissa, Greece

Anastasios Manolakis and Apostolos Koffas
Department of Gastroenterology, University Hospital of Larissa, Mezourlo 41110, Larissa, Greece

Vasiliki Pappi
Department of Hematology, General Hospital of Volos, Volos, Greece

Ryan T. Hoff, Ami Patel and Alan Shapiro
Department of Medicine, Division of Gastroenterology, Advocate Lutheran General Hospital, Park Ridge, USA

Toshi Murakami
Satsuki Naika Clinic, Okayama 703-8258, Japan

Katarzyna Ignasiak-Budzyńska, Mikołaj Danko and Janusz Książyk
Department of Paediatrics, Nutrition and Metabolic Diseases, Children's Memorial Health Institute, Al. Dzieci Polskich 20, Warsaw 04-730, Poland

Haritha Mopuru, Edward Mensah and Imran Siddiqui
Department of Medicine, St. Vincent's Medical Center, Bridgeport, CT, USA

Ahmed Elfiky and Asmaa Mokhtar
Department of Internal Medicine, Staten Island University Hospital-Northwell Health, New York, NY, USA

Mira Alsheikh, Hassan Almoussawi and Stephen Mulrooney
Department of Gastroenterology, Staten Island University Hospital-Northwell Health, New York, NY, USA

Joaquin Ponce-Zepeda, Wenchang Guo, Giorgioni Carmen, Vishal Suresh Chandan and Xiaodong Li
Department of Pathology and Laboratory Medicine, University of California-Irvine, Irvine, CA, USA

Daniel Moon Kim and Gregory C. Albers
Department of Internal Medicine, Gastroenterology, University of California-Irvine, Irvine, CA, USA

Khin San Aye, Thet Mar Win, Mya Thida Aye and Than Than Aye
Department of Gastroenterology, University of Medicine 2, Yangon, Myanmar

Lin Lin Htun
Department of Pathology, ingangyun General Hospital, Yangon, Myanmar

Drmyothettin Tin
Yangon General Hospital, Yangon, Myanmar

Giuseppe Macrì, Monica Milla, Tommaso Mello, Andrea Galli, Stefano Milani and Mirko Tarocchi
Department of Experimental and Clinical Biomedical Sciences "Mario Serio", University of Florence, Florence, Italy

Marek Cingel, Jakub Benko, Matej Samoš and Marián Mokáň
Clinic of Internal Medicine I of University Hospital Martin, Jessenius Faculty of Medicine, Comenius University, Bratislava, Slovakia

Bruno Besteiro, Filipa Gomes and Jorge Almeida
Internal Medicine Department, Centro Hospitalar e Universitário de São João, Oporto, Portugal

Cláudia Costa
Oncology Department, Instituto Português de Oncologia de Coimbra, Coimbra, Portugal

Raquel Portugal
Pathology Department, Centro Hospitalar e Universitário de São João, Oporto, Portugal

Isabel Garrido
Gastrenterology Department, Centro Hospitalar e Universitário de São João, Oporto, Portugal

Nicholas J. Corsi, Matthew P. Corsi and Murray N. Ehrinpreis
Wayne State University School of Medicine, Detroit, MI, USA

Ahmad A. Abu-Heija and Anand Kumar Ravi
Wayne State University School of Medicine, Detroit, MI, USA
John D. Dingell V.A. Medical Center, Detroit Medical Center, Wayne State University, Detroit, MI, USA

Siri A. Urquhart
Division of Internal Medicine, Mayo Clinic, Rochester, MN, USA

Nayantara Coelho-Prabhu
Division of Gastroenterology and Hepatology, Mayo Clinic, Rochester, MN, USA

Hsing Hwa Lee, Naveen Sritharan and Gabriela Strey
Department of Medicine, Hervey Bay Hospital, Pialba, Queensland, Australia

Daniel Bermingham
Department of Pharmacy, Hervey Bay Hospital, Pialba, Queensland, Australia

Ali Saleh Alshamrani
Internal Medicine Department, Armed Forces Hospital Southern Region, Khamis Mushayt, Saudi Arabia

Robert Dorrell and Katelyn Madigan
Department of Medicine, Wake Forest School of Medicine, Winston-Salem, USA

Swati Pawa and Rishi Pawa
Department of Medicine, Section on Gastroenterology, Wake Forest School of Medicine, Winston-Salem, USA

Chris Shamatutu
Department of Medicine, University of British Columbia, Vancouver, Canada

Daljeet Chahal, Isabella T. Tai and Peter Kwan
Department of Medicine, Division of Gastroenterology, University of British Columbia, Vancouver, Canada

Takahide Takahashi
Division of Medical Support, Okayama University Hospital, Okayama 700-8558, Japan

Tomohiro Toji
Department of Pathology, Okayama University Graduate School of Medicine, Dentistry, and Pharmaceutical Sciences, Okayama 700-8558, Japan

Sang Jin Lee
Department of Internal Medicine, University of Ulsan College of Medicine, Gangneung Asan Hospital, Gangneung, Republic of Korea

Werimo Pascal Kuka, Joe Rakiro, Joseph Gatheru, Felix Riunga
Aga Khan University Hospital Nairobi, 4th Floor East Tower Block, third Avenue Parklands, Nairobi 00100, GPO, Kenya

Hiroshi Yamazaki, Akinori Sasaki, Eriko Yamaguchi, Risa Okamoto and Yasuaki Motomura
Department of Gastroenterology, Tokyo Bay Urayasu Ichikawa Medical Center, 3-4-32 Toudaijima, Urayasu, 279-0001 Chiba, Japan

Kana Sawada and Kuniyasu Saigusa
Department of Neurosurgery, Tokyo Bay Urayasu Ichikawa Medical Center, 3-4-32 Toudaijima, Urayasu, 279-0001 Chiba, Japan

Mikheil Kalandarishvili, Ernst-Wolfgang Kolbe, Günther Winde and Michael Kaspari
University Clinic of General, Abdominal and oracic Surgery, Hospital of Herford, Herford, Germany

Courtney Stead
Department of Medicine, University of Massachusetts Medical School, 55 Lake Avenue North, Worcester, MA 01655, USA

Shahrad Hakimian
Division of Digestive Diseases, University of California Health, Los Angeles, CA, USA

Christina Luffman and Zendee Elaba
Department of Pathology, University of Massachusetts Medical School, Worcester, MA, USA

Gregory Orlowski
Department of Dermatology, University of Massachusetts Medical School, Worcester, MA, USA

Neil Marya
Division of Gastroenterology, University of Massachusetts Medical School, Worcester, MA, USA

Yusuke Kawai
Department of Gastroenterology, Mitoyo General Hospital, Kan'onji 769-1695, Japan

Mayu Uka, Yusuke Matsui and Takao Hiraki
Department of Radiology, Okayama University Graduate School of Medicine, Dentistry, and Pharmaceutical Sciences, Okayama 700-8558, Japan

Index

www.ingramcontent.com/pod-product-compliance
Lightning Source LLC
LaVergne TN
LVHW082156200926
848484LV00008B/2167